Intraoperative Echocardiography

PRACTICAL ECHOCARDIOGRAPHY SERIES

Look for these other titles in Catherine M. Otto's Practical Echocardiography Series

Linda Gillam & Catherine M. Otto
Advanced Approaches in Echocardiography

Mark Lewin & Karen Stout
Echocardiography in Congenital Heart Disease

Martin St. John Sutton & Susan E. Wiegers
Echocardiography in Heart Failure

Intraoperative Echocardiography

PRACTICAL ECHOCARDIOGRAPHY SERIES

Donald C. Oxorn, MD
Professor of Anesthesiology
Division of Cardio-Thoracic Anesthesia
Adjunct Professor of Medicine (Cardiology)
University of Washington Medical Center
Seattle, Washington

ELSEVIER
SAUNDERS

1600 John F. Kennedy Blvd.
Ste 1800
Philadelphia, PA 19103-2899

INTRAOPERATIVE ECHOCARDIOGRAPHY   ISBN: 978-1-4377-2698-5

Copyright © 2012 by Saunders, an imprint of Elsevier Inc.

Library of Congress Cataloging-in-Publication Data
Intraoperative echocardiography / [edited by] Donald C. Oxorn.—1st ed.
      p. ; cm.—(Practical echocardiography series)
   Includes bibliographical references and index.
   ISBN 978-1-4377-2698-5 (hardcover : alk. paper)
   I. Oxorn, Donald C.   II. Series: Practical echocardiography series.
   [DNLM: 1. Echocardiography—methods.   2. Intraoperative Care—methods.   3. Cardiovascular Diseases—ultrasonography.   4. Image Processing, Computer-Assisted. WG 141.5.E2]
   LC classification not assigned
   616.1′207543—dc23   2011033842

Senior Acquisitions Editor: Dolores Meloni
Editorial Assistant: Brad McIlwain
Publishing Services Manager: Pat Joiner-Myers
Senior Project Manager: Joy Moore
Designer: Steven Stave

Printed in China

Last digit is the print number: 9   8   7   6   5   4   3   2   1

Working together to grow
libraries in developing countries

www.elsevier.com | www.bookaid.org | www.sabre.org

ELSEVIER   BOOK AID International   Sabre Foundation

Contributors

Atilio Barbeito, MD
Assistant Professor of Anesthesiology, Duke University Medical Center; Staff Anesthesiologist and Intensivist, and Investigator, Patient Safety Center of Inquiry, Veterans Affairs Medical Center, Durham, North Carolina
Right-Sided Valvular Disease

Arthur A. Bert, MD
Clinical Professor of Surgery (Anesthesiology), Warren Alpert School of Medicine at Brown University, Brown University, Providence, Rhode Island; Associate Chief, Department of Anesthesiology, Rhode Island Hospital, Providence, Rhode Island; Director of Experimental Cardiac Surgery, Imaging and Anesthesia, Cardiac Surgery Research Laboratories, Children's Mercy Hospital, Kansas City, Missouri
Echocardiographic Evaluation of Prosthetic Valves

Albert T. Cheung, MD
Professor, Anesthesiology and Critical Care, University of Pennsylvania, Philadelphia, Pennsylvania
Diseases of the Aorta

James Drew, MBChB(UCT), FRCA, FANZCA
Simulation Instructor, Faculty of Medical and Health Sciences, Auckland University; Specialist Anaesthetist, Auckland City Hospital, Auckland, New Zealand
Intraoperative Echocardiography for Heart and Lung Transplantation

Mark Edwards, MBChB, FANZCA, DipPGEcho
Anaesthetist and Clinical Director, Department of Cardiothoracic and ORL Anaesthesia, Auckland City Hospital, Auckland, New Zealand
Intraoperative Echocardiography for Heart and Lung Transplantation

Kathryn E. Glas, MD, FASE, MBA
Associate Professor, Anesthesiology, Emory University School of Medicine, Atlanta, Georgia
Epiaortic Ultrasonography and Epicardial Echocardiography

Marjan Jariani, MD, FRCPC
Assistant Professor, Department of Anesthesia, University of Toronto; Staff Anesthesiologist, Toronto General Hospital, Toronto, Ontario, Canada
Aortic Valve and Aortic Root

Denise Joffe, MD
Associate Professor, Department of Anesthesiology, University of Washington; Attending Anesthesiologist, Seattle Children's Hospital and University of Washington Medical Center, Seattle, Washington
Congenital Heart Disease

Carol Kraft, BS, RDCS
Cardiac Sonographer Specialist, University of Washington Medical Center, Seattle, Washington
Introduction to Intraoperative Echocardiography

A. Stephane Lambert, MD, FRCP(C)
Assistant Professor of Anesthesiology, University of Ottawa; Attending Anesthesiologist, University of Ottawa Heart Institute, Ottawa, Ontario, Canada
Mitral Valve Diseases

Jonathan B. Mark, MD
Professor of Anesthesiology, Duke University Medical Center; Chief, Anesthesiology Service, and Principal Investigator, Patient Safety Center of Inquiry, Veterans Affairs Medical Center, Durham, North Carolina
Right-Sided Valvular Disease

Andrew D. Maslow, MD
Clinical Associate Professor in Anesthesiology, Warren Alpert School of Medicine, Brown University; Director of Cardiac Anesthesiology, Department of Anesthesiology, Rhode Island Hospital, Providence, Rhode Island
Echocardiographic Evaluation of Prosthetic Valves

Massimiliano Meineri, MD
Assistant Professor, University of Toronto; Staff Anesthesiologist, University Health Network, Toronto General Hospital, Toronto, Ontario, Canada
Masses and Devices

Patricia Murphy, MD, FRCPC
Associate Professor, University of Toronto; Staff Anesthesiologist, University Health Network, Toronto General Hospital, Toronto, Ontario, Canada
Masses and Devices

Alina Nicoara, MD
Assistant Professor, Duke University; Attending Physician, Duke University Medical Center, Durham, North Carolina
Ventricular Function

Donald C. Oxorn, MD
Professor of Anesthesiology, Division of Cardio-Thoracic Anesthesia, and Adjunct Professor of Medicine (Cardiology), University of Washington Medical Center, Seattle, Washington
Introduction to Intraoperative Echocardiography

Wendy L. Pabich, MD
Staff Anesthesiologist, Physicians Anesthesia Service, Swedish Medical Center, Seattle, Washington
Ventricular Function

Rebecca A. Schroeder, MD
Assistant Associate Professor of Anesthesiology, Duke University Medical Center; Staff Anesthesiologist, and Investigator, Patient Safety Center of Inquiry, Veterans Affairs Medical Center, Durham, North Carolina
Right-Sided Valvular Disease

Stanton K. Shernan, MD, FAHA, FASE
Associate Professor, Harvard Medical School; Director of Cardiac Anesthesia, Department of Anesthesiology, Perioperative and Pain Medicine, Brigham and Women's Hospital, Boston, Massachusetts
Epiaortic Ultrasonography and Epicardial Echocardiography

Madhav Swaminathan, MD
Associate Professor, Duke University; Attending, Duke University Hospital, Durham, North Carolina
Ventricular Function

Annette Vegas, MDCM, FRCPC, FASE
Associate Professor, University of Toronto; Staff Anesthesiologist, Toronto General Hospital, Toronto, Ontario, Canada
Aortic Valve and Aortic Root

Peter von Homeyer, MD
Assistant Professor, University of Washington; Assistant Professor, Department of Anesthesiology and Pain Medicine, University of Washington Medical Center, Seattle, Washington
Pericardial Disease

Stuart J. Weiss, MD, PhD
Department of Anesthesiology and Critical Care, University of Pennsylvania, Philadelphia, Pennsylvania
Diseases of the Aorta

Foreword

Echocardiography is a core component of every aspect of clinical cardiology and now plays an essential role in daily decision making. Both echocardiographers and clinicians face unique challenges in interpretation of imaging and Doppler data and in integration of these data with other clinical information. However, with the absorption of echocardiography into daily patient care, there are some voids in our collective knowledge base. First, clinicians caring for patients need to understand the value, strengths, and limitations of echocardiography relevant to their specific scope of practice. Second, echocardiographers need a more in-depth understanding of the clinical context of the imaging study. Finally, there often are unique aspects of data acquisition and analysis in different clinical situations, all of which are essential for accurate echocardiographic diagnosis. The books in the Practical Echocardiography Series are aimed at filling these knowledge gaps, with each book focusing on a specific clinical situation in which echocardiographic data are key for optimal patient care.

In addition to *Intraoperative Echocardiography*, edited by Donald C. Oxorn, MD, other books in the series are *Echocardiography in Congenital Heart Disease*, edited by Mark Lewin, MD, and Karen Stout, MD; *Echocardiography in Heart Failure*, edited by Martin St. John Sutton, MBBS, FRCP, FASE, and Susan E. Wiegers, MD, FASE; and *Advanced Approaches in Echocardiography*, edited by Linda Gillam, MD, and myself. Information is presented as concise bulleted text accompanied by numerous illustrations and tables, providing a practical approach to data acquisition and analysis, including technical details, pitfalls, and clinical interpretation, supplemented by web-based video case examples. Each volume in this series expands on the basic principles presented in the *Textbook of Clinical Echocardiography, Fourth Edition*, and can be used as a supplement to that text or can be used by physicians interested in a focused introduction to echocardiography in their area of clinical practice.

With advances in cardiac surgery and interventional cardiology, echocardiographic monitoring and guidance of therapeutic procedures has become an essential element in the procedure itself. These echocardiographic studies often are appropriately performed and interpreted by the anesthesiologist in conjunction with real-time review by the cardiac surgeon or interventional cardiologist. Other cardiologists and cardiac sonographers also often are asked to assist with imaging during these procedures. The optimal use of echocardiographic data in this setting requires specialized knowledge, as summarized in this book on intraoperative echocardiography.

The editor of this volume, Donald C. Oxorn, MD, is a Professor of Anesthesiology at the University of Washington Medical Center, where he is a key part of the echocardiography team in the operating room and interventional cardiology laboratory. He also is an Adjunct Professor of Medicine in recognition of his substantial clinical and teaching contributions in the Division of Cardiology. In this book, *Intraoperative Echocardiography*, Dr. Oxorn has built upon his extensive clinical experience and skills as an educator, along with the expertise of the chapter authors, to produce a truly practical guide to this area of clinical competence. This book introduced me to several new concepts in procedural imaging, as well as filling in many details about the use of echocardiography in the operating room. I hope you learn as much as I did.

Catherine M. Otto, MD

Preface

As the complexity of cardiac surgery and invasive cardiology has increased, so has the reliance on skilled interpretation of periprocedural echocardiography. As well as having a detailed knowledge of the pathophysiology of each disease process, the operative techniques available, and the validity of imaging information, the echocardiographer must be expert at knowing what information is critical, and the most expeditious way of obtaining it.

Intraoperative Echocardiography is one of four volumes contained within the Practical Echocardiography Series. Whereas most other textbooks of intraoperative echocardiography present an extensive review based on a detailed search of the literature, the focus in the current volume is practical aspects of image acquisition and interpretation in the operating room. The book is organized into 12 chapters covering all aspects of intraoperative echocardiography, including the aortic, mitral, tricuspid, pulmonic, and prosthetic heart valves; the pericardium; the aorta; and the right and left ventricles; as well as cardiac masses. In addition, chapters are dedicated to specialized procedures such as heart and lung transplantation, the surgical treatment of congenital heart disease, the complimentary technology of epicardial and epiaortic ultrasound, and intracardiac and intravascular devices, which are seen with increasing frequency both in the operating room and interventional suites.

The goal of this book is to provide content as concise text in a visually rich volume complimented by online video and case presentations. In each chapter, background information is followed by a step-by-step approach to patient examination. Information is conveyed in bulleted points, with each set of major principles followed by a list of key points. Potential pitfalls are identified and approaches to avoiding errors are provided. Data measurements and calculations are explained with specific examples. Numerous illustrations with detailed figure legends demonstrate each major point and guide the reader through the teaching points.

This atlas will be of interest to all health care providers involved in the acquisition and interpretation of perioperative echocardiograms. In addition to cardiac anesthesiologists, this book will be useful to cardiologists and cardiology fellows interested in expanding their knowledge of cardiac surgery and the important aspects of intraoperative imaging, cardiac sonographers who wish to participate as part of the intraoperative team, cardiac surgeons seeking to understand echocardiography, and individuals wishing to become more familiar with what actually transpires in the operating room.

This atlas is not a substitute for formal training in TEE performance and interpretation; instead it is designed to serve as an adjunct in furthering the skill required in the obtaining of relevant information critical for successful intraoperative interventions.

Donald C. Oxorn, MD

Acknowledgments

I wish to acknowledge the contributions and encouragement of my colleagues in Cardiothoracic Anesthesiology: T. Andrew Bowdle, Krishna Natrajan, Jorg Dziersk, Peter von Homeyer, Stefan Lombaard, Kei Togashi, Srdjan Jelacic, Erin Failor, and Sally Barlow; in Cardiothoracic Surgery: Edward Verrier, Gabriel Aldea, and Nahush Mokadam; and Starr Kaplan for her artwork. My appreciation extends to Natasha Andjelkovic at Elsevier and the production team who supported this project and helped make it a reality.

I would also like to acknowledge the guidance and encouragement provided by Catherine M. Otto in the preparation of this volume.

Finally, I wish to thank my wife Susan Murdoch and my children, Jonathan Oxorn, Sean Murdoch-Oxorn, and Alexandra Murdoch-Oxorn; their understanding and cheerful disposition was ever present and much appreciated.

I would like to thank two individuals from the University of Toronto: my friend and mentor Gerald Edelist, and Cam Joyner, my first and foremost teacher in echocardiography.

Contents

Video Contents

Glossary

2C two-chamber
2D two-dimensional
3D three-dimensional
4C four-chamber
5C five-chamber
A late diastolic ventricular filling velocity with atrial contraction
A' diastolic tissue Doppler velocity with atrial contraction
Ab abscess
AC atrial contraction
ACC American College of Cardiology
AHA American Heart Association
AI aortic insufficiency
AIDS acquired immunodeficiency syndrome
AL anterior leaflet
ALCAPA anomalous origin of the left coronary artery from the pulmonary artery
AML anterior mitral leaflet
AMVL anterior mitral valve leaflet
AO or Ao aorta
AoA effective orifice area-to-aortic area
APCs aortopulmonary collateral arteries
APV absent pulmonary valve
AR aortic regurgitation
AS aortic stenosis
ASD atrial septal defect
ASE American Society of Echocardiography
ASO arterial switch operation
AV aortic valve
AVA aortic valve area
AVC atrioventricular canal
AVR aortic valve replacement
AVR aortic valve repair
AVV atrioventricular valve
AVVR atrioventricular valve repair
BAV bicuspid aortic valve
BiVAD biventricular assist device
BLT bilateral lung transplant
BSA body surface area
BT Blalock-Taussig (shunt)
BVF biventricular flow
CABG coronary artery bypass graft
CAD coronary artery disease
CAVC common atrioventricular canal

CF color flow
CHD congenital heart disease
CHF congestive heart failure
CI cardiac index
cm centimeter(s)
cm/s centimeters per second
CO cardiac output
CPB cardiopulmonary bypass
CS coronary sinus
CSA cross-sectional area
CT computed tomography
CT connective tissue
CTGA complete transposition of the great arteries
CVA cerebrovascular accident
CVC central venous catheter
CVD cardiovascular disease
CVP central venous pressure
CW continuous wave
Cx circumflex coronary artery
dB decibel(s)
DCRV double-chamber right ventricle
DGC depth gain compensation
DILV double-inlet left ventricle
DKS Damus-Kaye-Stansel
DORV double-outlet right ventricle
dP/dt rate of change in pressure over time
DT deceleration time
D-TGA D-transposition of the great arteries
dT/dt rate of increase in temperature
DVI Doppler velocity index
E early diastolic peak velocity
E' early diastolic tissue Doppler velocity
EAU epiaortic ultrasonography
ECE epicardial echocardiography
ECG electrocardiogram
ECMO extracorporeal membrane oxygenation
EDD end-diastolic dimension
EF ejection fraction
EOA effective orifice area
ERO effective regurgitant orifice
EROA effective regurgitant orifice area
ESC European Society of Cardiology
ESD end-systolic dimension
ET ejection time

FAC fractional area of change
FL false lumen
FO fossa ovalis
FS fractional shortening
HACEK (group) haemophilus, aggregatibacter, cardiobacterium hominis, eikenella corrodens, kingella
HFNEF heart failure with a normal ejection fraction
HLHS hypertrophic left heart syndrome
HOCM hypertrophic cardiomyopathy
HPRF high pulse repetition frequency
HR heart rate
hr hour(s)
HV hepatic vein
HVF hepatic venous flow
Hz Hertz (cycles per second)
IABP intra-aortic balloon pump
IAS interatrial septum
IE infective endocarditis
iEOA indexed effective orifice area
IV innominate vein
IVC inferior vena cava
IVR isovolumic relaxation
IVRT isovolumic relaxation time
IVS interventricular septum
LA left atrium/left atrial
LAA left atrial appendage
LAD left anterior descending artery
LAE left atrial enlargement
LAP left atrial pressure
LAX long axis
LCA left coronary artery
LCC left coronary cusp
LCX left circumflex artery
LLPV left lower pulmonary vein
LMCA left main coronary artery
LPA left pulmonary artery
LPV left pulmonary vein
LSPV left superior pulmonary vein
LSVC left superior vena cava
LTGA left transposition of the great arteries
LUPV left upper pulmonary vein
LV left ventricle/left ventricular
LVAD left ventricular assist device
LVAd left ventricular area in end-diastole
LVAs left ventricular area in end-systole
LVDd left ventricular end-diastolic dimension
LVDs left ventricular end-systolic dimension
LVE left ventricular enlargement
LVEDP left ventricular end-diastolic pressure
LVEDV left ventricular end-diastolic volume
LVEF left ventricular ejection fraction
LVESV left ventricular end-systolic volume
LVH left ventricular hypertrophy
LVOT left ventricular outflow tract
LVOTO left ventricular outflow tract obstruction
LVP left ventricular pressure

M-mode motion display (depth versus time)
MAPCAs multiple aortopulmonary collateral arteries
ME midesophageal
MG mean valve gradient
min minute(s)
mL milliliter(s)
mPA or MPA main pulmonary artery
MR mitral regurgitation
MRI magnetic resonance imaging
MS mitral stenosis
MV mitral valve
MVA mitral valve area
MVR mitral valve replacement
MVR mitral valve repair
n number of subjects
NCC noncoronary cusp
NVE native valve endocarditis
NYHA New York Heart Association
OR operating room
PA pulmonary artery
PAC pulmonary artery catheter
PAIVS pulmonary atresia with intact ventricular septum
PAP pulmonary artery pressure
PAPVD partial anomalous pulmonary venous discharge
PBF pulmonary blood flow
PDA patent ductus arteriosus
PDA posterior descending artery
PE pericardial effusion
PFO patent foramen ovale
PHT pressure half-time
PHTN pulmonary hypertension
PI pulmonic insufficiency
PISA proximal isovelocity surface area
PL posterior leaflet
PLs paravalvular leaks
PM papillary muscle
PPM patient-prosthesis mismatch
PR pressure recovery
PR pulmonic regurgitation
PRF pulse repetition frequency
PS pulmonic stenosis
PulmV pulmonic valve
PV pulmonary vein
PVC pulmonary vein confluence
PVD pulmonary vascular disease
PVE prosthetic valve endocarditis
PVF pulmonary venous flow
PVR pulmonary vascular resistance
PW pulsed wave
RA right atrium/right atrial
RAA right atrial appendage
RAE right atrial enlargement
RAP right atrial pressure
RCA right coronary artery
RCC right coronary cusp

RF rapid filling
RLPV right lower pulmonary vein
RMPV right middle pulmonary vein
ROA regurgitant orifice area
RPA right pulmonary artery
RPV right pulmonary vein
RUPV right upper pulmonary vein
RV right ventricle/right ventricular
RVAD right ventricular assist device
RVAd right ventricular area in end-diastole
RVAs right ventriclular area in end-systole
RVDCA right ventricle-dependent coronary
  artery
RVE right ventricular enlargement
RVEDP right ventricular end-diastolic
  pressure
RVEDV right ventricular end-diastolic volume
RVESV right ventricular end-systolic volume
RVEF right ventricular ejection fraction
RVH right ventricular hypertrophy
RVOT right ventricular outflow tract
RVOTO right ventricular outflow tract
  obstruction
RVP right ventricular pressure
RVSP right ventricular systolic pressure
RWMA regional wall motion abnormality
s second(s)
SAM systolic anterior motion
SAX short axis
SBP systolic blood pressure
SCA Society of Cardiovascular Anesthesiologists
SF slow filling
SL septal leaflet
SLT single lung transplant
SOB shortness of breath
SoV sinus(es) of Valsalva
SR sarcoplasmic reticulum

STJ sinotubular junction
SV single ventricle
SV stroke volume
SV ASD sinus venosus atrial septal defect
SVC superior vena cava
SVR systemic vascular resistance
TA transapical
TAA thoracic aortic aneurysm
TAFS tricuspid annulus fractional shortening
TAPSE tricuspid annular plane systolic
  excursion
TAPVD total anomalous pulmonary venous
  discharge
TEE transesophageal echocardiography
TEVAR thoracic endovascular aortic repair
TF transfemoral
TG transgastric
TGA transposition of the great arteries
TGC time gain compensation
TL true lumen
TMF transmitral inflow
TOF tetralogy of Fallot
TR tricuspid regurgitation
TS tricuspid stenosis
TTE transthoracic echocardiography
TTF transtricuspid flow
TV tricuspid valve
TVR tricuspid valve repair
UE upper esophageal
Va aliasing velocity
VAD ventricular assist device
VC vena contracta
VOO asynchronous ventricular pacing
VS ventricular septum
VSD ventricular septal defect
VTI velocity time integral
WMAs wall motion abnormalities

Introduction to Intraoperative Echocardiography

Carol Kraft and Donald C. Oxorn

BACKGROUND

- The intraoperative setting can be daunting, even to experienced practitioners who do not spend the bulk of their clinical time in the operating room (OR).
- Factors that limit optimal image acquisition include bright lights and lots of noise.
- Time may be limited because several different physicians and nurses have responsibilities in surgical preparation and the surgical procedure.
- This chapter describes
  - The fundamentals of echocardiographic imaging in the OR.
  - Some basic physics and instrumentation.
  - Ultrasound artifacts that are particularly important for the intraoperative echocardiographer.
- Subsequent chapters delve into the details of image acquisition in specific clinical settings.

TRANSESOPHAGEAL ECHOCARDIOGRAPHY PROCEDURAL ISSUES

- After the induction of anesthesia, make sure the patient is being cared for by someone who is not distracted by the ultrasound examination.
- Start obtaining data as early as possible. This maximizes the available time for imaging before the surgical procedure starts.
- If feasible, request that the lighting be dimmed, or at a minimum, direct any overhead surgical lighting away from the echocardiography machine.
- Address any unresolved diagnostic imaging questions first.
  - For example, if the patient is known to have critical aortic stenosis and is scheduled for aortic valve replacement, it is unlikely that the intraoperative echocardiogram will alter that plan.

- Conversely, if the same patient has concurrent mitral regurgitation that has been difficult to quantify, and in which there is confusion regarding the underlying mechanism, this is something that needs to be clarified before the surgery begins.
- Know the preoperative data (transesophageal echocardiography [TTE], heart catheterization, computed tomography [CT], magnetic resonance imaging [MRI]), and review the images, if possible, to assess data quality.
- Speak to the surgeon and find out what information is needed from the intraoperative examination. If, as often occurs, you discover previously undiagnosed pathology, do not hesitate to share this information with the surgeon.
- Once the surgery begins, electrocautery will inevitably be used, which interferes with the two-dimensional (2D) and Doppler signals. Try to get crucial information before this situation exists.
- Electronic interference with the electrocardiogram (ECG) prevents appropriate triggering of cine loop recording from the QRS complex. Instead, set the echocardiography instrument to store data for a set length of time instead of a set number of beats.
- Record blood pressure and other parameters of loading conditions during echo acquisition so that pre- and postprocedure data can be interpreted in the context of the loading conditions.

KEY POINTS

- Most general anesthetic agents diminish vascular tone and depress myocardial contractility.
- Positive pressure ventilation has numerous hemodynamic effects that have the potential to alter echocardiographic findings.
- Cardiopulmonary bypass, especially when prolonged, has profound effects on vascular tone and systolic and diastolic function.

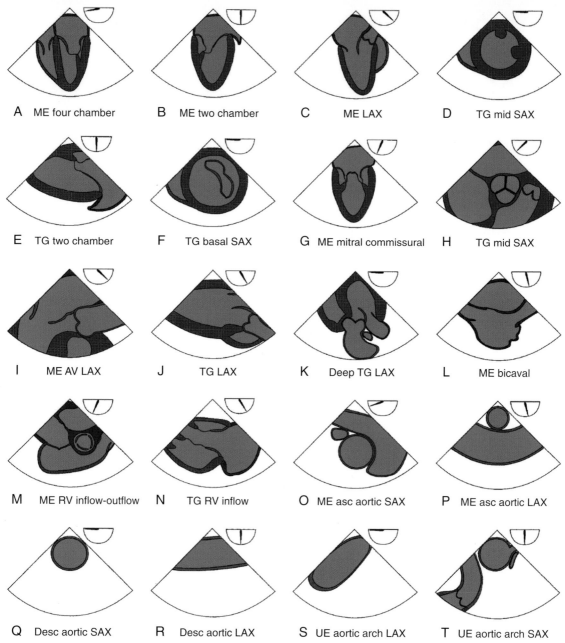

Figure 1-1. **A-T,** Twenty cross-sectional views composing the recommended comprehensive TEE examination. Approximate multiplane angle is indicated by the icon adjacent to each view. asc, ascending; AV, aortic valve; desc, descending; LAX, long axis; ME, midesophageal; RV, right ventricle; SAX, short axis; TG, transgastric; UE, upper esophageal. *A-T, From Shanewise JS, Cheung AT, Aronson S, et al. ASE/SCA guidelines for performing a comprehensive intraoperative multiplane transesophageal echocardiography examination: Recommendations of the American Society of Echocardiography Council for Intraoperative Echocardiography and the Society of Cardiovascular Anesthesiologists Task Force for Certification in Perioperative Transesophageal Echocardiography. Anesth Analg. 1999;88:870-874.*

TABLE 1-1   RECOMMENDED TRANSESOPHAGEAL ECHOCARDIOGRAPHY CROSS SECTIONS

Window (Depth from Incisors)	Cross Section (Panel in Figure 3)	Multiplane Angle Range	Structures Imaged
Upper esophageal (20-25 cm)	Aortic arch long axis (s)	0°	Aortic arch, left brachio v
	Aortic arch short axis (t)	90°	Aortic arch, PA, PV, left brachio v
Midesophageal (30-40 cm)	Four-chamber (a)	0°-20°	LV, LA, RV, RA, MV, TV, IAS
	Mitral commissural (g)	60°-70°	MV, LV, LA
	Two-chamber (b)	80°-100°	LV, LA, LAA, MV, CS
	Long axis (c)	120°-160°	LV, LA, AV, LVOT, MV, asc aorta
	RV inflow-outflow (m)	60°-90°	RV, RA, TV, RVOT, PV, PA
	AV short axis (h)	30°-60°	AV, IAS, coronary ostia, LVOT, PV
	AV long axis (i)	120°-160°	AV, LVOT, prox asc aorta, RPA
	Bicaval (l)	80°-110°	RA, SVC, IVC, IAS, LA
	Asc aortic short axis (o)	0°-60°	Asc aorta, SVC, PA, RPA
	Asc aortic long axis (p)	100°-150°	Asc aorta, right PA
	Desc aorta short axis (q)	0°	Desc thoracic aorta, left pleural space
	Desc aorta long axis (r)	90°-110°	Desc thoracic aorta, left pleural space
Transgastric (40-45 cm)	Basal short axis (f)	0°-20°	LV, MV, RV, TV
	Mid short axis (d)	0°-20°	LV, RV, pap mm
	Two-chamber (e)	80°-100°	LV, MV, chordae, pap mm, CS, LA
	Long axis (j)	90°-120°	LVOT, AV, MV
	RV inflow (n)	100°-120°	RV, TV, RA, TV chordae, pap mm
Deep transgastric (45-50 cm)	Long axis (k)	0°-20° (anteflexion)	LVOT, AV, asc aorta, arch

asc, ascending; AV, aortic valve; brachio v, brachiocephalic vein; CS, coronary sinus; desc, descending; IAS, interatrial septum; IVC, inferior vena cava; LA, left atrium; LAA, left atrial appendage; LV, left ventricle; LVOT, left ventricular outflow tract; MV, mitral valve; PA, pulmonary artery; pap mm, papillary muscles; prox, proximal; PV, pulmonary vein; RA, right atrium; RPA, right pulmonary artery; RV, right ventricle; RVOT, right ventricular outflow tract; SVC, superior vena cava; TV, tricuspid valve.
From Shanewise JS, Cheung AT, Aronson S, et al. ASE/SCA guidelines for performing a comprehensive intraoperative multiplane transesophageal echocardiography examination: Recommendations of the American Society of Echocardiography Council for Intraoperative Echocardiography and the Society of Cardiovascular Anesthesiologists Task Force for Certification in Perioperative Transesophageal Echocardiography. *Anesth Analg.* 1999;88:870-874.

INDICATIONS, CONTRAINDICATIONS, AND COMPLICATIONS OF INTRAOPERATIVE TRANSESOPHAGEAL ECHOCARDIOGRAPHY

- Shanewise's classic review[1] (Table 1-1; see also Figure 1-1) provides a common template on which to base an intraoperative TEE examination.
- Less traditional or "off-axis" views are often needed to adequately document abnormalities.
- The indications for intraoperative TEE have evolved, in keeping with a dramatic increase in surgical complexity; patients presenting for coronary revascularization are rarely without significant comorbidities.
- A number of recent documents relating to the local practice of, and training in, intraoperative echocardiography are referenced at the end of this chapter.[4-7]

Continued

- Patients having major noncardiac surgery who are at a high cardiac risk, including severe cardiac valve disease, severe coronary heart disease, or heart failure.
- TEE may be used in the critical care patient in whom severe or life-threatening hemodynamic disturbance is present and unresponsive to treatment or in patients in whom new or ongoing cardiac disease is suspected and who are not adequately assessed by transthoracic imaging or other diagnostic tests.

From European Association of Echocardiography. Recommendations for transoesophageal echocardiography: update 2010. *Eur J Echocardiogr*. 2010;11:557-576.

- The contraindications and complications of intraoperative TEE are described in Tables 1-2 and 1-3 and Figures 1-2 to 1-5. In general, these are the same as with TEE performed outside the OR with several caveats:
  - In the OR, the patient is under general anesthesia when the probe is introduced. Although these conditions facilitate probe insertion, patients are unable to indicate when excessive pressure is inapproriately applied.
  - In the OR, the probe may be left in the patient for extended periods of time.

IMAGE ACQUISITION

- Digital clip storage is the norm for all instruments on the market today.
- Most echocardiography systems can "slave" off the ECG of the anesthesia monitor
- Triggering should be time based and not ECG based. This will allow the choice of short or long clips and will not be affected by electrocautery interference with the ECG.

TABLE 1-2	SUGGESTED CONTRAINDICATIONS TO TRANSESOPHAGEAL ECHOCARDIOGRAPHY
Absolute Contraindications	**Relative Contraindications**
Perforated viscous	Atlantoaxial joint disease with restricted mobility
Esophageal pathology (stricture, trauma, tumor, scleroderma, Mallory-Weiss tear, diverticulum)*	Severe cervical arthritis with restricted mobility
Active upper GI bleeding	Prior radiation to the chest
Recent upper GI surgery	Symptomatic hiatal hernia
Esophagectomy, esophagogastrectomy	History of GI surgery Recent upper GI bleed Esophagitis, peptic ulcer disease Thoracoabdominal aneurysm Barrett's esophagus History of dysphagia Coagulopathy, thrombocytopenia

*TEE may be used for patients with oral, esophageal, or gastric disease if the expected benefit outweighs the potential risk, provided the appropriate precautions are applied. These precautions may include considering other imaging modalities (e.g., epicardial echocardiography), obtaining a gastroenterology consultation, limiting the examination, avoiding unnecessary probe manipulation, and using the most experienced operator.
GI, gastrointestinal.
From Hilberath JN, Oakes DA, Shernan SK, et al. Safety of transesophageal echocardiography. *J Am Soc Echocardiogr*. 2010;23:1115-1127.

TABLE 1-3	COMPLICATION RATE
Complication	**Incidence**
Dental injuries	0.03%*
Severe odynophagia	0.1%*
Minor pharyngeal bleeding	0.01%*
Endotracheal tube malposition	0.03%*
Perforation	0.01%*, 0.3%[†]
Major bleeding	0.03%*, 0.8%[†]
Mortality	0.004%*
Major morbidity	0.2%*, 1.2%[†]
Overall complication rate	0.2%*

*From Kallmeyer IJ, Collard CD, Fox JA, et al. The safety of intraoperative transesophageal echocardiography: A case series of 7200 surgical patients. *Anesth Analg*. 2001;92: 1126-1130.
[†]From Lennon MJ, Gibbs NM, Weightman WM, Leber J, Yusoff IF. Transesophageal echocardiography-related gastrointestinal complications in cardiac surgical patients. *Cardiothorac Vasc Anesth*. 2005;19:141-145.
From Hilberath JN, Oakes DA, Shernan SK, et al. Safety of transesophageal echocardiography. *J Am Soc Echocardiogr*. 2010;23:1115-1127.

SITES OF POTENTIAL INJURY

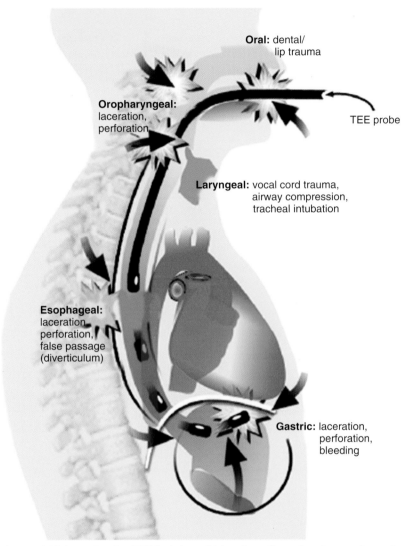

Figure 1-2. Sites of potential injury related to TEE include oral injury (e.g., lip or dental trauma), oropharyngeal injury (e.g., laceration, perforation), laryngeal injury (e.g., vocal cord trauma, compression of airway structures, inadvertent tracheal intubation), esophageal injury (e.g., laceration, perforation, false passage into diverticulum), gastric injury (e.g., lacerations or perforation, particularly of fundus or gastroesophageal junction), and gastric bleeding. *From Hilberath JN, Oakes DA, Shernan SK, et al. Safety of transesophageal echocardiography. J Am Soc Echocardiogr. 2010;23:1115-1127.*

BASIC PHYSICS PRINCIPLES

It is recommended that an in-depth review of basic ultrasound principles be completed before performing TEE.

- Speed of sound in tissue is 1540 m/s.
- The higher the frequency of the transducer the shorter the wavelength of the transmitted sound wave. This corresponds to better axial resolution, but a decrease in penetration.
- To detect two different points, they must be positioned further apart than the wavelength of the sound wave.
- Adult TEE transducers are usually between 7 and 3.5 MHz. Most TEE transducers have multiple frequencies to choose from on the same probe. Change the frequency to optimize what you are looking at.
- The angle of incidence will determine the intensity of the returned echo (a structure that is perpendicular to the sound wave will

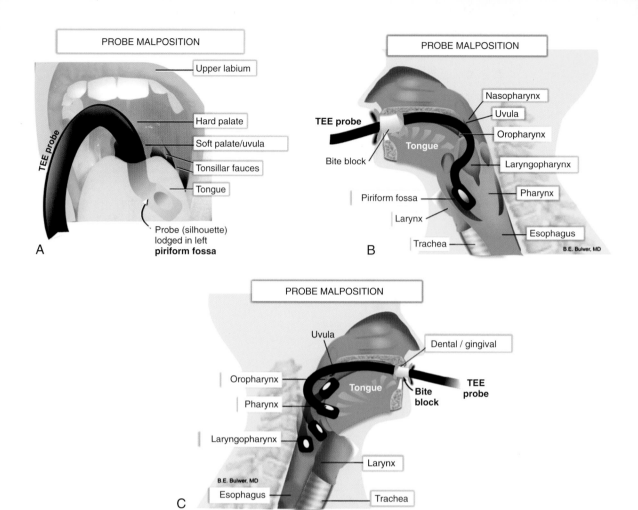

A

PROBE MALPOSITION

- Upper labium
- Hard palate
- Soft palate/uvula
- Tonsillar fauces
- Tongue
- Probe (silhouette) lodged in left **piriform fossa**

TEE probe

B

PROBE MALPOSITION

- Nasopharynx
- Uvula
- Oropharynx
- Laryngopharynx
- Pharynx
- Esophagus

TEE probe
Tongue
Bite block
Piriform fossa
Larynx
Trachea

B.E. Bulwer, MD

C

PROBE MALPOSITION

Uvula

- Oropharynx
- Pharynx
- Laryngopharynx
- Larynx
- Esophagus

Dental / gingival
Tongue
Bite block
TEE probe
Larynx
Trachea

B.E. Bulwer, MD

Figure 1-3. **A** and **B,** Probe malposition. Difficulty during probe insertion can be encountered if the TEE probe is lodged into one of the pyriform sinuses. **C,** In addition to causing mucosal injury to the oropharynx, the TEE probe can occasionally become distorted in extreme flexion. Attempts to withdraw a TEE probe in this configuration before advancing into the stomach and unfolding the kink can lead to severe esophageal injury. *A-C, From Hilberath JN, Oakes DA, Shernan SK, et al. Safety of transesophageal echocardiography. J Am Soc Echocardiogr. 2010;23:1115-1127.*

Figure 1-4. Gastric probe manipulations. Gastric injury typically occurs in the gastric fundus during deep transgastric probe manipulation, especially when requiring extreme anteflexion to bring the probe in line and in contact with the apex of the heart (e.g., deep transgastric aortic outflow view). The gastroesophageal junction is a vulnerable zone because probe manipulation at this level may place the relatively fixed tissues under considerable tension. *From Hilberath JN, Oakes DA, Shernan SK, et al. Safety of transesophageal echocardiography. J Am Soc Echocardiogr. 2010;23:1115-1127.*

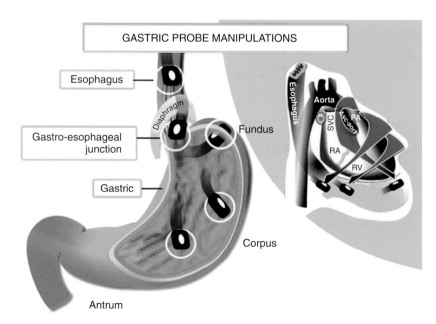

GASTRIC PROBE MANIPULATIONS

- Esophagus
- Gastro-esophageal junction
- Gastric

Diaphragm
Fundus
Corpus
Antrum

Esophagus
Aorta
SVC
Asc-aorta
PA
RA
RV

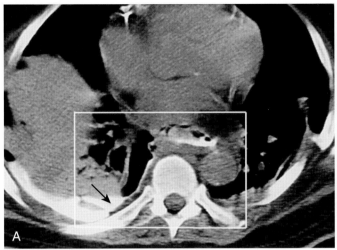
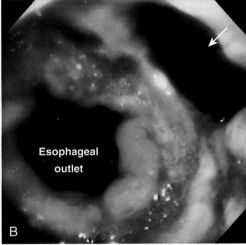

Figure 1-5. After a CT scan that was diagnostic for aortic dissection, this 67-year-old patient underwent ascending aortic repair, during which diagnostic TEE was performed. There was no premorbid history of symptoms related to esophageal dysfunction. Postoperatively, he became clinically septic. A right pleural effusion was drained and was cultured for a heavy growth of *Candida albicans*. Because of the suspicion of gastrointestinal contamination, a CT scan was obtained after barium swallow, which demonstrated extravasation of dye into the right pleural space (**A,** *arrow*). An upper gastrointestinal endoscopy was performed that revealed esophageal perforation through a preexisting diverticulum at the gastroesophageal junction (**B,** *arrow*). The patient was taken to the OR for right thoracotomy and esophageal resection. Postoperatively, the patient made an uneventful recovery.

give a stronger/brighter signal in return than one that is at a 45-degree angle).

- The higher the decibel (dB) level the less sensitive the azimuthal (side beam/lateral) resolution, that is, it makes it harder for a system to tell the difference between two different structures.
- The Nyquist limit is the maximum velocity of blood flow that a system can display. Once you have hit the maximum velocity, your signal will alias in both color and pulsed wave (PW) Doppler.

Setting Up for Two-Dimensional Imaging (Figure 1-6 and Table 1-4)

All systems will come with preset or default settings. It is important to know what each of these settings mean so you can adjust the image to your needs.

- Setting up preprocessing refers to adjustments made to the image before freezing it.
- Postprocessing: Can be changed either before you freeze the image or after the image is frozen. This can be helpful to use when you are trying to define a mass.

An ideal 2D image is one that allows for a strong border between the blood pool and the myocardium but still allows for myocardial fill-in and the ability to see textural differences in the tissue.

- If an image is undergained, it may be difficult to appreciate structures in the farfield (Figure 1-7).
- The gray scale or decibel level will affect the amount of gain you will use. If an image does not have enough gray scale, it will appear very black and white. This may be helpful when the lights are on in the OR, but it will not allow for visualizing subtleties on an examination.
- All systems will have proprietary terms or names for different processing features. Always ask your applications person for all of their functions.

Setup for Spectral Pulsed or Continuous Wave Doppler (Table 1-5)

- PW Doppler: There is a limit to the highest velocity that may be recorded. This is called the *Nyquist limit.* This limit is based upon the frequency of the transducer and depth that you are sampling from.
- You can maximize the velocity displayed by adjusting the baseline and velocity scale. All systems will allow you to move the

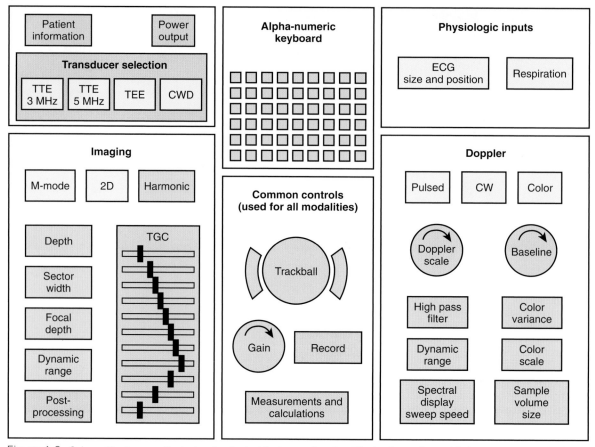

Figure 1-6. Schematic diagram illustrates the typical features of a simplified echocardiographic instrument panel. Many instrument controls affect different parameters depending on the imaging modality. For example, the trackball is used to adjust the position of the M-mode and Doppler beams, sample volume depth, and the size and position of the color Doppler box. The trackball also may be used to adjust 2D image depth and sector width and the position of the zoom box. The gain control adjusts gain for each modality, imaging, PW, or CW Doppler. Only a simplified model of an instrument panel is shown. The transducer choices are examples; other transducers are available depending on the system. In addition to the time gain compensation (TGC) controls, a lateral control scale may also be present. TTE, transthoracic echocardiography. *From Otto CM, Schwaegler RG. Echocardiography Review Guide. Philadelphia: Saunders; 2008:15.*

TABLE 1-4	SYSTEM CONTROLS INCLUDE DEPTH, OVERALL GAIN, POWER, DYNAMIC RANGE, TIME GAIN COMPENSATION/DGC. RECOMMENDED OR SUGGESTED SYSTEM SETUP FOR THE BEGINNING OF EACH TRANSESOPHAGEAL ECHOCARDIOGRAPHY EXAMINATION
Depth	15-16 cm
Overall gain	0 (some systems may have automatic gain compensation)
Dynamic range	65-70 dB
TGC/DGC (slide pots)	Midline or slightly lower
Focal zone	8-10 cm

DGC, depth gain compensation; TGC, time gain compensation.

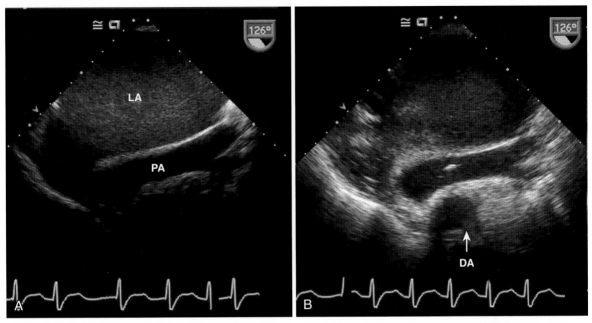

Figure 1-7. Transgastric images in a patient with a giant left atrium (LA). **A,** The pulmonary artery (PA) is seen, but nothing distal to it is visualized. **B,** With increased gain, the descending thoracic aorta (DA) comes into view.

TABLE 1-5	SUGGESTED PRESET DOPPLER SETTINGS AT THE BEGINNING OF AN EXAMINATION					
	Velocity Scale	Wall Filters	Baseline	Sample Volume Size	Sector Width	Gain
Pulsed Doppler	Maximum	Medium to medium-low	Centered	2-5 mm	N/A	Low enough to give strong outline without blooming of edges of tracing
CW Doppler	~3 m/s on either side of baseline	Medium-high to high	Centered	N/A	N/A	Low enough to give strong outline without blooming of edges of tracing
Color Doppler	Maximum for depth of color box	Medium	Centered	Small to medium	~30 to 45 degrees	Turn down gain just a bit from where you get extra speckling in the background

CW, continuous wave; N/A, not applicable.

baseline and increase or decrease the velocity scale.

- The area you are sampling or measuring is called the *sample volume*. The sample volume size is adjustable. Some systems may also call this the "gate."
- Continuous wave (CW) Doppler is used to measure peak velocities to help determine pressure gradients, for example, in cases of stenosis or measuring pulmonary artery pressures.
  - There is no adjustment of the area you are "listening" to. You will detect flow velocities along the entire length of the line displayed.

KEY POINTS
• *Pitfalls for PW Doppler:* You need to be parallel to flow to record the highest velocity flow. Blood flow velocity is often higher than the Nyquist limit.
• *Pitfalls for CW Doppler:* You need to be parallel to the flow to record the highest velocity of flow. You pick up the Doppler signals along the entire length of the sound beam; therefore, you may pick up two signals at the same time.

Setup for Color Doppler Imaging
(see Table 1-5)

Color Doppler is similar to PW Doppler in how it detects the blood flow; however, instead of "listening" or sampling to one spot at a time, the ultrasound system has many "sample volumes listening" in the selected area at the same time.

- The Nyquist limit also affects color Doppler the same way it affects PW Doppler. You can overestimate the size of a regurgitant jet if you do not have the color map set to the maximum velocity scale (Figure 1-8).
- Most equipment will use a red/blue "map" or a red/blue and green variance "map."
  - Red represents blood flow moving toward the transducer and blue is blood flow moving away from the transducer.

- Green variance shows high velocity or turbulent blood flow in green (Figure 1-9).

KEY POINTS: COLOR DOPPLER PITFALLS
• Wide color sector = • Low frame rate = • Low velocity scale increases aliasing =   • Slow frame rate • Decreased sensitivity to detect small jets • Falsely increases size of a regurgitant jet

Imaging Artifacts

A complete discussion of ultrasound artifacts is beyond the scope of this chapter. Several excellent references are listed at the end of this chapter.[10,11] Some artifacts commonly encountered in intraoperative practice are presented.

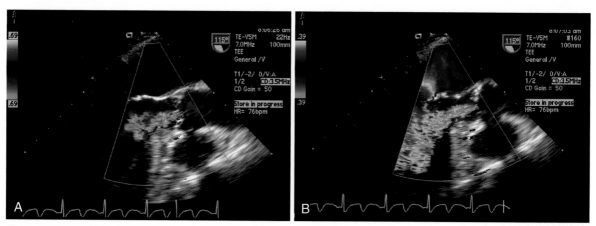

Figure 1-8. Both images are from the same patient with different color velocity scale settings (**A,** 69 cm/s; **B,** 39 cm/s) illustrating how the velocity scale can falsely make a regurgitant jet appear larger and, thus, potentially affect the diagnostic outcome for a patient.

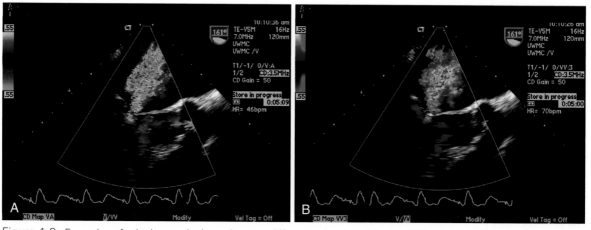

Figure 1-9. Examples of mitral regurgitation using two different color maps. **A,** A red/blue "map" or red/blue. **B,** A green variance "map."

This is a very important topic, especially in the intraoperative setting, where complex surgical procedures may be undertaken on the basis of findings in the prebypass TEE.

- Ultrasound artifacts are an incorrect representation of anatomic structures or the way in which they move. They occur because of problems in imaging technique, and the result is a breach in one of the basic assumptions of 2D imaging (Table 1-6):
  - Most artifacts seen in the OR are a result of the presence of strong reflectors that accompany most patients coming for surgery—calcified structures, prosthetic valves, intravascular catheters and devices.
  - As will be seen, the interface of great vessels such as the aorta and the main or branch pulmonary arteries also present strong reflecting surfaces. The frequent presence of linear artifacts may be mistaken for aortic dissection.

Acoustic Shadowing

Acoustic shadowing occurs when a strongly reflecting structure attenuates the ultrasound beam distal to it and thereby leads to an inability to obtain meaningful images distal to the reflecting structure (Figures 1-10 to 1-13)

- In echocardiography, acoustic shadowing occurs most commonly in the setting of heavily calcified structures such as the aorta and stenotic valves, with prosthetic valves, and in the presence of intracardiac and intravascular devices such as intra-aortic balloon pumps. It can occur with both 2D and Doppler imaging.
- Imaging the "shadowed" structure may be possible by using different angles of interrogation.
- Techniques such as epicardial echocardiography may allow approaching the "shadowed" structure from the other side of the reflector.

TABLE 1-6	2D IMAGING PRINCIPLES AND THE RESULTANT ARTIFACTS WHEN BREACHED	
Principle	**Artifact**
Transmitted wave is a single dimension; it reflected echo travel in a straight line path to and from the transducer	Refraction
Beam width is infinitesimally small in lateral and slice thickness dimensions. Echoes originate in the line of the transducer	Side lobe, beam width
Distance is proportional to round trip travel time. 1540 m/s. Each reflector contributes a single echo	Reflection, mirror image

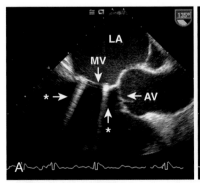
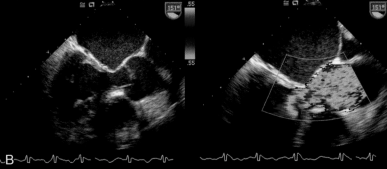

Figure 1-10. **A,** A bileaflet mechanical mitral valve prosthesis (MV) prevents imaging of the left ventricular outflow tract. The *asterisks* indicate the "comet tail" phenomenon secondary to multiple reverberations from the sewing ring of the mitral prosthesis. **B,** Between these is an area of acoustic shadowing. Changing the angle of interrogation allows adequate 2D and color Doppler imaging of the left ventricular outflow tract. AV, aortic valve; LA, left atrium.

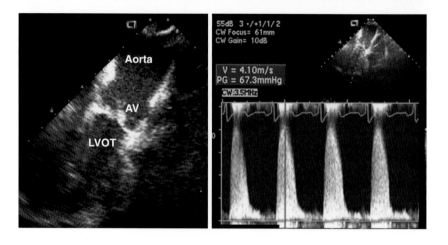

Figure 1-11. Epiaortic imaging of the calcified and stenotic aortic valve (AV) minimizes the attenuation of the Doppler signal that would have occurred with transgastric TEE imaging. LVOT, left ventricular outflow tract.

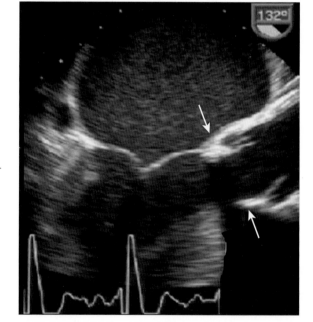

Figure 1-12. The stents *(arrows)* of an aortic valve tissue prosthesis produce distal acoustic shadowing.

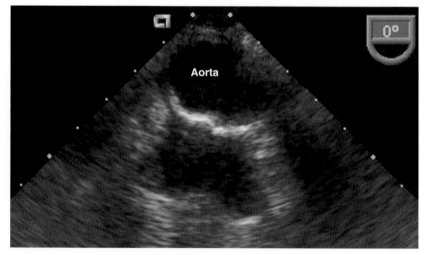

Figure 1-13. Calcification in the descending aorta produces distal acoustic shadowing.

Reverberation

Reverberation occurs in the presence of a strong reflector. A substantial amount of the ultrasound beam moves back and forth between the reflector and the transducer, so that at twice the distance from the transducer to the reflector, an artifactual image is displayed.

In addition, the presence of two parallel strong reflectors may allow the reflected energy to reverberate off the second reflector. This can be especially problematic around the ascending aorta where reverberations may lead to an erroneous diagnosis of aortic dissection (Figures 1-15 and 1-16).

- Recognize situations in which there are strong reflectors.
- Motion is congruent with cause of the artifact; use M-mode for temporal resolution.
- Color Doppler can overlie the artifact.
- Obtain multiple views.
- Use alternate imaging techniques, for example, epiaortic scanning.
  - A particular form of reverberation is the "comet tail." Two closely spaced reflective surfaces can produce a series of discrete and closely spaced echoes.
  - Figure 1-17 shows a series of images from a bileaflet mitral prosthesis. If there is the suspicion that one leaflet is stuck, multiple angles, depths, and probe rotations combined with color Doppler must be employed.

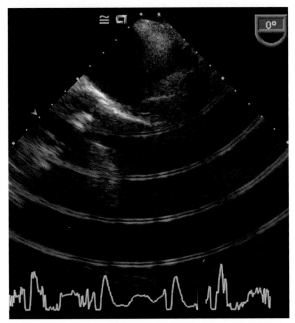

Figure 1-14. Surgical electrocautery. The four-chamber view is difficult to interpret. The clip frequency was left at 2 beats; interference with the ECG signal made the clip length extremely short.

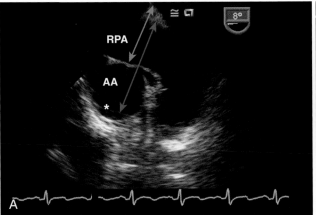
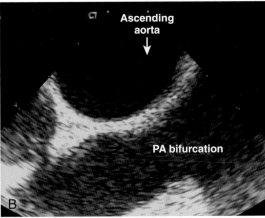

Figure 1-15. **A,** In this high esophageal short axis image, ultrasound is emitted and reflects off the interface of the anterior wall of the right pulmonary artery (RPA) and the posterior wall of the ascending aorta (AA), with most echoes returning to the transducer *(blue line)*. Some echoes, however, reflect off the posterior wall of the RPA *(red line)* and move toward the interface of the anterior wall of the RPA and the posterior wall of the ascending aorta. When these echoes return to the transducer from that interface, they are interpreted as coming from a distance equal to the sum of the distances covered by both red and blue lines. This artifact (*) may be erroneously interpreted as an aortic dissection flap. **B,** With epiaortic ultrasound, the artifact is no longer seen.

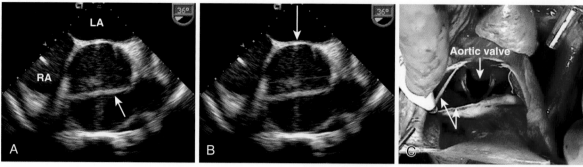

Figure 1-16. **A,** An aortic dissection *(short arrow)* is suspected. **B,** It is shown that, if the suspected flap is more than twice the distance *(red line)* from the transducer to the posterior wall of the aorta *(long arrow)*. **C,** At surgery, a dissection is confirmed *(double arrow)*.

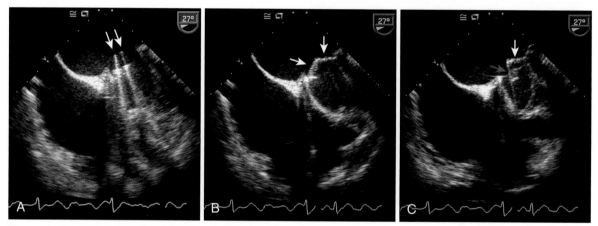

Figure 1-17. **A,** Both leaflets *(arrows)* open normally in diastole. **B,** They close normally during systole. **C,** There is the appearance that one leaflet is closing normally during systole *(white arrow)*, but that the other leaflet *(red arrow)* is not. In fact, the image indicated by the *red arrow* is not one of the leaflets, but a comet tail arising from the strut of the valve.

Mirror Image, Refraction

- These phenomena occur when an image is incorrectly visualized on the other side of a strong reflector (mirror image) or when the ultrasound beam is distorted by intervening tissue with inhomogeneous acoustic impedances (refraction) (Figures 1-18 to 1-20).

Side Lobe and Beam Width Artifacts

- Side lobes are progressively weaker ultrasound signals that radiate away from the main ultrasound beam.
- When a side lobe meets a reflective surface, a weaker image appears where the main ultrasound beam is at that time directed.
- The result is a series of artifacts on both sides of the actual structure. All images, artifactual and true, are equidistant from the transducer (Figures 1-21 and 1-22).

  Beam width artifacts occur because ultrasound beams are three-dimensional (3D) cone-shaped structures, such that a highly reflective structure

—such as a calcified aortic valve, or aortic atheroma—that is within the cone may be displayed in the imaging plane (Figure 1-23).
- Recognize strong reflectors, both in and adjacent to the imaging plane.
- Side lobes are always weaker than the source
  - Look for source.
  - Scan adjacent planes.
  - Decrease imaging intensity.
- Side lobes are always at the same depth as the source
  - Note depths.
  - Use different windows (artifact moves or disappears) or techniques (e.g., epiaortic or epicardial scanning; Figure 1-24).

Range Ambiguity

- Aliasing of PW Doppler occurs when the velocity of the jet being interrogated is too high relative to the Nyquist limit.
- In order to circumvent this problem, the pulse repetition frequency (PRF) may be increased.

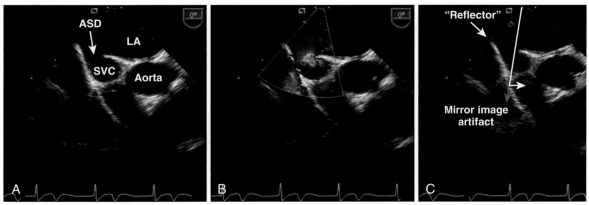

Figure 1-18. **(A and B)** A sinus venosus ASD is demonstrated. **(C)** Emitted ultrasound strikes the lateral border of the superior vena cava (SVC) and is reflected to the right, thereby imaging part of the right atrium *(white arrowhead)*. The *red arrowhead* shows the path the ultrasound would have taken, so that a portion of the right atrium also appears "outside" the heart as a mirror image artifact. ASD, atrial septal defect.

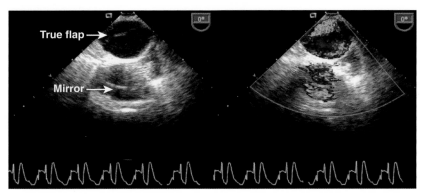

Figure 1-19. Another example of a mirror image artifact. The aorta, dissection flap, and differential color Doppler flow are duplicated on either side of the aorta-lung interface—a very strong reflecting surface.

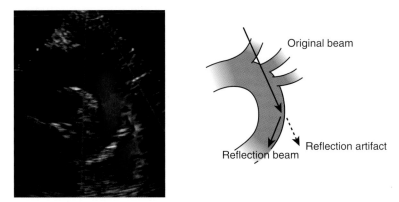

Figure 1-20. In this suprasternal view, a reflection artifact is demonstrated with color Doppler. *Courtesy of David Linker, MD.*

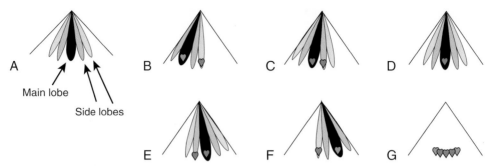

Figure 1-21. **A,** The strong main lobe and progressively weaker side lobes. **B-F,** One sweep of the sector is achieved. **G,** The result is the actual image, darkest and in the center, flanked by progressively weaker side lobes. **A-G,** *Courtesy of Stephane Lambert, MD.*

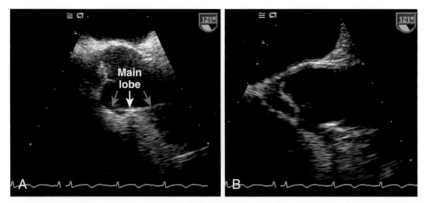

Figure 1-22. Some calcium near the right coronary sinus of Valsalva results in progressively weaker side lobes (**A,** *blue arrows*), which give the appearance of an aortic dissection. Acoustic shadowing is also present. **B,** When the image gain is decreased, the side lobes disappear.

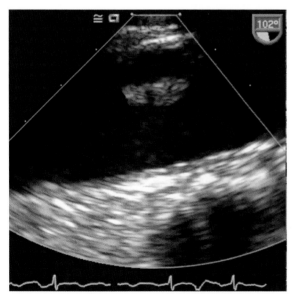

Figure 1-23. Example of beam width artifact in the descending aorta. A plaque that appears to be "floating" in the aorta is actually a beam width artifact.

However, this may lead to the problem of range ambiguity.

- In essence, increasing the PRF leads to the situation in which echoes from a first transmit burst return to the transducer after the next transmit burst has been sent out.
- The overlap of returning echoes from the two different scatterers leads to confusion as to the depth from which they originate (Figure 1-25).
- A similar problem can occur with 2D echocardiography, when high pulse repetition frequencies (HPRFs) are used, and there are strong reflectors in the distance. In the OR, problems typically occur when strong reflectors such as intravascular devices are present (Figure 1-26).
  - Recognize situations in which there are strong reflectors.
  - Increasing the imaging depth should make the artifact disappear.

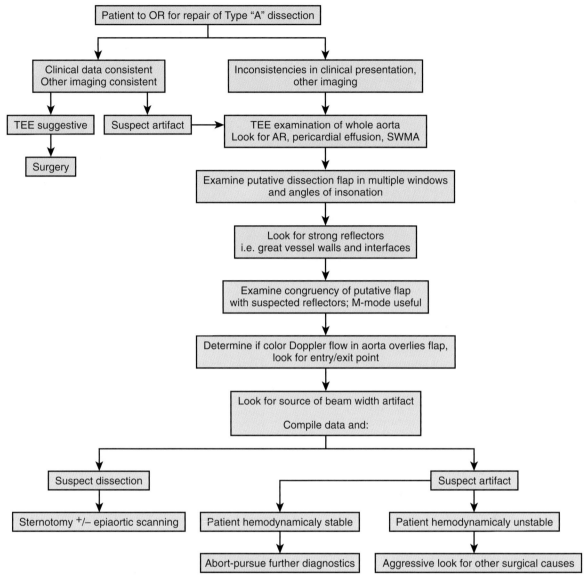

Figure 1-24. Flow chart for a patient in the OR for repair of a type A aortic dissection with suspected artifact.

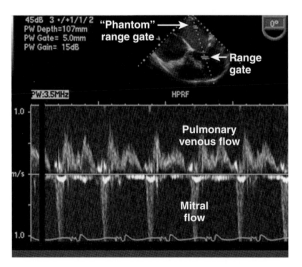

Figure 1-25. In this patient being ventricularly paced, the increased PRF used to avoid aliasing of the mitral inflow has led to HPRF and the creation of a second gate ("phantom") in the LA. Pulmonary vein flow velocities are simultaneously displayed.

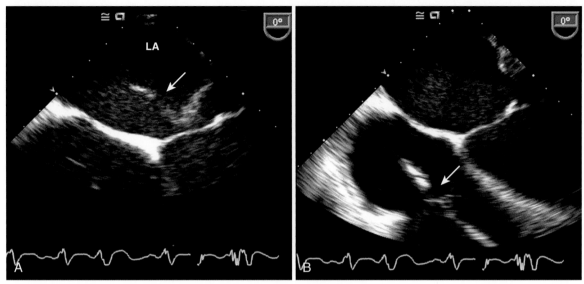

Figure 1-26. **A,** An unexpected mass is seen in the LA *(arrow).* **B,** The depth is increased and the PRF thereby decreases; the artifact disappears, and it can be seen that its origin was a collection of right-sided catheters/pacing wires *(arrow).*

- Motion is congruent with cause of the artifact; use M-mode for temporal resolution.
- Change the approach to interrogation to minimize the number of potentially confounding scatterers.

Suggested Readings

1. Shanewise JS, Cheung AT, Aronson S, et al. ASE/SCA guidelines for performing a comprehensive intraoperative multiplane transesophageal echocardiography examination: Recommendations of the American Society of Echocardiography Council for Intraoperative Echocardiography and the Society of Cardiovascular Anesthesiologists Task Force for Certification in Perioperative Transesophageal Echocardiography. *Anesth Analg.* 1999;88:870-874.
   The foundation for an intraoperative program.
2. Béïque F, Ali M, Hynes M, et al. Canadian guidelines for training in adult perioperative transesophageal echocardiography. Recommendations of the cardiovascular section of the Canadian Anesthesiologists' Society and the Canadian Society Echocardiography. *Can J Cardiol.* 2006;22:1015-1027.
3. Kneeshaw JD. Transoesophageal echocardiography (TOE) in the operating room. *Br J Anaesth.* 2006;97:77-84.
4. European Association of Echocardiography. Recommendations for transoesophageal echocardiography: update 2010. *Eur J Echocardiogr.* 2010;11:557-576.
   An extremely well-written and illustrated document written from a European perspective. Indications, contraindications, complications, and recommended training for those practicing perioperative TEE are discussed.
5. ANZCA—Australian and New Zealand College of Anaesthetists. Recommendations for Training and Practice of Diagnostic Perioperative Transoesophageal Echocardiography in Adults—2004 (PS46). Available at ANZCA website: WWW.anzca.edu
6. American Society of Anesthesiologists and the Society of Cardiovascular Anesthesiologists. Practice guidelines for perioperative transesophageal echocardiography. *Anesthesiology.* 2010;112:1084-1096.
7. Cahalan MK, Stewart W, Pearlman A, et al. American Society of Echocardiography and Society of Cardiovascular Anesthesiologists Task Force guidelines for training in perioperative echocardiography. *J Am Soc Echocardiogr.* 2002;15:647-652.
8. Hilberath JN, Oakes DA, Shernan SK, et al. Safety of transesophageal echocardiography. *J Am Soc Echocardiogr.* 2010;23:1115-1127.
9. Kallmeyer IJ, Collard CD, Fox JA, et al. The safety of intraoperative transesophageal echocardiography: A case series of 7200 surgical patients. *Anesth Analg.* 2001;92:1126-1130.
10. Kremkau FW. *Diagnostic Ultrasound.* 7th ed. St. Louis: Elsevier/Saunders; 2006.
    A superb resource.
11. Hedrick WR, Peterson CL. Image artifacts in real-time ultrasound. *J Diagn Med Sonogr.* 1995;11:300-308.
12. ASE/SCA recommendations and guidelines for continuous quality improvement in perioperative echocardiography. *J Am Soc Echocardiogr.* 2006;19:1303-1313.
    Recommendations and guidelines for a continuous quality improvement (CQI) program specific to the perioperative environment. Using the prior American Society of Echocardiography (ASE) publication on CQI as the foundation, this article (1) presents a rationale for CQI in the perioperative period; (2) defines the components of a perioperative echocardiography service; (3) establishes the principles of CQI as they relate to the practice of perioperative echocardiography; and (4) assesses whether CQI programs are effective in the perioperative period.

Mitral Valve Diseases

2

A. Stephane Lambert

INTRODUCTION: THE ROLE OF INTRAOPERATIVE TRANSESOPHAGEAL ECHOCARDIOGRAPHY IN MITRAL VALVE SURGERY

> ### KEY POINTS
>
> The major roles of intraoperative transesophageal echocardiography (TEE) in mitral valve (MV) surgery are as follows:
> - Confirm the preoperative diagnosis.
> - Evaluate the progression of MV disease since the last preoperative investigation.
> - Evaluate the valve in its dynamic state.
> - Assist in planning surgical intervention.
> - Evaluate associated cardiac dysfunction that may need attention (specifically tricuspid regurgitation).
> - Rarely, detect unsuspected MV disease, which may require intervention.
> - Evaluate repair in the operating room before chest closure, allowing further intervention if required.
>
>   When used in that fashion, intraoperative TEE has been shown to improve outcome.

INDICATIONS

The 2003 ACC/AHA/ASE (American College of Cardiology/American Heart Association/American Society of Echocardiography) Guideline Update for the Clinical Application of Echocardiography lists the various indications for TEE.[1] Several of them apply specifically to the MV and they are listed in Table 2-1.

MITRAL VALVE ANATOMY
(Figure 2-1)

- The mitral apparatus consists of
  - Left atrial (LA) walls
  - Mitral annulus
  - Mitral leaflets
  - Chordae tendinae
  - Papillary muscles
  - Left ventricular (LV) walls, which support the papillary muscles.
- Mitral annulus
  - It is saddle shaped.
  - It is a dynamic structure that changes its shape and diameter during the cardiac cycle.
  - It plays a crucial role in proper MV coaptation.
  - Dilatation of the annulus also leads to a loss of its saddle shape, which contributes to mitral dysfunction.
- Mitral leaflets (Figure 2-2)
  - The anterior leaflet is larger and covers two thirds of the surface area of the MV.
  - The posterior leaflet is smaller but it accounts for two thirds of the circumference of the MV.
  - The two leaflets join at the anterolateral and posteromedial *commissures*.
  - Coaptation between the two leaflets is *curvilinear*.
  - The posterior leaflet has distinct *scallops*, separated anatomically by little indentations at the leaflet edges.
  - The anterior leaflet does not have scallops, but is divided into *segments* for purposes of description.
- Chordae tendinae
  - There are three types
    - *Primary:* attach to the edges of the leaflets
    - *Secondary:* attach to the body of the leaflets
    - *Tertiary:* attach to the base of the posterior leaflet
  - (Some authors describe quaternary chordae, which attach to the LV wall, not the valve, and they play a role in maintaining LV geometry.)

TABLE 2-1   INDICATIONS FOR MITRAL VALVE ASSESSMENT BY TRANSESOPHAGEAL ECHOCARDIOGRAPHY

Class I Conditions for which there is evidence for and/or general agreement that a procedure be performed or a treatment is of benefit.	• Surgical *repair* of valvular lesions • "Complex" valve replacement (e.g., homograft) • Surgical repair of congenital lesions (including mitral valve lesions) • Surgery for endocarditis • Placement of intracardiac devices (which may affect mitral valve function)
Class IIa Conditions for which there is a divergence of evidence and/or opinion about the treatment. Weight of evidence/opinion is in favor of usefulness or efficacy.	• Surgery in patients at high risk of myocardial ischemia/infarction or hemodynamic disturbances (often includes ischemic MR) • Routine valve replacement • Cardiac aneurysm repair (may affect mitral valve and/or papillary muscle geometry/function) • Resection of cardiac tumors (LA myxomas can disrupt mitral valve function)
Class IIb Conditions for which there is a divergence of evidence and/or opinion about the treatment. Usefulness/efficacy is less well established by evidence or opinion.	• Evaluation of suspected cardiac trauma • Evaluation of regional myocardial function during off-pump coronary artery bypass (includes the diagnosis of acute ischemic mitral regurgitation)

LA, left atrium; LA, left atrial; MR, mitral regurgitation.
From the 2003 ACC/AHA/ASE Guideline Update for the Clinical Application of Echocardiography.

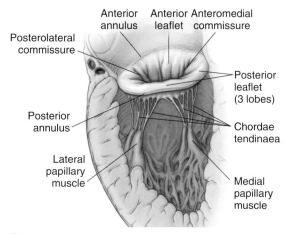

Figure 2-1. MV anatomy. *Adapted from Otto CM. Evaluation and management of chronic mitral regurgitation. N Engl J Med. 2001;345:740-746. Reproduced with permission.*

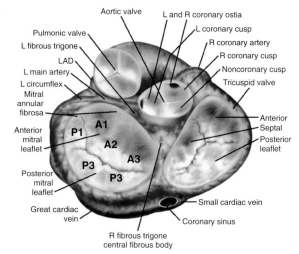

Figure 2-2. Cross section through the base of the heart shows the MV from the surgeon's perspective in the LA. It demonstrates the relationship of the valve with other major cardiac structures. The MV segments are labeled according to the Carpentier nomenclature (see text for details). LAD, left anterior descending. *Modified from Otto CM. Textbook of Clinical Echocardiography. 4th ed. Philadelphia: Elsevier/Saunders; 2009:40. With permission.*

• Papillary muscles
  • The LV has two: anterolateral and posteromedial, roughly aligned with the mitral commissures.
  • Each papillary muscle supplies *both* leaflets with chordae tendinae.
  • By contracting in systole, they play an important role in MV competence.
  • Papillary muscle ischemia, infarct, or rupture may lead to acute mitral regurgitation (MR).

• The posterior papillary muscle is more prone to infarction/rupture owing to its single blood supply (right coronary artery [RCA]) in most patients.
• Chronic LV dysfunction leads to posterior and apical displacement of the papillary muscles, which also can lead to MR (see section on "Functional MR")

MITRAL VALVE NOMENCLATURE

- Three nomenclatures of the MV exist in the literature.
- It is important to know which nomenclature is used by the surgical team to avoid confusion
  1. Classic anatomic
     - The posterior leaflet scallops are identified as anterolateral, middle, and posteromedial according to their anatomic location.
     - The anterior leaflet has no subdivisions.
  2. **Carpentier's nomenclature** (this is the most commonly used and was adopted by the ASE/Society of Cardiovascular Anesthesiologists)
     - The three posterior leaflet scallops are named P1, P2, and P3, from anterolateral to posteromedial.
     - The corresponding segments of the anterior leaflet are named A1, A2, and A3, respectively (note that the anterior leaflet does *not* have scallops and the various areas are referred to as *segments*).
  3. Duran's nomenclature
     - Used in some centers.
     - The three posterior leaflet scallops are named P1 (anterolaterally), P2 (posteromedially), and PM (middle). PM is further divided into PM1 (lateral half) and PM2 (medial half).
     - The anterior leaflet is divided into two segments, A1 laterally and A2 medially.
     - The commissural *areas* are named C1 (anterolateral) and C2 (posteromedial).
     - All segments of the MV that attach to the anterolateral papillary muscle receive the number 1 and all segments that attach to the posteromedial papillary muscle receive the number 2

SYSTEMATIC EXAMINATION OF THE MITRAL VALVE

Regardless of the type of MV disease, the TEE assessment always begins with a systematic two-dimensional (2D) examination of the valve. Using an organized sequence of cross sections, each scallop/segment of the MV is carefully examined for structure and function. The next section describes one sequence of views of the MV. *It is important to remember that only the basic views are described here. With increasing experience, echocardiographers make great use of transition images, or images between standard views.*

Sequence of Views (Table 2-2 and Figure 2-3)

- The examination begins in the *mid-esophageal (ME) four-chamber view* at 0 degrees. Identify the MV and zoom in on it by decreasing the depth of scanning.
  - Slight anteflexion/withdrawal of the probe will reveal *anterior* aspects of the valve (A1-P1 and A2-P2).
  - Slight retroflexion/insertion of the probe will reveal the *posterior* aspects of the valve (A2-A3 and P2-P3).
- Rotation of the transducer to about 60 degrees reveals the *ME commissural view*: P3-A2-P1 are seen from left to right.
- Further rotation of the transducer to about 90 degrees reveals the *ME two-chamber view*. In this view, the plane of the scan passes through the posteromedial commissure and provides a good view of P3. Slight rotation of the probe to the left demonstrates increasing amounts of the posterior leaflet, mostly the base of P2.
- Finally, rotation of the transducer to about 130 to 150 degrees reveals the *ME long axis view*: If lined up with the *center* of the valve, the plane of this view should cut through the middle of A2 and P2.

KEY POINTS

- Pitfall: As a general rule, angles of rotation are reliable only if the scanning plane is in the *center* of the valve. In the long axis view, one can ensure that the scan passes through the center of the valve by turning the probe slightly from left to right. Only then can one be certain that one is looking at A2-P2.
- Intentionally "scanning" the valve from lateral to medial is an advanced technique that can be very useful to pinpoint the location of a lesion. This technique can be applied to the commissural view, two-chamber view, and long axis view.

- Returning to 0 degrees and advancing the probe into the stomach demonstrates the *transgastric (TG) short axis view* of the MV. In this projection, the anterior leaflet appears on the *left* of the screen and the posterior leaflet appears on the *right* (as if the observer were looking at the MV from the *LV apex*). This view is useful to diagnose mitral clefts. Color flow Doppler in this view also helps to localize the *origin* of the regurgitant jet.

TABLE 2-2   THE SYSTEMATIC MITRAL VALVE EXAMINATION

Name of view	Description of the view	Picture
ME four-chamber view (0 degree)	• The AML is on the left hand side, adjacent to the aortic valve. The PML is on the right hand side. • The area of PML visible is mostly P2 (see Figure 2-3A).	
ME bicommissural view (60 degrees)	• Two apparent coaptation points. • From left to right, the visible mitral segments are P3, A2, and P1 (see Figure 2-3B).	
ME two-chamber view (90 degrees)	• Small P3 on left hand side and large AML on right hand side. The segment that coapts with P3 is A3. The rest of the visible AML is variable (see Figure 2-3C).	
ME long axis view (130–150 degrees)	• PML on the left hand side and AML on the right hand side. • If the plane of the scan is centered, P2 and A2 visible. May scan from side to side (see Figure 2-3D).	
TG short axis view (0 degree)	• AML on the left hand side, PML on right hand side. • Posteromedial commissure at top, anteromedial commissure at bottom (see Figure 2-3E).	
TG long axis view (90 degrees)	• Inferior wall at top. • Anterior wall at bottom. • Slight movement from side to side will reveal both papillary muscles (see Figure 2-3F).	

TABLE 2-2 THE SYSTEMATIC MITRAL VALVE EXAMINATION—cont'd

Name of view	Description of the view	Picture
3D LA view	• This view looks "down" at the valve from the LA and is closest to the surgeon's actual view of the valve. • By convention, the AML is at the top, and the PML is at the bottom (see Figure 2-3G).	
3D LV view	• This view looks "up" at the valve from the LV apex • The AML is at the top, and the PML is at the bottom (see Figure 2-3H).	

AML, anterior mitral leaflet; LA, left atrium; LA, left atrial; LV, left ventricle; LV, left ventricular; ME, midesophageal; PML, posterior mitral leaflet; 3D, three-dimensional; TG, transgastric.

• Finally, rotating the transducer to 90 degrees demonstrates the *TG basal long axis view.* This view is particularly useful to examine the subvalvular apparatus.

Three-Dimensional Echocardiography

Three-dimensional (3D) TEE provides exceptional images of the heart. Instead of a plane of information, the computer acquires a volume of data, which can then be reconstructed and viewed from any angle (Figure 2-4). Moreover, the data set can be sliced in any desired plane, much like a computed tomography (CT) scan, in order to re-create 2D images sometimes impossible to obtain by standard 2D echocardiography (Figure 2-5).

The MV, because of its proximity to the TEE transducer, lends itself particularly well to 3D imaging. At this time, 3D remains an adjunct to 2D, but as more centers gain experience with this technology, 3D imaging will become an integral part of intraoperative MV assessment.

The mechanism of MR is usually readily apparent on 3D imaging. Furthermore, off-line MV analysis software packages allow detailed quantification of MV disease, including dimensions, prolapses, and restriction (Figure 2-6). This is very useful in planning the surgical management of MR and may help to identify patients who require specialized surgical care. Moreover, the

TABLE 2-3 ETIOLOGY OF MITRAL REGURGITATION

Structural MR	• Congenital disease • Fibroelastic disease • Myxomatous degeneration • Rheumatic disease • Infectious disease
Functional MR	• Ischemic heart disease • Non-ischemic dilated cardiomyopathy
MR due to LVOT obstruction	• In association with HOCM • As a result of underfilled/hyperdynamic LV (rare without HOCM) • Post-mitral valve repair (usually in the setting of underfilling/hyperdynamic states)

HOCM, hypertrophic obstructive cardiomyopathy; LV, left ventricle; LVOT, left ventricular outflow tract; MR, mitral regurgitation.

development of leaflet stress analysis packages opens the door to the possibility of predicting, in the immediate post-bypass stage, the durability of some MV repairs.

MITRAL REGURGITATION

MR can be due to a structural problem in the valve itself or it may be due to distortion of the valve by external factors, described in Table 2-3.

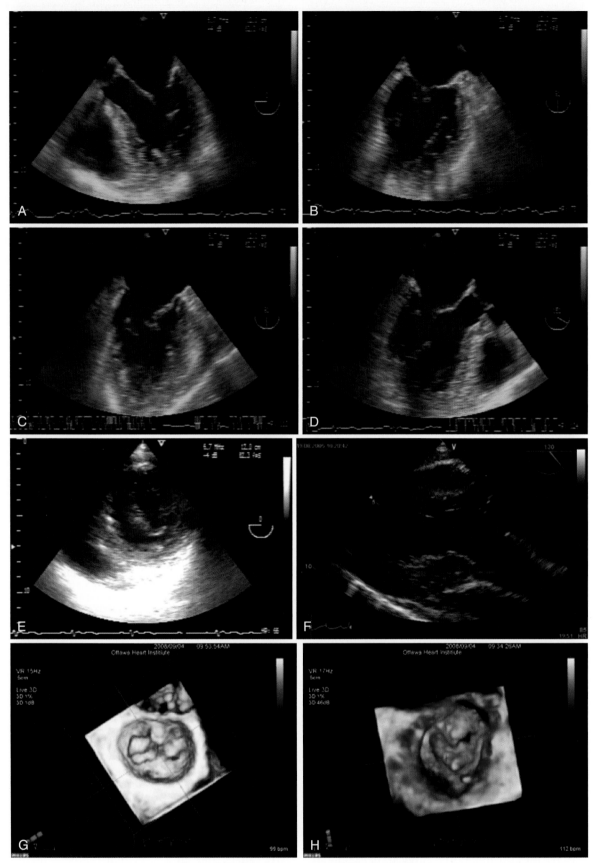

Figure 2-3. **A-H,** The systematic MV examination.

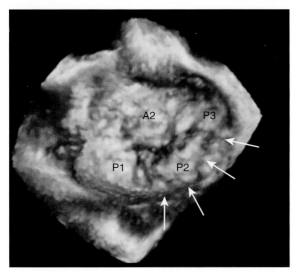

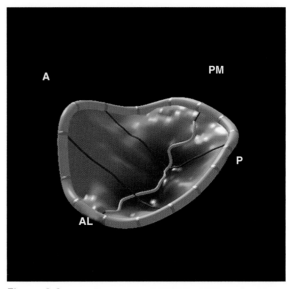

Figure 2-4. Real-time 3D TEE image of an MV prolapse from the LA perspective. Note the prolapsed area of the posterior leaflet, involving P2 and P3 *(arrows)*.

Figure 2-6. 3D MV analysis. Off-line analysis software allows detailed quantitative measurements of the MV, like annular dimensions, leaflet area and elevation, and tenting volumes.

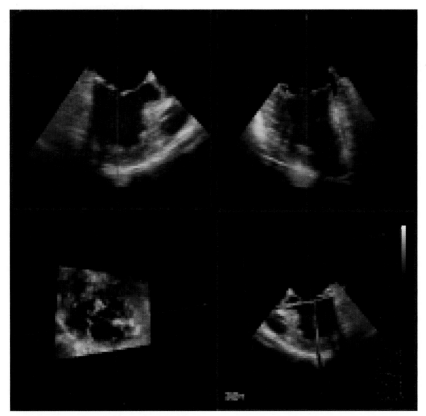

Figure 2-5. Multiplane reconstruction. This is a 3D data set of the heart, focusing on the MV. Once the data set is acquired, multiple planes can be displayed simultaneously and the scan lines can be adjusted to show any 2D cross section of the heart.

Classification of Mitral Regurgitation

KEY POINTS

- The three categories of MR as enunciated by Carpentier are normal, excessive, and restricted leaflet motion.
- **Pitfall:** Some mechanisms of MR do not fall in any specific category. This is the case of MR resulting from systolic anterior motion (SAM) of the anterior leaflet. Other conditions may span more than one mechanism, as is true for many cases of ischemic MR: those patients usually have some degree of annular dilatation (type 1) *and* some tethering of the leaflets (type 3b).
- Note that the differentiation between *severe prolapse* and *flail* is often academic and depends on whether ruptured chordae tendinae can be visualized or not. The surgical treatment is often the same.
- *Chronic* MR of any type almost always leads to some degree of secondary annular dilatation. However, pure annular dilatation without any other pathology is relatively infrequent.

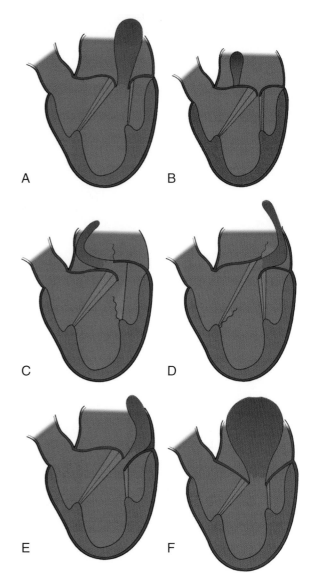

Figure 2-7. Carpentier's classification of MR based on leaflet motion. **A** and **B,** In type 1, the leaflet motion is normal and the jet tends to be central. The cause of MR is usually annular dilatation (**A**) or leaflet perforation (**B**). **C** and **D,** In type 2, there is excessive leaflet motion and the jet is directed away from the diseased leaflet. **E** and **F,** In type 3 lesions, the leaflet motion is restricted. Type 3 lesions are further subdivided into 3A and 3B. The jet can be directed toward the affected leaflet or it can be central if both leaflets are equally affected. *Modified from Perrino and Reeves' The Practice of Perioperative Transesophageal Echocardiography. Philadelphia: Lippincott Williams & Wilkins; 2003; Chapter 8, Fig. 8.7. With permission.*

- Popularized by Carpentier
- Based on *leaflet motion:* normal, excessive or restricted (Figure 2-7).
  - **Type 1: normal leaflet motion.** In type 1 lesions, the MR is usually due to pure annular dilatation or leaflet perforation.
  - **Type 2: excessive leaflet motion.** In type 2 lesions, part or all of a mitral leaflet extends past the plane of the mitral annulus (into the left atrium [LA]) in systole. There are different degrees of severity of type 2 lesions:
    - *Billowing or scalloping:* refers to a situation in which the *body* of the leaflet protrudes above the annular plane in systole but the *point of coaptation* remains below the annular plane. Often this is not associated with significant MR.
    - *Prolapse:* refers to a state in which the *tip* of the leaflet extends above the annular plane during systole, leading to failure of coaptation and MR. This is usually the result of redundant leaflet tissue or elongated chordae tendinae.
    - *Flail:* when the edge of the mitral leaflet flows freely into the LA during systole. This is usually the result of one or many ruptured chordae tendinae, which may be visible in the LA.
  - **Type 3: restricted leaflet motion.** In type 3 lesions, part of one or both mitral leaflets is prevented from reaching the proper coaptation point, resulting in MR. Two subtypes exist:

- **Type 3a:** the restriction occurs in *systole* and *diastole*, meaning that the leaflet does not close properly and does not open fully. This is often the result of a structural leaflet problem, most commonly rheumatic valve disease. It may also be associated with some degree of mitral stenosis.
- **Type 3b:** the leaflet restriction occurs in *systole* only. The leaflet opening is not affected. Most commonly in type 3b lesions, the leaflets are *structurally normal*, but are tethered, hence the term "functional" MR. The mechanism is usually multifactorial and it is discussed in a later section of this chapter.

Evaluation of Mitral Regurgitation

Step 1: Determine the Mechanism and Localization of Lesions and Etiology

The TEE evaluation of MR requires a comprehensive structural examination of the MV, to determine the mechanism of MR and localization of lesions. This involves a detailed 2D examination described previously. In each cross section, the appearance and integrity of the leaflets is noted: Are the leaflets thickened or calcified? Are they redundant (too much tissue)? Are they intact? One also looks at leaflet motion: Is it normal, excessive, or restricted? The coaptation point is then examined; is it below, at, or above the annular plane? Is there lack of coaptation?

One then proceeds to color Doppler evaluation of the regurgitant jet(s) and spectral Doppler measurements. When available, 3D echocardiography is useful to supplement a comprehensive 2D examination, but in the vast majority of cases, it is not essential to making a diagnosis.

KEY POINTS

- *Pitfall:* The echocardiographic appearance of MR is highly dependent on the loading conditions (preload and afterload), which can change during the course of an intraoperative examination. Moreover, *general anesthesia* is well known to decrease the apparent severity of MR by as much as one full grade (e.g., 4+ → 3+ or 3+ → 2+) owing to its effects on loading conditions.
- *Pitfall:* The appearance of MR by color Doppler is highly dependent on the *gain* and *Nyquist limit* of the transducer. Setting the gain too high or the Nyquist limit too low can make the MR appear more severe.

KEY POINTS—cont'd

- Very eccentric jets are usually structural in nature. Functional MR with posterior leaflet tethering often results in a slightly eccentric, posteriorly directed jet. The rest of the overall mitral evaluation allows differentiation between the two. Jet direction is only one of a number of factors used in the evaluation of MR.
- It is very important to establish whether MR is *structural* or *functional:* In the context of coronary artery bypass surgery, MR due to a structural leaflet problem is highly unlikely to improve after revascularization alone. Such mitral lesions should be addressed separately.

Examination of the Mitral Annulus

- As stated previously, the mitral annulus is a saddle-shaped, dynamic structure, intimately involved in MV competence. The systematic 2D evaluation of the valve includes a careful look at the annulus. Its diameter should be measured in both major axes, bicommissural (~60 degrees) and anteroposterior (ME long axis view at ~150 degrees). The normal MV measures 28 to 32 mm in diameter.
- The anterior leaflet and the commissural areas are well supported by the fibrous trigones. Conversely, the posterolateral mitral annulus is relatively poorly supported. For that reason, the MV annulus tends to dilate predominantly in the anteroposterior axis, in a posterior direction.

Flow chart of MR severity (Figure 2-8).

Severity of Mitral Regurgitation

- Except in cases of severe valve prolapse, no single view or sign is enough by itself to make a diagnosis of severe MR. However, taken as a group, the following signs have a high diagnostic accuracy.

Step 2: Qualitative Assessment
Color Flow Doppler

Color flow Doppler remains the best screening method to diagnose MR. It also allows a semiquantitative assessment of the severity of regurgitation and can provide clues to the mechanism of MR. *Pitfall:* The appearance of MR by color Doppler is highly dependent on the *gain* and *Nyquist limit* of the transducer. Setting the gain too high or the Nyquist limit too low can make the MR appear more severe.

- Total jet area:
  - All else being equal, small jets tend to be mild and large jets tend to be more severe (see Pitfall, earlier).
  - A surface area of the aliasing jet of 10 cm² has been associated with severe MR.
  - (As stated previously, the size of the MR jet is dependent on gain and Nyquist limit.)
- Jet area/LA area ratio
  - When taken as a percentage of the LA area, the specificity of the jet surface area as an index of severity of MR increases.
  - Jet surface area/LA surface area greater than 40% is associated with severe MR on cardiac catheterization.
- Eccentricity of the jet
  - The term *eccentric jet* refers to a jet that has a greater than 45-degree angle of incidence from the mitral annular plane.
  - Central jets can be structural or functional.

- Eccentric jets *tend to be* more structural than functional.
- Wall hugging jets
  - The term *wall hugging jet* refers to an eccentric MR jet that hits the LA wall, then follows it for some distance thereafter (Figure 2-9)
  - Wall hugging jets should be considered hemodynamically significant until proven otherwise and they *always* warrant careful examination:
    - It takes a high energy jet to follow the LA wall for some distance.
    - Owing to a physical phenomenon called the *coanda effect*, these jets appear smaller on color flow Doppler than they actually are.
    - They are almost always due to a *structural* leaflet problem.
- Direction of the MR jet (see Figure 2-7)
  The direction of the jet can provide useful clues about the mechanism of MR and the location of regurgitant lesions.
  - **In type 1 lesions** (normal leaflet motion), the origin and the direction of the jet are usually *central*.
  - **In type 2 lesions** (excessive leaflet motion), the direction of the jet is usually *away from* the diseased leaflet. If both leaflets are equally prolapsed, the resulting jet may be mostly central.
  - **In type 3a lesions** (restricted leaflet motion), the direction of the jet is usually *toward* the diseased leaflet. As in type 2 lesions, if both mitral leaflets are equally affected, the resulting regurgitant jet may be central.
  - **In type 3b lesions** (functional MR), because the posterior papillary muscle attaches to both leaflets, the regurgitant jet is typically *central* or slightly posteriorly directed.

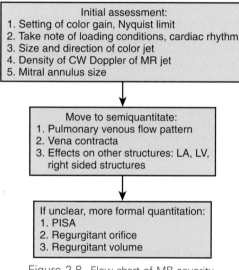

Initial assessment:
1. Setting of color gain, Nyquist limit
2. Take note of loading conditions, cardiac rhythm
3. Size and direction of color jet
4. Density of CW Doppler of MR jet
5. Mitral annulus size

Move to semiquantitate:
1. Pulmonary venous flow pattern
2. Vena contracta
3. Effects on other structures: LA, LV, right sided structures

If unclear, more formal quantitation:
1. PISA
2. Regurgitant orifice
3. Regurgitant volume

Figure 2-8. Flow chart of MR severity.

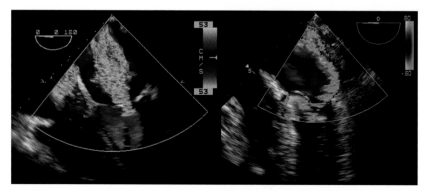

Figure 2-9. Central *(left)* vs. wall hugging *(right)* jet. Note how the latter hits the LA wall, then follows it all the way up to the top of the atrium.

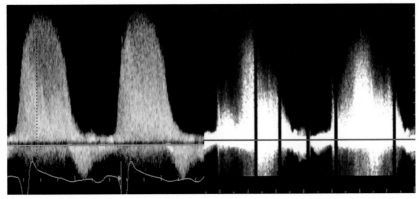

Figure 2-10. CW Doppler in severe and mild MR. **Left,** The image demonstrates a dense CW signal with a complete envelope (contour), associated with severe MR. **Right,** The envelope is faint and indistinct. This is seen with mild MR.

Spectral Doppler

Spectral Doppler provides additional qualitative signs of the severity of MR
- Density of the continuous wave (CW) Doppler signal (Figure 2-10)
  - The *peak velocity* of the MR jet on CW is determined by the LV-to-LA gradient.
  - The *density* of the MR jet is proportional to the number of blood cells crossing the mitral regurgitant orifice in systole.
  - A dense signal with a sharp, complete envelope (contour) is associated with more severe MR.
  - A faint signal with an indistinct, incomplete envelope is associated with less severe MR.
- Pulmonary venous flow (Figures 2-11 and 2-12)
  - Owing to the absence of valve between the pulmonary veins and the LA, blood can freely flow backward into the pulmonary veins under certain circumstances.
  - Once the pulmonary veins have been identified, the flow pattern is evaluated by placing the pulsed wave (PW) sample volume about 1 to 2 cm inside the pulmonary vein.
  - The normal flow pattern in the pulmonary veins is *forward* in systole (the S wave) and *forward* in diastole (the D wave), with a short period of flow reversal after the atrial contraction (the A wave).
  - The S wave is often *biphasic:* the first deflection (called S_1) corresponds to atrial relaxation whereas the second deflection (called S_2) corresponds to the descent of the atrial floor during systole.
  - The S, D, and A waves can be affected by many factors, including filling pressures, diastolic LV function, and MV disease.

- In the context of MR, increasing amounts of MR will lead to progressive *blunting* and eventually *reversal* of the S wave.
- In the presence of MR, systolic blunting or reversal of pulmonary venous flow suggests hemodynamically significant MR.
- In severe, central MR, the pulmonary systolic flow tends to be reversed in all pulmonary veins. However, when a jet is very eccentric, there can be situations in which there is flow reversal in only one set of pulmonary veins (left or right). That is why it is important to always check the pulmonary venous flow on both sides.

Step 3: Quantitative Assessment

There are few true quantitative methods for assessing the severity of MR. They tend to be time-consuming and require various calculations. Because of this, their intraoperative use tends to be limited to research and borderline clinical cases, in which the surgical management depends on the immediate echocardiographic assessment.

Vena Contracta (Figure 2-13)
- This is probably the exception to the previous rule, a quantitative measurement that can be performed relatively quickly in the operating room.

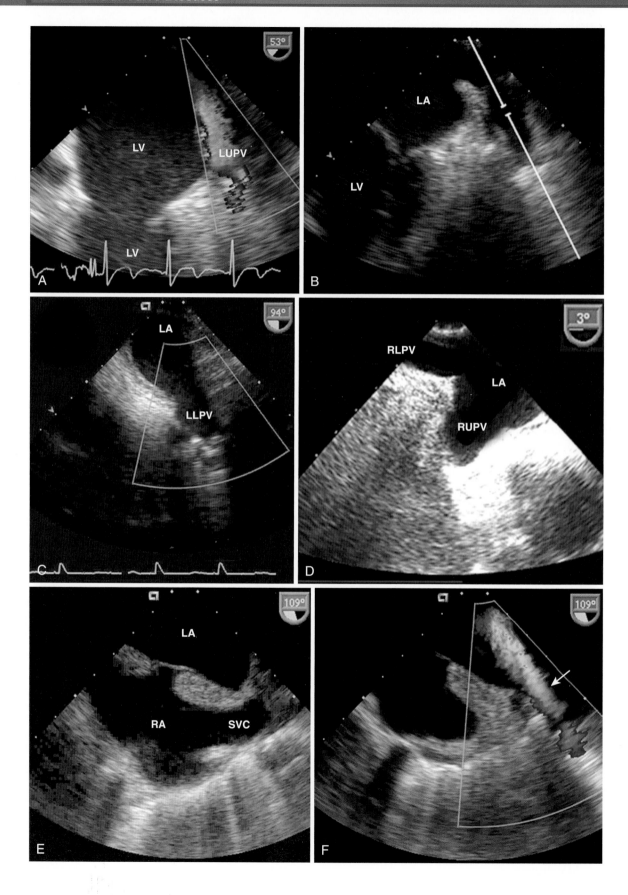

Figure 2-11. Imaging the pulmonary veins (PVs): Finding all four PVs can be a challenge owing to anatomic variations between patients. **A** and **B,** The easiest PV to image is the *left upper* (LUPV). It can be found by rotating the transducer to approximately 50 to 90 degrees and slightly withdrawing the probe until it is visible in the upper right region of the echocardiography screen. **C,** The left lower pulmonary vein (LLPV) can be imaged at an interrogation angle of approximately 90 to 100 degrees, with the probe rotated toward the patient's left and advanced slightly. Moving the probe in and out slightly will allow one to switch from one PV to the other, which may facilitate identification of those structures. **D,** With the probe at 0 to 30 degrees and rotated to the patient's right from the ME four-chamber view, the right upper (RUPV) and right lower (RLPV) PVs may be seen. After rotating to the right, the probe may need to be withdrawn slightly to image the RUPV and advanced slightly to image the RLPV. Alternatively, the RUPV may be reliably imaged by starting from the bicaval view (**E**) and rotating the probe further to the patient's right (**F**). Note that in all those views, color flow Doppler *(arrow)* can be used to help identify the vein (**A** and **F**). Once the desired PV is identified, the PW cursor is positioned about 1 to 2 cm inside the vein to obtain the spectral Doppler signal.

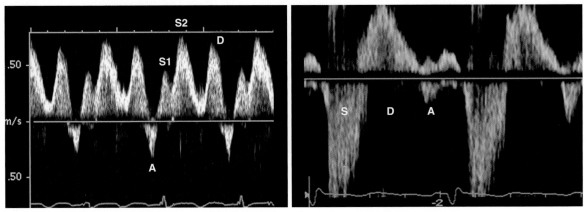

Figure 2-12. Pulmonary venous flow pattern. **Left,** The normal pattern: forward flow (upright) in systole (S1 atrial relaxation, S2 ventricular systole) and diastole (D), with brief backward flow (inverted) following atrial contraction (A). **Right,** Systolic reversal of flow can be seen in severe MR.

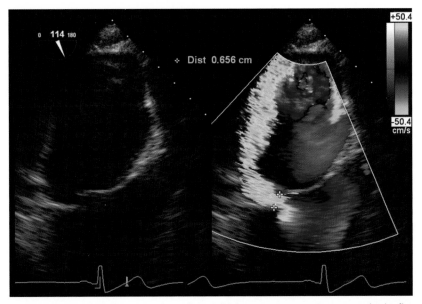

Figure 2-13. Vena contracta. This ME long axis view of the MV demonstrates a severe anterior leaflet prolapse. **Left,** Severe prolapse with obvious failure of coaptation. **Right,** The MR jet is seen by color flow Doppler. The narrowest point of the jet, corresponding to the coaptation gap in the MV, is measured. A diameter greater than 7 mm is associated with severe MR.

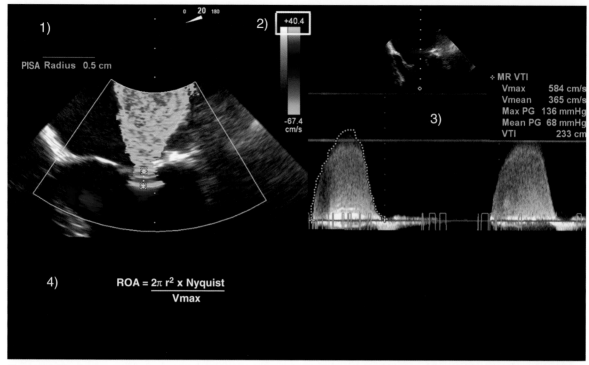

Figure 2-14. PISA demonstration. This figure summarizes the calculation of the regurgitant orifice by the PISA method. (**1**) Identify the flow convergence area and freeze the image. Measure the radius of the PISA shell where the color shifts from red to blue. (**2**) Identify the Nyquist limit. (**3**) Measure the peak systolic velocity across the mitral valve by CW. (**4**) Calculate the regurgitant orifice using the equation.

- The term *vena contracta* refers to the *narrowest* point of the mitral regurgitant jet.
- Because of the shape and orientation of the mitral coaptation line, this measurement should be made in the ME *long axis view*.
- The Nyquist limit should be approximately 55 cm.
- The *zoom* mode should be used to decrease the measurement error.
- The width of the vena contracta correlates with the size of the regurgitant orifice and the severity of the MR.
- A diameter less than 3 mm correlates with mild MR on cardiac catheterization, whereas a diameter greater than 7 mm is generally accepted as severe.

KEY POINTS

- *Pitfall:* If the vena contracta is not circular (as is often the case), the various axes in which it can be measured will yield different numbers. This is why the standardized measurement should be performed in the ME long axis view. This is also the reason why the width of the vena contracta *alone* is not enough to determine the severity of MR.

KEY POINTS—cont'd

- In order to measure the vena contracta, the entire color Doppler jet itself must be visible in continuity, from the zone of flow convergence to the vena contracta and the MR jet itself (see Figure 2-13).
- Recent studies suggest that the *surface area* of the vena contracta, measured using color 3D echocardiography, may be more reliable than the *diameter* of the 2D color jet.

PISA (*Proximal Isovelocity Surface Area*) Method (Figure 2-14)

- This technique is based on the physics of flow acceleration and the continuity equation.
- As blood accelerates from a large chamber into a small orifice, the blood cells accelerate along a series of concentric hemispheres within an area of flow acceleration.
- If a jet is severe enough, this area of flow acceleration (also called the *flow convergence area* or the *PISA shell*) will be visible by color flow Doppler (see Figure 2-14).
- The aliasing velocity can be adjusted to facilitate visualization of the PISA shell.

- Within the flow convergence area, the color Doppler displays the acceleration of blood cells toward the mitral orifice as progressive shades of dark red, brighter red, orange, yellow, and eventually *blue* (according to generally accepted color Doppler mapping conventions, beyond the scope of this discussion).
- When the color changes to blue, the velocity at that point in space is known with certainty: it is the aliasing velocity or Nyquist limit (displayed on the color map on the right side of the echo screen).
- The *radius* (r) of the PISA shell defined by that point is measured from the mitral regurgitant orifice.
- Because **flow = area × velocity**, one can calculate the flow at that particular point in space (**Flow = $2\pi r^2$ × Nyquist limit**).
- The continuity equation dictates that flow is constant along the regurgitant jet; therefore, one knows the flow at the regurgitant orifice.
- Once the *flow* is known at the regurgitant orifice, one can then measure the *peak velocity* (V_{max}) of the MR jet by CW Doppler and calculate the *regurgitant orifice area*.

In summary, one can calculate the regurgitant orifice area (ROA) using the following formula:

$$ROA = \frac{2\pi r^2 \times Nyquist}{V_{max}}$$

- ROA greater than 40 mm^2 is consistent with severe MR.
- Angle correction: When the PISA shell is incomplete (<180 degrees) because it is restricted laterally by a ventricular wall or a mitral leaflet, one must use an *angle correction*. This means estimating the angle width (α) of the PISA shell and dividing by 180.
- The complete PISA equation then becomes:

$$ROA = \frac{2\pi r^2 \times Nyquist \times \alpha}{V_{max}\,180}$$

Regurgitant Volume

- Using the method described previously, one calculates the ROA.
- Once the ROA is known, the regurgitant volume (RV) is obtained by measuring the velocity time integral (VTI) of the regurgitant jet on the CW Doppler

$$RV = VTI \times ROA$$

- RV > 60 mL is consistent with severe MR. Modern echocardiography machines automatically calculate the RV and regurgitant fraction (RF).

Regurgitant Fraction

- The RF is obtained by dividing the RV by the total volume ejected by the heart in systole (RV plus forward stroke volume, which can be calculated using the surface area and the VTI of the left ventricular outflow tract [LVOT]).
- RF greater than 50% is consistent with severe MR.

A summary of the methods used to quantify is shown in Table 2-4.

TABLE 2-4   QUALITATIVE AND QUANTITATIVE PARAMETERS USEFUL IN GRADING MITRAL REGURGITATION SEVERITY

	Mild	Moderate		Severe
Structural Parameters				
LA size	Normal*	Normal or dilated		Usually dilated[†]
LV size	Normal*	Normal or dilated		Usually dilated[†]
Mitral Leaflets or Support Apparatus	Normal or abnormal	Normal or abnormal		Abnormal/flail leaflet/ruptured papillary muscle
Doppler Parameters				
Color flow jet area[‡]	Small, central jet (usually <4 cm^2 or <20% of LA area)	Variable		Large central jet (usually >10 cm^2 or >40% of LA area) or variable size wall-impinging jet swirling in LA
Mitral inflow—PW	A wave dominant[§]	Variable		E wave dominant[§] (E usually 1.2 m/s)
Jet density—CW	Incomplete or faint	Dense		Dense
Jet contour—CW	Parabolic	Usually parabolic		Early peaking—triangular
Pulmonary vein flow	Systolic dominance[‖]	Systolic blunting[‖]		Systolic flow reversal**
Quantitative Parameters[¶]				
VC width (cm)	<0.3	0.3-0.69		≥0.7
R Vol (mL/beat)	<30	30-44	45-59	≥60
RF (%)	<30	30-39	40-49	≥50
EROA (cm^2)	<0.20	0.20-0.29	0.30-0.39	≥0.40

*Unless there are other reasons for LA or LV dilation. Normal 2D measurements: LV minor axis ≤ 2.8 cm/m^2, LV end-diastolic volume ≤ 82 ml/m^2, maximal LA antero-posterior diameter ≤ 2 cm/m^2, maximal LA volume ≤ 36 ml/m^2.
[†]Exception: acute mitral regurgitation.
[‡]At a Nyquist limit of 50-60 cm/s.
[§]Usually above 50 years of age or in conditions of impaired relaxation, in the absence of mitral stenosis or other causes of elevated LA pressure.
[‖]Unless other reasons for systolic blunting (e.g., atrial fibrillation, elevated left atrial pressure).
[¶]Quantitative parameters can help sub-classify the moderate regurgitation group into mid-to-moderate and moderate-to-severe.
**Pulmonary venous systolic flow reversal is specific but not sensitive for severe MR.
CW, continuous wave; EROA, effective regurgitant orifice area; LA, left atrium; LV, left ventricle; PW, pulsed wave; RF, regurgitant fraction; R Vol, regurgitant volume; VC, vena contracta.

Functional Mitral Regurgitation

Functional MR describes a situation in which the mitral leaflets are *structurally* normal, but failure of coaptation still occurs, resulting in MR. It includes a variety of pathologic states, which have in common LV *dilatation* and *decreased systolic function*. The term *functional MR* is often used interchangeably with *ischemic MR*, because ischemic heart disease is by far the most common cause of functional MR, but strictly speaking, they are not the same: not all functional MR is ischemic in nature (e.g., idiopathic dilated cardiomyopathy), whereas not all ischemic MR is functional (e.g., a ruptured papillary muscle following a myocardial infarct).

Mechanism of Functional Mitral Regurgitation

- Usually multifactorial, but the final mechanism is *tethering* (or *tenting*) of the MV leaflets, preventing proper coaptation.
- Pathophysiologically, *dilatation* and *change in geometry* of the LV, especially the posterior wall, results in *posterior* and *apical* displacement of the papillary muscles. The chordae tendinae then cause tenting of the mitral leaflets, preventing proper coaptation.
- Poor systolic function may also decrease the "closing" forces on the MV and this is believed to play some role in functional MR.
- The tenting of the valve is most pronounced in the anterior leaflet in most patients and it is readily visible on TEE, especially in the ME long axis view. It appears as though the "hinge point" of the MV is somewhere along the leaflet itself, rather than at its insertion point in the annulus (an appearance that has been termed "seagull deformity").
- Severe papillary muscle displacement (indicative of worse LV remodeling) is a predictor of recurrence after surgical repair of functional MR.
- The extent of papillary dislocation can be determined by measuring the *tethering* (or *tenting*) *height* and the *tethering* (or *tenting*) *area* (Figure 2-15).
- The *tethering height* is measured by drawing a perpendicular line from the mitral annular plane to the coaptation point in systole. Eleven millimeters or more is considered significant.

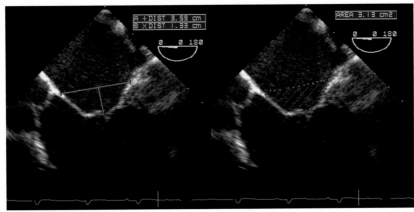

Figure 2-15. Functional MR with tenting of the MV. This ME four-chamber view of the valve in systole demonstrates how to measure the tenting height and tenting area. **Left,** A perpendicular line is drawn from the annular plane to the coaptation point. **Right,** One then measures the surface area defined by the annular plane and the mitral leaflets.

- The tethering area is the area defined by the mitral leaflets (in systole) and the annular plane. A value of 2 cm² or more is generally considered to be indicative of significant tethering.
- 3D echocardiography studies have confirmed the tenting deformity of the MV in ischemic/functional MR.
- MV tethering is almost always accompanied by some degree of mitral annular dilatation and flattening, which compound the problem.

KEY POINTS

- Functional MR is a disease of *ventricular remodeling*, not a problem with the MV leaflets per se. This is important to remember when considering potential surgical treatment of functional MR.
- In the context of ischemic heart disease, the presence of functional MR is a *poor prognostic marker*. Patients presenting for coronary artery bypass graft (CABG) surgery who have severe functional MR have a significantly worse perioperative mortality and lower survival rates.

Echo Evaluation of Functional Mitral Regurgitation
- Anatomy is paramount!
- Once the screening color images establish the presence of significant MR, the evaluation of MV structure and function is done mostly in 2D.
- A comprehensive MV examination is performed to exclude structural mitral disease (e.g., prolapse or perforation).

- Tethering of the leaflets is noted (especially the anterior leaflet),
- The tenting height and area are measured,
- The mitral annular dimensions are measured in both the anteroposterior and commissural diameters.
- Ventricular function is noted, paying particular attention to dilatation and/or dysfunction of the inferior and posterior walls.

Management of Functional Mitral Regurgitation
- Because MR is only one element of the syndrome of dilated cardiomyopathy, a *multimodal* approach is recommended, including:
  - Revascularization, percutaneous or surgical.
  - Aggressive medical therapy (e.g., β-blocker, angiotensin-converting enzyme inhibitors [ACEIs], statins).
  - Resynchronization therapy if indicated.
  - Treatment of atrial fibrillation.
  - Surgical intervention on the MV (see next section).

Left Ventricular Outflow Obstruction, Systolic Anterior Motion, and Mitral Regurgitation

- Dynamic LVOT obstruction with SAM of the MV can result in MR.
- In the context of hypertrophic cardiomyopathy (HOCM), ventricular septal hypertrophy results in high velocity jets, which pulls the MV into the LVOT.
- More commonly in the *intraoperative setting,* dynamic LVOT obstruction occurs as a result

of *MV repair*, especially when it involves an undersized annuloplasty ring.

- The coaptation point of the MV occurs too far anteriorly, with the redundant mitral tissue being dragged into the LVOT in systole, causing a progressive increase in the gradient over systole.
  - This can be because the posterior leaflet is left too long, which brings the coaptation point too far anteriorly.
  - If the ring annuloplasty is made too small, excess anterior leaflet will be available to be pulled in the LVOT during systole.
- Regardless of the cause, the final mechanism is the same: as the anterior mitral leaflet gets pulled into the LVOT, there is failure of coaptation and MR.
- MR caused by SAM is typically directed *slightly posteriorly.*
- *Anatomic* factors that predispose the patient to dynamic LVOT obstruction include a small LV cavity and a relatively long posterior leaflet.
- *Hemodynamic* factors that contribute to the dynamic outflow obstruction include
  - Underfilling.
  - Low afterload.
  - Tachycardia/hyperdynamic state.

Echocardiographic Signs of Left Ventricular Outflow Tract Obstruction (Figure 2-16)
- 2D: characteristic SAM of the MV.
- Color flow Doppler: systolic aliasing in the LVOT.
- Spectral Doppler: pathognomonic appearance of the CW Doppler signal across the LVOT.

The signal has a typical "dagger shape," with the peak velocity occurring in late systole. This is because the LVOT gradient builds up throughout systole, with increasing obstruction from the MV. The best views to measure the LVOT gradient are the TG mid long axis view of the LV or the deep TG view of the LV, depending on the orientation of the LVOT relative to the probe.

MITRAL STENOSIS

Mitral stenosis (MS) is a relatively rare disease in developed countries but it is still the cause of substantial morbidity and mortality worldwide. It was the first cardiac disease to be diagnosed by echocardiography and the first valve disease to be successfully treated surgically.

Etiology

Step 1: Determine the Etiology
Acquired
- *Rheumatic disease* is by far the most common cause. Rheumatic fever is becoming rare in developed countries but it is still widely prevalent in the developing world. Half the patients do not recall having had rheumatic fever. The rate of progression and time to diagnosis correlate with the number of episodes of rheumatic fever.
- *Calcific stenosis* is most often seen in elderly or dialysis-dependent patients, who have severe mitral annular calcification encroaching on the leaflets and causing effective stenosis.

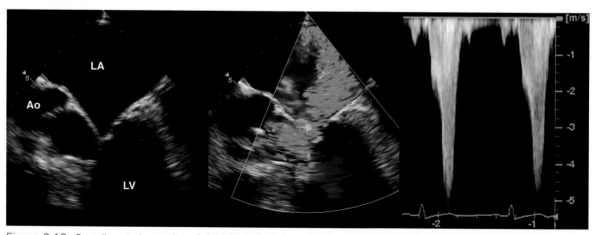

Figure 2-16. Systolic anterior motion of the MV. **Left,** A four-chamber view of the MV in 2D shows systolic displacement of the valve into the LVOT. **Center,** The same four-chamber view of the valve with color Doppler demonstrates the flow acceleration in the LVOT and the severe MR resulting from the failure of coaptation. **Right,** The pathognomonic CW Doppler signal shows the LVOT gradient peaking late in systole.

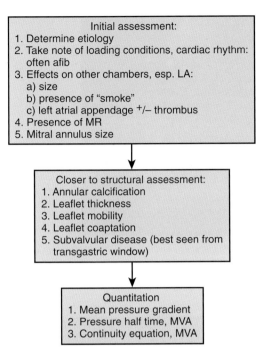

Initial assessment:
1. Determine etiology
2. Take note of loading conditions, cardiac rhythm: often afib
3. Effects on other chambers, esp. LA:
   a) size
   b) presence of "smoke"
   c) left atrial appendage +/– thrombus
4. Presence of MR
5. Mitral annulus size

Closer to structural assessment:
1. Annular calcification
2. Leaflet thickness
3. Leaflet mobility
4. Leaflet coaptation
5. Subvalvular disease (best seen from transgastric window)

Quantitation
1. Mean pressure gradient
2. Pressure half time, MVA
3. Continuity equation, MVA

Figure 2-17. Flow chart of MS severity.

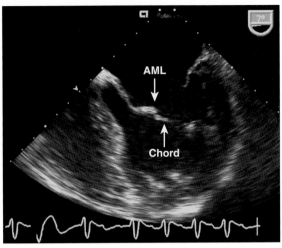

Figure 2-18. MS. This ME four-chamber view of the MV in diastole shows typical *doming* of the anterior mitral leaflet (AML), as well as thickening, shortening, and calcification of the chordae tendinae.

- Physical obstructions: tumor (most often myxoma), thrombus, vegetation.
- *Carcinoid* (rare).
- *Radiation-induced* stenosis.
- *Stenosis after MV repair:* see section on "Mitral Regurgitation."

Congenital
- Congenital MS.
- Parachute MV.
- Double orifice MV.
- Supravalvular ring; cor triatriatum
- Infiltrative disease (e.g., mucopolysaccharidoses)

"Functional" Mitral Stenosis
- Severe aortic insufficiency resulting in apparent poor opening and/or early closure of the MV. This is rarely associated with any significant mitral gradient.
  Flow chart on MS severity (Figure 2-17).

Evaluation of Mitral Stenosis

Pathophysiologically, chronic inflammation causes leaflet thickening and commissural fusion, leading to the classic "fish mouth" appearance of the valve. Concomitantly, there is fusion and shortening of the subvalvular apparatus results in further decrease in valve mobility. These features are readily visible by echocardiography.

Step 1: 2D Appearance
Because rheumatic MS tends to affect the entire valve, pinpointing the location of disease is often not necessary. Still, a detailed systematic examination of the MV should be performed. Technically, these patients are often difficult to examine: they commonly have severe LA enlargement, which causes rotation of the heart and brings the MV out of alignment with the ultrasound beam. This makes classic TEE cross sections difficult to obtain. The typical 2D echocardiographic findings include
- Thickened, nodular appearance of the leaflets.
- Restricted leaflet motion.
- The leaflet tips are often more affected than the base, leading to the typical "doming" or "hockey stick" appearance in diastole (Figure 2-18).
- There is commissural calcification and/or fusion (readily appreciated on TG basal short axis views and with 3D echocardiography).
- There may be extensive annular calcification.
- The subvalvular apparatus (chordae tendinae ± papillary muscle heads) is often calcified and thickened. This is best viewed in the TG long axis view. (Figure 2-19)
- The LA is usually enlarged (sometimes massively), especially in patients with atrial fibrillation.
- Spontaneous contrast (known in the echocardiography jargon as "smoke") is visible in the LA. This is due to

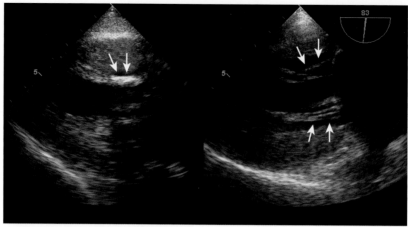

Figure 2-19. Shortened chordae tendinae. **Left,** The chordae tendinae *(arrows)* are shortened, thickened, and calcified. **Right,** This is in contrast to the normal chordae tendinae *(arrows)*.

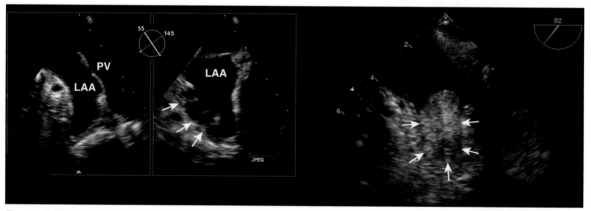

Figure 2-20. LAA thrombus. Patients with MS are at high risk of developing an LAA thrombus, especially if they have concomitant atrial fibrillation. The LAA appears crescent-shaped and contains trabeculations *(short arrows)*, which can make the detection of clots difficult. The image on the *left* shows a normal LAA in two planes, whereas the image on the **right** demonstrates a large LAA thrombus *(long arrows)*.

slow-swirling blood flow causing the formation of red blood cell "rouleaux," which become visible by echocardiography.

- Patients with slow flow in an enlarged LA are at very high risk of developing LA thrombus, especially in the left atrial appendage (LAA). A careful examination of the LAA is mandatory in every patient with MV stenosis (Figure 2-20).
- The LAA is best visualized in ME views between 60 and 90 degrees of transducer rotation, by pulling out slightly from the mitral position. It appears crescent shaped and contains multiple trabeculations, which may make the diagnosis of LAA thrombus difficult.

KEY POINTS

- *Pitfall:* The presence of pericardial fluid *outside* the LAA may sometimes create the illusion that the LA wall with its trabeculations is an intra-atrial mass. It is usually possible to distinguish the two by carefully imaging the appendage and by identifying a pericardial effusion on other views.

Step 2: Color Flow Doppler

- Aliasing diastolic flow is seen through the MV (Figure 2-21).
- With significant flow restriction, an area of flow convergence (PISA shell) can be seen on the atrial side of the MV.

Step 3: Spectral Doppler
- Diastolic gradients (Figure 2-22)
  - The peak and mean gradients are best measured by CW Doppler, because the velocity is often too high for PW Doppler. Another reason to use CW is that it eliminates potential error in positioning the sample window: indeed, the narrowest point of a stenotic MV may not be at the valve leaflets. In some cases, the narrowest point may be in the subvalvular apparatus.

- The peak and mean diastolic gradients are typically elevated.
- A mean gradient greater than 10 to 12 mm Hg is consistent with severe MS.

KEY POINTS
• Remember that mitral gradients are dependent on the cardiac output and loading conditions at the time of the examination.

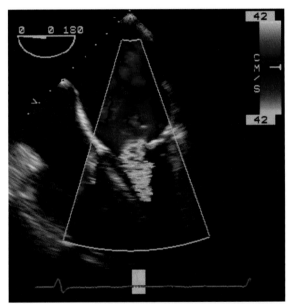

Figure 2-21. Color flow Doppler of MS. Note the aliasing flow across the MV in diastole and the flow convergence area, visible on the LA side of the valve. Note also the large LA.

- Pressure half time (see Figure 2-22)
  - The *pressure half-time (PHT)* is defined as the time it takes for the diastolic pressure gradient across the MV to decrease by half (the pressure gradient, NOT the velocity).
  - A smaller mitral orifice is associated with a greater PHT.
  - Once the PHT is measured, the empirical formula: MVA = 220/PHT is used to calculate the mitral valve area (where MVA = mitral valve area).
- PISA (see the section on "Mitral Regurgitation" for additional details) (Figure 2-23)
  - The same technique, described in the section on "Mitral Regurgitation," applies to the evaluation of MS, except that the flow (in the ME four-chamber view) is *away* from the TEE transducer. Typically, as blood accelerates toward the MV orifice, the color changes from dark blue to lighter blue to yellow/red.

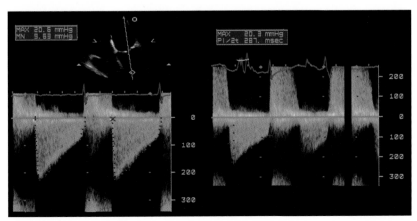

Figure 2-22. Spectral Doppler in MS. **Left,** The peak and mean diastolic gradients are measured by tracing the CW Doppler envelope. **Right,** The PHT is calculated by placing the cursor at the peak of the CW Doppler; if the deceleration slope is nonlinear, use of the midportion of the velocity profile is preferred. The MVA is the constant 220 divided by the PHT in milliseconds.

- Note that, owing to the shape of the MV (V-shaped pointing toward the LV), an angle correction must almost always be used because the PISA shell is usually restricted by the mitral leaflets.
- Continuity equation
  - The continuity principle states that, unless there is an intracardiac shunt, the *flow* of blood is constant throughout the heart. What changes is the *velocity* of the blood, depending on the *cross-sectional area* of the chamber through which it flows. (By extension, the volume of blood that travels through the heart during one systole—the stroke volume—is the same throughout the heart.)
  - We know that **Flow = Velocity × Area.**
  - Therefore, $V_1 \times A_1 = V_2 \times A_2$.
  - Similarly, **Stroke volume = VTI × Area.**
  - Therefore, $VTI_1 \times A_1 = VTI_2 \times A_2$.
  - If one calculates the flow in the LVOT or the pulmonary artery, *assuming there is no*

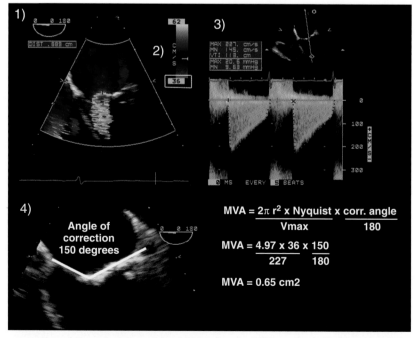

Figure 2-23. Demonstration of the calculation of the MVA using the PISA method. (**1**) After identifying the flow convergence area, the radius of the PISA shell is measured. (**2**) The Nyquist limit is noted, in the direction of flow. (**3**) The peak velocity of the mitral flow is measured using CW. (**4**) Next, the angle of correction is estimated. Finally, the MVA is calculated using the same equation used for MR (discussed previously). In this example, r = 0.89 cm, Nyquist = 36 cm/s, V_{max} = 227 cm/s, angle of correction 150 degrees. Note that all the measurements are in cm.

major valvular regurgitation or intracardiac shunt, one can calculate the MVA using one of these two formulas.

THE REST OF THE HEART: NONVALVULAR INDICATORS OF SEVERE VALVULAR DISEASE

MV disease, especially when chronic, has repercussions throughout the heart, usually in the form of LV and LA volume overload as well as pulmonary hypertension and right ventricular (RV) volume/pressure overload. In the context of mitral disease, the following echocardiographic signs suggest significant longstanding valve disease:

- LV dilatation.
- LA dilatation.
- Dilated pulmonary arteries.
- RV dilatation.
- RV hypertrophy.
- RV dysfunction.
- Tricuspid dilatation
- Tricuspid regurgitation.
- Elevated peak TR velocity (right ventricular systolic pressure [RVSP]).
- RA enlargement.

Mitral Valve Endocarditis

- This is a rare but serious condition. Despite modern antibiotic therapy, MV endocarditis still carries an overall mortality rate of 20% to 30%.
- MV endocarditis is usually caused by a bacteremia, the source of which may not be known.
- Although it can occur on normal valves, endocarditis tends to develop much more commonly on *previously abnormal* valves, at a site of turbulent blood flow.
- Prosthetic valves are also especially vulnerable to the development of endocarditis.
- The type of microorganism often determines the aggressiveness of the disease and its complications.
- TEE is the gold standard for the diagnosis of vegetations.
- TEE has a much better sensitivity (86-98%) than transthoracic echocardiography for the diagnosis of vegetations.
- TEE is also sensitive (76-100%) and specific (95%) in detecting *complications* of endocarditis, such as abscesses and fistulas.

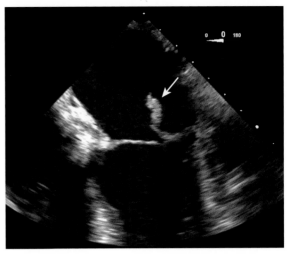

Figure 2-24. MV endocarditis. This ME four-chamber view shows a large vegetation *(arrow)* attached to the posterior mitral leaflet.

- In *native* MV endocarditis, the disease process most often involves the *leaflets*, whereas in patients with *prosthetic* valve endocarditis, extension of the infection to the *perivalvular tissues* (with dehiscence of the prosthesis) is much more common.
- Echocardiographically, the presence of a *vegetation* is the hallmark finding in endocarditis and it confirms the diagnosis (Figure 2-24).
  - Vegetations are accumulations of microorganisms, platelets, and fibrin, which attach to the MV.
  - The echo density of *fresh* vegetations is that of soft tissue or thrombus (making the distinction difficult in certain cases). *Older* vegetations are often dense and calcified. Comparison with the surrounding tissues is important.
  - Vegetations tend to be located on the *upstream* side of a valve. MV lesions usually occur on the LA side.
  - They can be pedunculated (narrow base) or sessile (broad base). Unless completely sessile, most vegetations tend to move in an erratic fashion, independent of the movement of adjacent tissue.
  - The leaflet edges can be destroyed by vegetations, leading to failure of coaptation and *intravalvular* regurgitation. Sometimes, the vegetation results in perforation and the MR jet is seen *through* the leaflet. Multiple mechanisms can coexist in the same valve.

- The clinical management of MV endocarditis includes intravenous antibiotic therapy and supportive treatment.
- Although the approach should be individualized, indications for early surgical treatment include
  - The development of congestive heart failure (class I indication).
  - Persistent bacteremia despite appropriate antibiotic therapy (class I indication).
  - Fungal endocarditis or endocarditis with aggressive organisms or evidence of embolization (class I indication).
  - Large vegetations (>10 mm in size). These respond less well to antibiotic therapy and present a much higher risk of embolization. This is a class IIa indication for early surgery.
  - The echocardiographic detection of complications of endocarditis, such as abscess and fistulas (class I indication) (Figure 2-25).
- If surgery is undertaken, systematic literature reviews demonstrate that MV repair is preferable to replacement owing to

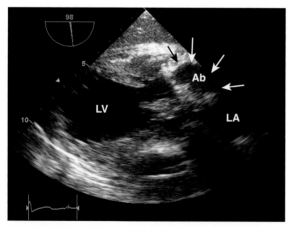

Figure 2-25. Complications of mitral endocarditis: This TG long axis view of the MV shows a large posterior mitral annular abscess (marked by the *arrows*). Ab, abscess cavity.

- Lower early and late mortality.
- Low recurrence of MR and good overall long-term functional results.
- Echocardiography plays an important role in surgery for MV endocarditis.
  - It allows a detailed assessment of the location and extent of vegetations.
  - It reveals the presence of significant leaflet destruction, which will make successful repair much less likely.
  - It demonstrates accompanying lesions in the perivalvular tissues, as described previously.
  - It confirms competence of the valve after successful repair/replacement and directs further intervention, if necessary.

SURGICAL MANAGEMENT OF MITRAL VALVE DISEASE

Surgical Management of Mitral Regurgitation

The surgical management of MR is surgeon dependent. The current expert consensus is that MV repair is always the treatment of choice for mitral degenerative disease. In experienced hands, it is highly successful with low complication rates and good long-term results. For rheumatic valve disease, the success rate of mitral repair varies among surgeons, but it is still the treatment of choice *if feasible*. MV replacement is much more common in this patient population. Finally, the surgical management of functional MR is controversial, as described later.

Specifically:

- Type 1 MR is generally treated with an undersized *annuloplasty ring*. Surgeons advocate different types of rings/bands based on their own personal preference. In the case of leaflet perforation, a primary closure or pericardial patch is commonly used.
- Type 2 MR is addressed with a variety of repair techniques depending on the location and type of disease
  - Triangular or quadrangular leaflet resection. This procedure involves resection of the prolapsed/flail segment. It also often includes a "sliding annuloplasty," a technique by which the base of posterior leaflet is detached from the annulus for some distance and reattached in a different location (Figure 2-26).
  - Chordal transfers.
  - Artificial chordal replacement.

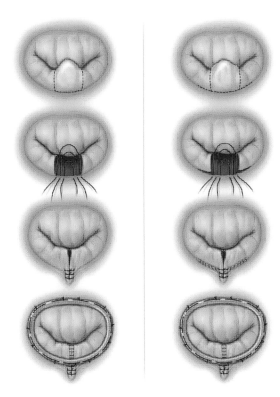

Figure 2-26. Quadrangular posterior leaflet resection. This is one of the most commonly performed MV repair procedures. The prolapsed scallop is resected and the surrounding leaflets are detached from the annulus. The remaining valve segments are sewn together, with varying amounts of "sliding" of the leaflets along the mitral annulus. Then a supportive annuloplasty ring is inserted. *Modified from Verma S, Mesana TG. Mitral-valve repair for mitral-valve prolapse. N Engl J Med. 2009;361:40-48. With permission.*

- Note that, in such cases, an annuloplasty ring or band is always inserted to support the repair.
- Type 3a MR: here, chordal release and/or decalcification can be attempted, but such valves have the lowest rate of successful repair and often end up needing replacement.
- Type 3b MR: the treatment of functional MR is controversial.
  - If the etiology is ischemia, revascularization alone may or may not lead to improvement in MR.
  - Undersized annuloplasty is the favored treatment at the moment, using a variety of rings, some of which re-create the saddle shape of the annulus.
  - Because the primary cause of functional MR is LV dysfunction/dilatation, some surgeons advocate ventricular remodeling techniques to treat this type of MR.

KEY POINTS

- It is important to remember that the long-term prognosis of MV repair generally depends in large part on the *etiology* of the disease: myxomatous degeneration is a *leaflet* problem. A good repair is usually curative. Rheumatic mitral disease is an *inflammatory* disease: after repair, the prognosis depends on the progression of the inflammatory process. Finally, functional MR is essentially a *ventricular* disease: the long-term success of a repair depends mainly on the progression or regression of ventricular remodeling.

POST-BYPASS ASSESSMENT IN MITRAL VALVE PROCEDURES

Mitral Repair for Mitral Regurgitation

- Following surgery, MV evaluation involves the same systematic examination of the valve.
- The immediate post-bypass evaluation of MR can be challenging owing to rapid changes in
  - Hemodynamics.
  - Loading conditions.
  - LV compliance and contractility (post ischemia).
- The quality and length of coaptation is noted in 2D (and 3D if available).

KEY POINTS

After mitral repair, the triad of important elements in the TEE examination are
- Residual MR—quantity, mechanism, clinical significance.
- Creation of MS.
- SAM and LVOT obstruction.

- Three important elements:
  - Residual MR
    - It is important to understand how much MR and what the mechanism of the residual MR is.
    - Color Doppler is used to identify the presence and severity of MR. It is important to pinpoint the location of any residual MR jet.
    - 2D echocardiography is important to demonstrate the mechanism of MR
    - More than mild MR is associated with worse outcome and should be revised.

- Inadvertent creation of MS
  - Peak and mean gradients are load dependent.
  - PHT is unreliable owing to changes in LV compliance.
  - Planimetry may not be reliable if restriction is not at the level of the annulus.
- SAM and LVOT obstruction
  - Anatomic predisposing factors (see previous section).
  - Hemodynamic exacerbating factors (see previous section).

Mitral Replacement
(See Chapter 5)

- More common in MS than in MR.
- A thorough evaluation of mitral prostheses immediately post bypass
  - Ensures stability of the valve and proper "forward" function of the valve: the valve is well seated and the leaflets open well. Diastolic peak and mean gradients are measured (to be interpreted in light of the loading conditions at the time).
  - Ensures proper "backward" function of the valve: assess normal backwash jets and rule out significant paravalvular leaks.
  - Documents the "baseline" appearance of the valve immediately post-insertion. These images can be referred to if the patient presents with suspected complications in the future.

Evaluation of Surrounding Structures

After any mitral procedure, one must carefully check the surrounding structures and the other cardiac valves. All valves are intimately related and a procedure involving one valve may cause disruption of another valve.

- The aortic valve shares a common attachment to the fibrous body of the heart with the anterior leaflet of the MV. Sutures in the mitral annulus may disrupt the aortic valve.
- Similarly, the tricuspid valve annulus can be distorted by sutures in the MV.
- Overenthusiastic decalcification of the mitral annulus may result in fistula formation into a number of adjacent structures.
- Finally, the circumflex artery runs in the atrioventricular groove, immediately

posterior to the mitral annulus. Annuloplasty sutures may cause kinking or obstruction of the artery, resulting in new wall motion abnormalities after bypass. Patients with a left-dominant coronary circulation, owing to a shorter distance between the artery and the mitral annulus, are at increased risk of this complication.

Suggested Readings

1. Quiñones MA, Douglas PS, Foster E, et al. ACC/AHA Clinical Competence Statement on Echocardiography: A Report of the American College of Cardiology/American Heart Association/American College of Physicians–American Society of Internal Medicine Task Force on Clinical Competence. *J Am Coll Cardiol.* 2003;41:687-708.
2. Shanewise JS, Cheung AT, Aronson S, et al. ASE/SCA guidelines for performing a comprehensive intraoperative multiplane transesophageal echocardiography examination: Recommendations of the American Society of Echocardiography Council for Intraoperative Echocardiography and the Society of Cardiovascular Anesthesiologists Task Force for Certification in Perioperative Transesophageal Echocardiography. *Anesth Analg.* 1999;89:870-884.
   This consensus paper established the standards for performing a comprehensive intraoperative TEE examination. The document also contains recommendations on how to examine the mitral valve by TEE.
3. Lambert AS, Miller JP, Merrick SH, et al. Improved evaluation of the location and mechanism of mitral valve regurgitation with a systematic transesophageal echocardiography examination. *Anesth Analg.* 1999;88:1205-1212.
   This study describes how a systematic TEE examination of the mitral valve can improve the localization of mitral valve regurgitant lesions.
4. Cheitlin MD, Armstrong WF, Aurigemma GP, et al. ACC/AHA/ASE 2003 guideline update for the clinical application of echocardiography: A report of the American College of Cardiology/American Heart Association Task Force on Practice Guidelines (ACC/AHA/ASE Committee to Update the 1997 Guidelines for the Clinical Application of Echocardiography). *J Am Coll Cardiol.* 2003;42:954-970.
   This is an update of the 1997 extensive guidelines for the clinical application of echocardiography, including TEE. This document updates the various recommended indications for perioperative TEE.
5. Zoghbi WA, Enriquez-Sarano M, Foster E, et al. Recommendations for evaluation of the severity of native valvular regurgitation with two-dimensional and Doppler echocardiography: A report from the American Society of Echocardiography's Nomenclature and Standards Committee and The Task Force on Valvular Regurgitation. *J Am Soc Echocardiogr.* 2003;16:777-802.
   As its name implies, this is a set of recommendations, based on expert consensus, on how to evaluate regurgitant lesions by echocardiography, both transthoracic and transesophageal.
6. Baumgartner H, Hung J, Bermejo J, et al. Echocardiographic assessment of valve stenosis: EAE/ASE recommendations for clinical practice. *Eur J Echocardiogr.* 2009;10:1-25.
   These are the latest recommendations of the European Association of Echocardiography (EAE) and American Society of Echocardiography (ASE) for the echo assessment of stenotic valve lesions. They are not specific to TEE.

7. Bonow RO, Carabello BA, Chatterjee K, et al. ACC/AHA 2006 guidelines for the management of patients with valvular heart disease: A report of the American College of Cardiology/American Heart Association Task Force on Practice Guidelines. *J Am Coll Cardiol.* 2006;48:e1-e148.
   This set of guidelines, although not specifically focused on echocardiography, provides the reader with context on the presentation, non-echocardiographic evaluation, and clinical management of congenital and acquired mitral valve disease. A section is also devoted to endocarditis.

8. Zoghbi WA, Chambers JB, Dumesnil JG, et al. Recommendations for evaluation of prosthetic valves with echocardiography and Doppler ultrasound: A report from the American Society of Echocardiography's Guidelines and Standards Committee and the Task Force on Prosthetic Valves. *J Am Soc Echocardiogr.* 2009;22:975-1014.
   Although not specifically covered in this chapter, a good understanding of prosthetic valves and their evaluation by echocardiography is essential when dealing with mitral valve disease.

9. Baddour LM, Wilson WR, Bayer AS, et al. Infective endocarditis: Diagnosis, antimicrobial therapy, and management of complications. *Circulation.* 2005;111:3167-3184.
   This comprehensive set of recommendations were endorsed by the Committee on Rheumatic Fever, Endocarditis, and Kawasaki Disease, the Council on Cardiovascular Disease in the Young, and the Councils on Clinical Cardiology, Stroke, and the Societies of Cardiovascular Surgery and Anesthesia, as well as the American Heart Association.

10. Ayres NA, Miller-Hance W, Fyfe DA, et al. Indications and guidelines for performance of transesophageal echocardiography in the patient with pediatric acquired or congenital heart disease: A report from the Task Force of the Pediatric Council of the American Society of Echocardiography. *J Am Soc Echocardiogr.* 2005;18:91-98.
    This extensive document contains guidelines on the performance of TEE in the pediatric congenital heart population, including intraoperative TEE. It includes indications, contraindications, and technical and cognitive skills necessary to safely perform TEE in this population, as well as recommendations about maintenance of skills.

11. Roberts BJ, Grayburn PA. Color flow imaging of the vena contracta in mitral regurgitation: Technical considerations. *J Am Soc Echocardiogr.* 2003;16:1002-1006.
    This manuscript discusses the technical considerations and potential pitfalls surrounding the measurement of the vena contracta in MR.

12. Kahn RA, Mittnacht AJ, Anyanwu AC. Systolic anterior motion as a result of relative "undersizing" of a mitral valve annulus in a patient with Barlow's disease. *Anesth Analg.* 2009;108:1102-1104.
    This report presents a case of SAM after MV repair and contains a discussion of the various pathophysiologic mechanisms involved in SAM post MV repair.

Aortic Valve and Aortic Root

Annette Vegas and Marjan Jariani

3

ANATOMY AND FUNCTION

> ### KEY POINTS
>
> - Aortic root is a dynamic system that maximizes blood flow through the aortic valve (AV) with no structure fixed in position or dimension during the cardiac cycle.
> - The AV lacks a true anatomic annulus (ring-shaped); instead, it is supported by a crown-shaped base at the aortoventricular junction.
> - Named for the coronary artery arising from the corresponding sinus of Valsalva, the three AV cusps include the anterior right coronary cusp (RCC), noncoronary cusp (NCC) near the interatrial septum (IAS), and left coronary cusp (LCC) associated with the left atrium (LA).
> - Normal AV cusps are soft, pliable, unequal in size (NCC > RCC > LCC) and have geometric dimensions that ensure competent AV function (Figure 3-1).
> - Sinuses of Valsalva are three outpouches of the aorta that give rise to the coronary ostia, the upper portions of which join with the superior AV cusps at the aorta in the nonlinear sinotubular junction (STJ).

Normal Aortic Valve and Root Anatomy and Function

- The aortic root is a three-dimensional structure composed of the aortic annulus, AV cusps, sinuses of Valsalva, STJ, and proximal ascending aorta (see Figure 3-1).
- Cusp attachment forms the hemodynamic junction between the left ventricle (LV) and the aorta. The proximal structures are subjected to left ventricular (LV) pressure (diastolic expansion and systolic contraction) whereas distal structures exposed to aortic pressures expand during systole, facilitating AV opening.
- The aortic root is joined to the LV (see Figure 3-1) with 45% of its circumference attached to ventricular muscle (muscular

interventricular septum [IVS] and LV free wall) and 55% to fibrous tissue (aortomitral membrane and membranous IVS).
- Each cusp free margin has a central thickening, the nodule of Arantii, and on either side, the lunula, which form an overlapping closure line (or commissure) during diastole.
- Lambl's excrescences are degenerative filamentous structures on the AV ventricular free margin.

Congenital Anomalies of Cusp Number

- Congenital absence of the AV is very rare; abnormalities in the number of AV cusps can range from unicuspid to hexacuspid.
- These valves can be regurgitant or stenotic at birth or develop functional impairment later in life.

Bicuspid Aortic Valve
- Bicuspid aortic valve (BAV) is a common congenital abnormality affecting 2% to 3% of adults.
- In children, a BAV may be stenotic at birth without calcification, whereas in adults, it is from superimposed calcification.
- Characteristic midesophageal (ME) AV short axis (SAX) and long axis (LAX) transesophageal echocardiography (TEE) views (see Case 3-1 on the companion website) show two slightly thickened cusps with two commissures, a raphe, an elliptical systolic orifice and an asymmetrical closure line.
- Possible coexisting anomalies with a BAV can be identified by echocardiography: coarctation of the aorta, post-stenotic aortic dilatation, aortic dissection and patent ductus arteriosus (PDA).
- RCC and LCC (80%) fusion form larger anterior and smaller posterior cusps with both

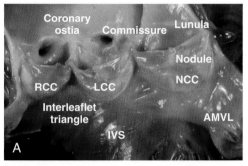 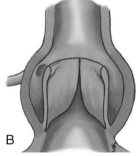 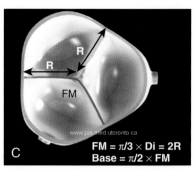

Figure 3-1. Aortic root anatomy. **A** and **B,** The aortic root is a complex, dynamic three-dimensional (3D) structure that forms the transition from the muscular LV to the elastic aorta. Composed of the AV, sinuses of Valsalva, STJ, and proximal ascending aorta, it extends from the base of the AV cusps to the STJ. Coaptation of each cusp edge with a 2- to 3-mm overlap forms the commissures and prevents aortic regurgitation. **C,** Individual cusps have a semilunar shape with a height of 12 to 18 mm. The free margin (FM) length is twice the measured cusp edge (R) and approximates the annulus diameter (Di). The cusp base is roughly 1.5 times the FM length. **C,** *Courtesy of pie.med.utoronto.ca with permission.*

coronary arteries arising from the anterior cusp. RCC and NCC (20%) fusion has a larger right than left cusp with one coronary artery arising from each cusp. Fusion of the LCC and NCC is rare.

- The two cusps have unequal size and are described by the location of the cusp opening, commissures, coronary ostia, and a raphe that may be present at 90 degrees to the commissure.

Unicuspid and Quadracuspid Aortic Valve

- Unicuspid AV is rare and consists of two types: either acommissural with a central orifice or, more commonly, a posterior commissure with an eccentric elliptical-shaped orifice (Figure 3-2).
- Quadracuspid AV is the rarest and appears as four equal cusps (see Figure 3-2). It may have associated coronary anomalies and present with aortic regurgitation (AR).

ECHOCARDIOGRAPHIC IMAGING OF THE AORTIC VALVE AND ROOT

- Echocardiography documents complete anatomic and functional assessment of the AV, including cusp morphology, mobility, coaptation and aortic root size.
- Color Doppler evaluates flow through the AV to demonstrate AR or aortic stenosis (AS).
- Continuous wave (CW) Doppler alignment is best in the transgastric (TG) views with the spectral trace used to assess antegrade (AS) and retrograde (AR) flow (Table 3-1).

AORTIC STENOSIS

KEY POINTS

- Obstruction can occur at the valvular level, below the valve (fixed, dynamic), or above the valve.
- Important associated findings include mitral regurgitation (MR), left ventricular hypertrophy (LVH) and aortic root dilation. There is often significant diastolic dysfunction.
- Severe MR or low cardiac output (CO) reduces the transaortic flow rate, causing a low gradient even with severe AS and obliges aortic valve area (AVA) calculation. Falsely low gradients can also occur in the presence of a high ejection fraction with a low stroke volume (SV).
- High CO and low systemic vascular resistance (SVR) falsely elevate pressure gradients, which may misdiagnose severe AS as with a dynamic left ventricular outflow tract (LVOT) obstruction.
- Pressure recovery (PR) is greatest from a small orifice (native AV or prosthesis) with gradual distal widening; compared with abrupt widening to the larger aorta.

Etiology of Aortic Stenosis

Step 1: Determine the Etiology

- Obstruction can occur below, above, or at the AV level. It is easily differentiated based on the site of increased velocity seen with color or spectral Doppler and local anatomy.

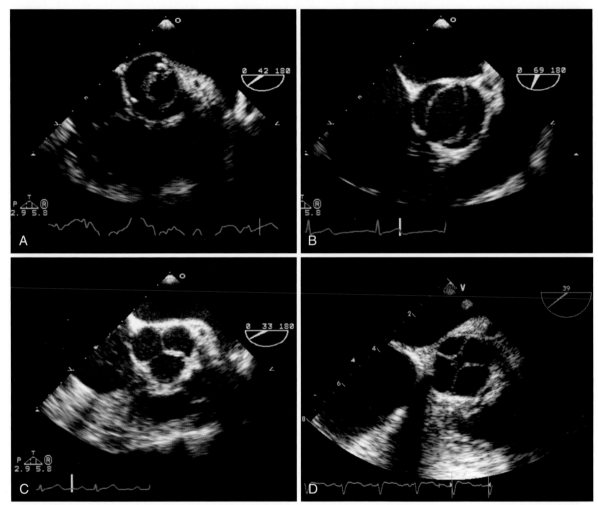

Figure 3-2. Cusp variations. ME AV SAX views of different AVs show a variable number of cusps. **A,** A unicuspid valve shown during systole has an elliptical orifice with a posterior commissure. **B,** A bicuspid valve during systole has an elliptical orifice with two commissures. **C,** A normal AV with three cusps forms a "Mercedes Benz" sign during diastole. **D,** A quadracuspid valve shown during diastole has four cusps that fail to coapt centrally and commissures that make the valve appear X-shaped.

TABLE 3-1   BEST VIEWS FOR ASSESSING THE AORTIC VALVE

Description of View	How Best to Achieve
ME AV SAX view	• Relative to the heart, the AV plane is oblique. A 30- to 60-degree transducer angle is necessary to show symmetrical imaging of all valve cusps (Figure 3-3). • During systole, cusp opening is normally unrestricted with the orifice shape identifying the number of cusps and planimetry of the edges determining the anatomic AVA. • During diastole, the three cusps of the normal AV close to resemble a Mercedes Benz sign with color Doppler used to show AR. • Withdrawing the probe reveals the left and right coronary ostia, whereas advancing the probe yields a SAX view of the LVOT.
ME AV LAX view	• Rotating the transducer angle to 120 to 140 degrees from the SAX view with slight probe advancement aligns the LVOT, AV, and ascending aorta on the display right (see Figure 3-3). • The normal AV appears during systole as two thin, parallel lines within the sinuses of Valsalva, the RCC is always anterior adjacent to the RVOT and the posterior cusp is either the LCC or, more often, the NCC. • Aortic root dimensions are measured during systole (Figure 3-4), whereas color Doppler demonstrates the presence and site of turbulent flow related to obstruction or AR.
TG views	• The TG LAX view at 90 to 120 degrees images the AV on the display right, and the deep TG view at 0 degrees locates the AV in the center of the display (Figure 3-5). • Although assessment of AV anatomy may be imprecise in these views, they are especially useful for spectral Doppler alignment to measure optimal transvalvular velocity.
3D echocardiography	• Real-time 3D TEE compared with 2D TTE can assess valvular morphology and provide additional information regarding AS severity with accurate planimetry of the anatomic AV orifice.

AR, aortic regurgitation; AV, aortic valve; AVA, aortic valve area; LAX, long axis; LCC, left coronary cusp; LVOT, left ventricular outflow tract; ME, midesophageal; NCC, noncoronary cusp; RCC, right coronary cusp; RVOT, right ventricular outflow tract; SAX, short axis; 3D, three-dimensional; TEE, transesophageal echocardiography; TG, transgastric; TTE, transthoracic echocardiography; 2D, two-dimensional.

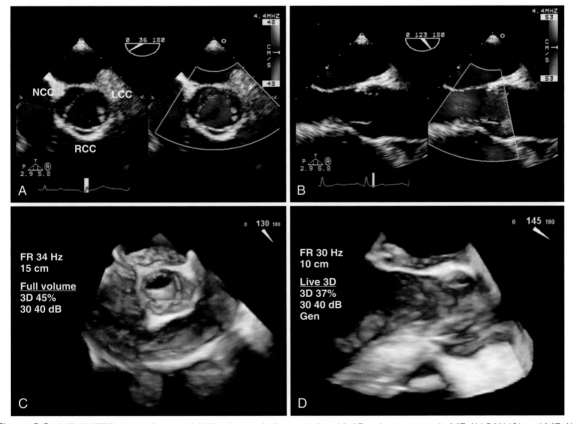

Figure 3-3. ME AV TEE views. A normal AV is shown during systole with 2D color compare in ME AV SAX (**A**) and ME AV LAX (**B**) views. Real-time 3D TEE views of the AV are shown in SAX using the full-volume mode (**C**) and in LAX using the 3D live mode (**D**). In the ME AV SAX, identify the NCC near the IAS, the anterior RCC and the LCC adjacent to the LA.

- Valvular AS is a common valvular lesion caused by congenital (bicuspid 38%), rheumatic (24%), or degenerative calcification in the elderly (33%).
- Supravalvular stenosis is uncommon arising from a congenital condition, such as Williams' syndrome with persistent or recurrent obstruction in adulthood.
- There are two types of subvalvular obstruction: (1) fixed from a subaortic

membrane or muscle band with similar hemodynamics to valvular AS, or (2) dynamic from septal hypertrophy, with variable systolic ejection and a predominantly late peaking velocity.

Features of Valvular AS

Anatomic AV evaluation is based on a combination of echocardiographic ME AV SAX and LAX images to identify cusp number, mobility, calcification and commissural fusion.

Calcific AS is typified by calcification within the central part of each cusp without commissural fusion, resulting in a stellate-shaped systolic orifice (Figure 3-6).

Rheumatic AS is characterized by commissural fusion with thickening and calcification along the cusp edges resulting in a triangular systolic orifice, almost always accompanied by rheumatic mitral valve (MV) changes (see Figure 3-6).

A predictor of clinical outcome, calcification severity is graded semiquantitatively, as mild (few areas of dense echogenicity with little acoustic shadowing), moderate, or severe (extensive thickening and increased echogenicity with a prominent acoustic shadow).

Associated findings with AS (Figure 3-7) are important to identify including MR, LVH with variable ventricular function, and aortic root dilatation. Their presence may affect the type and timing of intervention.

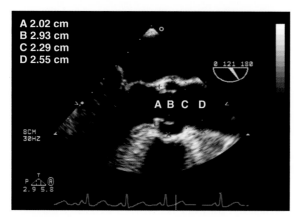

A. Annulus	1.8–2.5 cm
B. Sinus of valsalva	2.4–3.9 cm
C. Sino-tubular junction	2.2–2.9 cm
D. Ascending aorta	2.2–3.4 cm
Aortic root height	<2.2 cm
Ratio annulus/root height	<0.8

Figure 3-4. Aortic root measurements. The largest aortic root measurements are made in the ME AV LAX view during midsystole at the basal valvular attachments (annulus), widest portion of the sinuses, STJ, and ascending aorta. Accurate measurements require symmetrical cusp alignment and optimal gain to minimize excessive tissue thickness. Representative values are shown. The aortic root height is the distance from the AV annulus to the STJ. The aortic root height-to-STJ ratio is greater than 1.0 if the STJ dilates from Marfan syndrome but is preserved at less than 1.0 in hypertensive aortopathy.

Quantitative Assessment of Aortic Stenosis

Step 2: Assess AS Jet Velocity
- CW Doppler parallel alignment with flow direction (or within 15 degrees) may be difficult using TEE. It aims to record the

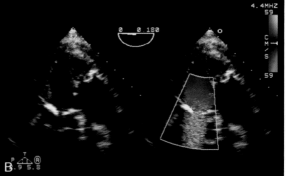
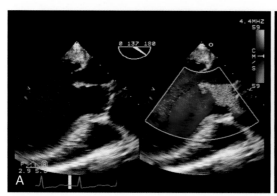

Figure 3-5. TG AV views. TG views are well suited for spectral and color Doppler interrogation of the AV. TG LAX view shows AR (**A**) and deep TG view demonstrates AS (**B**) using color Doppler in two different patients.

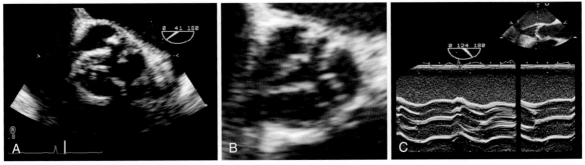

Figure 3-6. AS etiology. Standard 2D imaging for AS assesses cusp: number, mobility, and calcium location. Shown here are calcific (**A**) and rheumatic (**B**) AVs in zoomed ME AV SAX views. The number of cusps may be difficult to distinguish owing to shadowing from the calcium. **C,** Restricted cusp mobility, reduced cusp separation less than 15 mm is seen in ME AV LAX by M-mode.

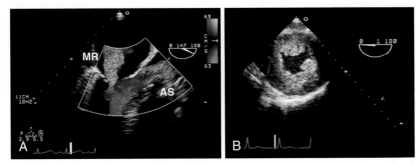

Figure 3-7. Associated findings in AS. **A,** Color Doppler shows turbulence at the level of obstruction from a calcified AV in the ME AV LAX view. MR may occur from LV dysfunction, SAM, or intrinsic MV disease. Functional MR arises from elevated LV pressures and may improve after AVR without MV intervention. **B,** Concentric LVH (wall thickness > 12 mm) with a small noncompliant cavity requires higher filling pressures to maintain SV. The LV is prone to diastolic dysfunction and systolic posterobasal hypokinesis segmental wall motion abnormality. A hypertrophied septum may result in SAM of the AMVL after AVR.

highest AS jet velocity, which is the strongest predictor of clinical outcome.

- The gray scale spectral Doppler signal is optimized with a velocity scale to fit the signal, a 100-mm/s time scale, high wall filters, and reduced gain to record a smooth velocity curve with a dense outer edge and clear maximum velocity (Figure 3-8).
- Usually, three or more beats are averaged in sinus rhythm, and at least five consecutive beats are mandatory with irregular rhythms using care to avoid post-extrasystolic beats.
- The CW Doppler velocity curve shape distinguishes the level, severity and dynamics of obstruction (see Figure 3-8).

Step 3: Assess Transaortic Pressure Gradient

- CW Doppler quantifies AS by measuring blood velocity across the AV and calculating the transaortic pressure gradient (ΔP) using the simplified Bernoulli equation: $\Delta P = 4V^2$.

- The simplified Bernoulli equation assumes that the proximal velocity can be ignored. This is a reasonable assumption when it is less than 1 m/s, but if greater than 1.5 m/s or the aortic velocity is less than 3.0 m/s, it is included when calculating maximum gradients: $\Delta P = 4(V^2_{max} - V^2_{proximal})$.
- The mean pressure gradient has potential advantages over the peak gradient determined from the peak velocity. It is obtained by averaging instantaneous gradients during the entire systole and not from the mean velocity (see Figure 3-8).
- There is good correlation between mean and peak gradients though this depends on the velocity curve shape, which varies with stenosis severity and flow rate.

Pitfalls: Factors Affecting the Pressure Gradient

- Underestimation of aortic velocity causes an even greater underestimation in pressure gradients, owing to the squared relationship between velocity and pressure.

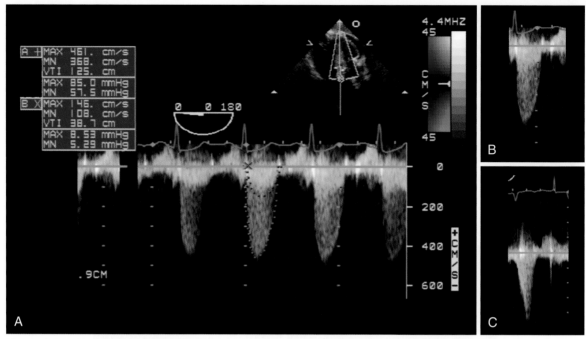

Figure 3-8. CW Doppler. **A,** CW spectral Doppler trace is obtained by careful alignment of the sampling line through the stenotic AV orifice using an appropriate velocity scale. Tracing the Doppler profile identifies the peak and mean velocity and pressure gradients. AVA by the continuity equation using the double envelope technique involves a single CW trace through the LVOT and AV. The inner envelope represents LVOT and the outer envelope the AV velocity measurements. **B,** Fixed obstruction at any level has a similar-shaped velocity curve. Severe obstruction has a rounder shape from the midsystolic peak velocity. Mild obstruction has an early systolic peak (shown here) and a triangular-shaped velocity curve. **C,** Dynamic subaortic obstruction has a characteristic late-peaking velocity curve, often with a concave curve in early systole.

- Pressure gradient underestimation occurs with high SVR, low CO and MR, whereas overestimation occurs with low SVR, high CO and AR.
- Peak Doppler pressure gradients represent the maximum instantaneous pressure difference across the aortic valve. This pressure is typically greater than the unphysiologic peak-to-peak LV and aortic pressures, which do not occur at the same time point at cardiac catheterization.
- Measures of AS severity (Vmax, mean gradient, AVA) remain accurate when severe AR accompanies AS but will be higher than expected for a given AVA.
- LVH commonly accompanies AS and typically results in a small LV cavity with thick walls, diastolic dysfunction, and small SV with a lower than expected AS velocity and mean gradient, for a given AVA (see Figure 3-7).

Pressure Recovery
- PR is the increase in pressure (decrease in velocity) that occurs shortly after the vena contracta as kinetic energy is reconverted into potential energy.

- PR is greatest from a small orifice (native AV or prosthesis) with gradual distal widening, compared with abrupt widening to the larger aorta yielding a lower PR (Figure 3-9).
- In AS, PR (in mm Hg) is related to the effective orifice area (EOA)-to-aortic area (AoA) ratio; a small AoA (diameter < 30 mm) favors PR. The initial pressure drop across the stenosis from LV to vena contracta by Doppler may be significantly higher (overestimate) than the relevant actual net pressure drop (see Figure 3-9).

Left Ventricular Systolic Dysfunction
- LV systolic dysfunction with severe AS reduces the AS velocity and pressure gradient despite a small AVA. This is a condition termed *low-flow low-gradient AS*, commonly defined by
  - EOA < 1.0 cm^2
  - Left ventricular ejection fraction (LVEF) < 40%
  - Mean pressure gradient < 30 to 40 mm Hg
- Dobutamine stress echocardiogram alters stroke volume (or ejection fraction [EF]) and

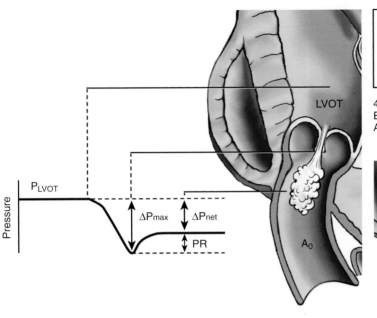

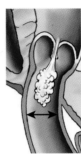

$$PR = P_{distal} - P_{VC}$$

$$PR = 4v^2 \times \frac{2\ EOA}{AoA} \times \left(1 - \frac{EOA}{AoA}\right)$$

$4v^2$ = initial pressure drop across AV
EOA = effective orifice area stenotic AVA
AoA = ascending aorta area

Figure 3-9. Pressure recovery (PR). Shortly after the vena contracta (VC), kinetic energy is reconverted into potential energy with a corresponding increase in pressure (decrease in velocity), the PR. CW Doppler measures the maximal pressure difference (ΔPmax) at the VC. The pressure difference between the LVOT and the PR is the net transvalvular pressure (ΔPnet). In native AS, PR is significant only if the aorta diameter is less than 30 mm.

changes aortic velocity, mean gradient, and AVA as flow rate increases. This helps differentiate these clinical situations.

1. LV systolic dysfunction from severe AS results in a moderate transaortic peak velocity and mean pressure gradient and a small AVA usually with improvement in LV function after aortic valve replacement (AVR).
2. Moderate AS with another cause of LV dysfunction (e.g., myocardial infarct) has insufficient LV energy to maximally open the AV; thus, a small AVA is calculated and an AVR may not improve LV systolic function.

- Stress echocardiography is not indicated in a patient with a low EF and resting AS velocity of 4.0 m/s or mean gradient of 40 mm Hg. This represents a normal LV response to high afterload, not a poor LV, and will improve after relief of stenosis.
- The velocity ratio $(VTI)_{LVOT}/VTI_{AV}$ less than 0.25 is a dimensionless number, independent of CO, that can be used to assess severe AS.

Step 4: Calculate Valve Area

- Planimetry of the anatomic AVA is tracing the smallest orifice and can be technically challenging to obtain using TEE (Figure 3-10).
- Careful TEE probe manipulation locates the smallest orifice at maximal cusp separation in

the ME AV LAX view that, after angle rotation to a ME AV SAX view, identifies this orifice with all cusps and a circular aortic wall visualized.

- Doppler velocity and pressure gradients are flow dependent. Calculation of the functional AVA is helpful when flow rates are very low or very high because the AVA remains constant despite the flow across the valve.
- Functional AVA is calculated based on the continuity equation, which represents the equal SV ejected through the LVOT and stenotic AV:

$$SV_{AV} = SV_{LVOT}$$

- Volume flow rate through any cross-sectional area (CSA) is equal to the CSA times flow velocity over the ejection period (VTI). This equation can be rewritten as

$$AVA \times VTI_{AV} = CSA_{LVOT} \times VTI_{LVOT}$$

- Solving for AVA yields the continuity equation, which requires three measurements (see Figure 3-10):

$$AVA = CSA_{LVOT} \times VTI_{LVOT}/VTI_{AV}$$

- AS jet velocity by CW Doppler
- LVOT diameter for calculation of a circular CSA
- LVOT velocity recorded with pulsed Doppler.

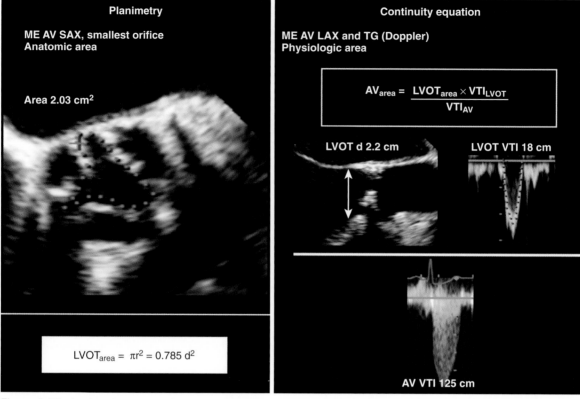

Figure 3-10. Aortic valve area (AVA). AVA can be assessed using either the anatomic AVA measured by planimetry or the functional AVA calculated from the continuity equation.

Grading Aortic Stenosis

Step 5: Assessing Aortic Stenosis Grading
- Limitations with clinical implications are summarized in Table 3-2.

Step 5a: No Discrepancies in Aortic Stenosis Quantification
- General guidelines (Table 3-3) have been established by the American College of Cardiology/American Heart Association (ACC/AHA) and European Society of Cardiology (ESC) for categorizing AS severity as mild, moderate, or severe to provide guidance for clinical decision making.
- If during cardiac surgery for other reasons TEE reveals evidence of AS, quantitation may be attempted, but if the intercept angle is inadequate, epiaortic scanning should be performed (Figure 3-11).

Step 5b: Resolving Discrepancies of Aortic Stenosis Quantification
- In clinical practice, many patients have an apparent discrepancy in AS severity as defined by maximum velocity (and mean gradient) compared with the calculated AVA, which can be resolved (Figure 3-12).

AORTIC REGURGITATION

KEY POINTS
• AR is a disease of either the valve itself, the aortic root, or the ascending aorta.
• Advanced techniques of quantitation may be difficult in the operating room (OR), where AR is usually assessed by measurement of the vena contracta, pulsed Doppler of the descending aorta and the secondary effects on other structures (e.g., LV).
• The degree of jet penetration into the LV is unreliable in the quantitation of AR. The pressure half-time (PHT) of the AR jet is extremely dependent on the LV compliance.
• Acute AR is a surgical emergency.

Etiology of Aortic Regurgitation

Step 1: Determine the Etiology
- AR results from either intrinsic cusp disease (rheumatic, infectious, traumatic, congenital) or secondarily from diseases

TABLE 3-2   LIMITATIONS AND IMPLICATIONS IN ASSESSING AORTIC STENOSIS

	Limitations	Implications
Etiology	Calcium, acoustic shadowing	Difficulty determining cusp number
AS jet velocity (CW Doppler)	Poor Doppler alignment Flow dependent	Underestimate velocity
AS pressure gradient (CW Doppler)	Underestimate (high SVR, low CO, MR) Overestimate (low SVR, high CO, AR) Pressure recovery Severe LVH (low stroke volume) LV systolic dysfunction	Low flow and gradient, calculate AVA High flow and gradient, calculate AVA Only if small aorta (<30 mm) Underestimate velocity, gradients Consider dobutamine stress
Velocity ratio (VR = V_{LVOT}/V_{AV})	Doppler-only measurement	Ignores LVOT size variability Less variability than EOA by continuity
AVA planimetry Anatomic AVA	Asymmetrical AV view Heavily calcified valve, pinhole AS	Overestimates AVA Difficult to assess AVA
AVA continuity Measures EOA	Doppler alignment (eccentric jet) Inaccurate LVOT measurement Arrhythmias (atrial fibrillation) Flow rate dependence	Underestimate AVA Underestimate AVA Average Inaccurate AVA

AS, aortic stenosis; AV, aortic valve; AVA, aortic valve area; CO, cardiac output; CW, continuous wave; EOA, effective orifice area; LV, left ventricular; LVH, left ventricular hypertrophy; LVOT, left ventricular outflow tract; MR, mitral regurgitation; SVR, systemic vascular resistance.
From Baumgartner H, Hung J, Bermejo J, et al. Echocardiographic assessment of valve stenosis: EAE/ASE recommendations for clinical practice. *J Am Soc Echocardiogr.* 2009;22:1-23.

TABLE 3-3   GRADING AORTIC STENOSIS SEVERITY

	Mild	Moderate	Severe
Aortic jet velocity (m/s)	2.6-2.9	3.0-4.0	>4.0
Mean gradient (mm Hg)	<20 (<30*)	20-40[†] (30-50*)	>40[†] (>50*)
AVA (cm^2)	1.5	1.0-1.5	<1.0
Indexed AVA (cm^2/m^2)	>0.85	0.60-0.85	<0.6
Velocity ratio	>0.50	0.25-0.50	<0.25

ACC, American College of Cardiology; AHA, American Heart Association; AVA, aortic valve area; ESC, European Society of Cardiology.
*ESC guidelines.
[†]AHA/ACC guidelines, normal AVA 3.0-4.0 cm^2.
From Baumgartner H, Hung J, Bermejo J, et al. Echocardiographic assessment of valve stenosis: EAE/ASE recommendations for clinical practice. *J Am Soc Echocardiogr.* 2009;22:1-23.

affecting the aortic root and ascending aorta.
- AV competence depends on the normal anatomic relationships in the aortic root. Conditions such as aortic dissection or dilatation may lead to AV incompetence despite normal AV cusps.
- Analogous to the Carpentier classification of MV disease, El Khoury and coworkers[4] described a classification of aortic root pathology that provides a simple guide to aid in diagnosis and choice of corrective surgical techniques (Figure 3-13).
- This functional classification describes three classes of abnormalities based primarily on cusp function and secondarily on aortic root

anatomy by combining TEE data and visual examination.
- Type I pathologies have structurally and functionally normal AV cusps, but has enlargement of an area supporting the cusps, with four additional subcategories (Figure 3-14).
- Type II lesions involve prolapse of one or more cusps below the normal coaptation level as a result of degenerative cusp changes, acute aortic dissection, subaortic ventricular septal defect (VSD) or previous cardiac surgery (Figure 3-15).
- Type III lesions describe restricted cusp mobility with inadequate coaptation from thickened cusps, usually from calcific

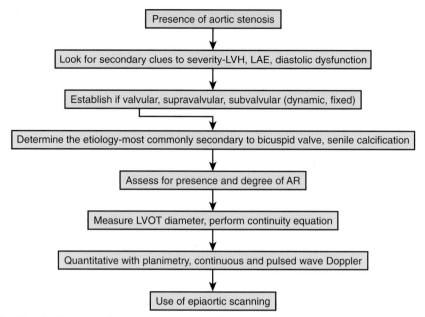

Figure 3-11. Algorithm for intraoperative assessment of AS discovered during other cardiac surgery. LAE, left atrial enlargement.

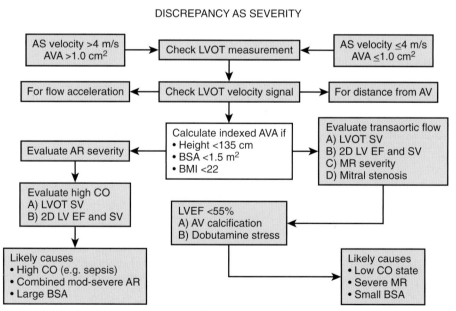

Figure 3-12. Algorithm used to resolve discrepancies in AS severity. BMI, body mass index.

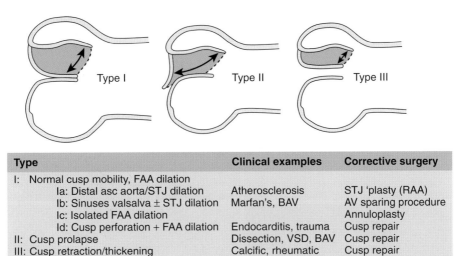

Type	Clinical examples	Corrective surgery
I: Normal cusp mobility, FAA dilation		
Ia: Distal asc aorta/STJ dilation	Atherosclerosis	STJ 'plasty (RAA)
Ib: Sinuses valsalva ± STJ dilation	Marfan's, BAV	AV sparing procedure
Ic: Isolated FAA dilation		Annuloplasty
Id: Cusp perforation + FAA dilation	Endocarditis, trauma	Cusp repair
II: Cusp prolapse	Dissection, VSD, BAV	Cusp repair
III: Cusp retraction/thickening	Calcific, rheumatic	Cusp repair

The functional aortic annulus (FAA) is defined as the region between the STJ and the aorta-ventricular junction (AVJ).

Figure 3-13. El Khoury classification for aortic root pathology. This classification is based on cusp mobility and root size.

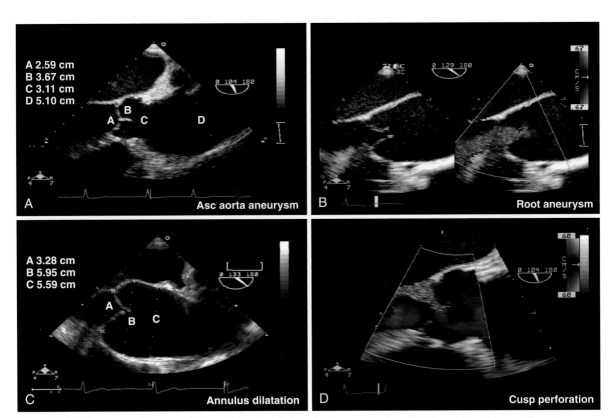

Figure 3-14. Type 1 aortic root pathology. Type 1 pathology is diagnosed when the dimension of any aortic root component exceeds the upper limit of normal with normal cusp mobility. Examples of type 1 aortic root pathology include an ascending (asc) aorta aneurysm (**A**), root aneurysm (**B**), annuloaortic ectasia (**C**), and root dilatation with cusp perforation (**D**).

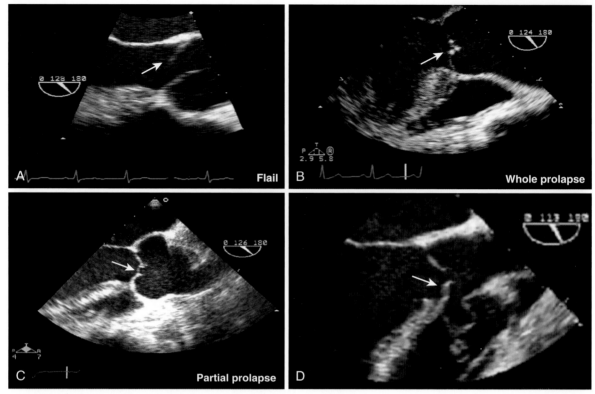

Figure 3-15. Type 2 aortic root pathology. Type 2 excessive cusp motion or prolapse has three subtypes and occurs when the cusp free edge overrides the aortic annulus plane resulting in eccentric AR. **A,** Flail cusp has an everted cusp tip which points toward the LVOT. **B,** Whole prolapse of the entire cusp has the cusp tip pointing toward the aorta. **C,** Partial prolapse has only part of the aortic cusp below the annular plane. **D,** RCC prolapse through a perimembranous VSD. The arrows show individual cusp pathology.

degenerative changes or rheumatic disease (see Figure 3-6).

Quantification of Aortic Regurgitation

Step 2: Assess Aortic Regurgitation Severity

- AR assessment is based on the comprehensive utilization of two-dimensional (2D), color, pulsed and CW Doppler techniques. Although more time consuming and difficult to obtain reliably using TEE, quantitative measures are essential for clinical evaluation.
- LV dilatation (Figure 3-16) with variable function accompanies significant chronic AR but may be absent in significant acute AR as from endocarditis.

Step 2a: Color Doppler

- Color Doppler visualizes the three components of the regurgitant jet (Figure 3-17): (1) the jet origin (flow convergence),

(2) jet width (vena contracta), and (3) spatial orientation in the LV (jet area).
- Regurgitation jet size and its temporal resolution are significantly affected by transducer frequency and instrument settings such as gain, output power, Nyquist limit, size and depth of the image sector.
- A standard technique uses a Nyquist limit (aliasing velocity) of 50 to 60 cm/s and a color gain that just eliminates random color speckle from nonmoving regions.
- Eccentric jets should alert to the possibility of valvular structural abnormalities (e.g., prolapse, flail, or perforation), frequently affecting the cusp opposite to the jet direction (Figure 3-18).

Jet Size and Area

- Regurgitant jet area in the LV and jet size in the LVOT provide rapid screening for the presence, direction, and a semiquantitative assessment of AR severity (Figure 3-19).
- The length of AR jet penetration into the LV is an unsatisfactory indicator of AR severity,

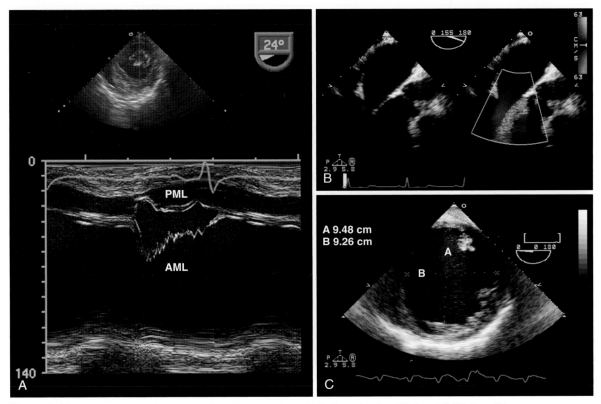

Figure 3-16. Associated findings in AR. The MV may show AML fluttering in a TG basal SAX view (**A**) or reverse doming and premature closure with diastolic mitral regurgitation in a ME AV LAX view (**B**). **C,** The LV may become dilated with variable function. AML, anterior mitral leaflet; PML, posterior mitral leaflet.

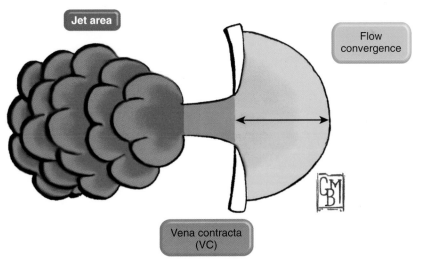

Figure 3-17. AR jet components. The AR regurgitant jet comprises three regions: (1) flow convergence has the highest velocity, (2) vena contracta (VC) has the narrowest portion of the jet, and (3) jet area is the largest portion with flow into the LV. Assessment of different components of the jet help grade AR severity.

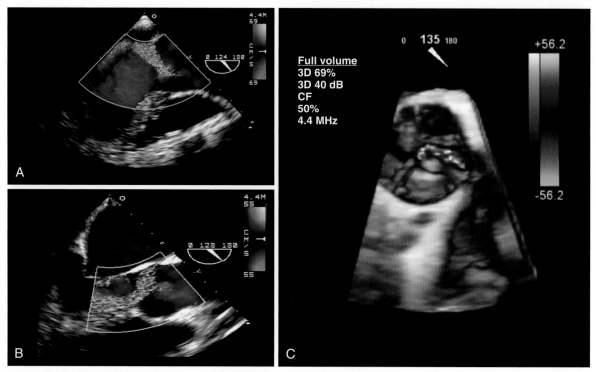

Figure 3-18. AR jet direction and location. The origin and directionality of the AR jet can help establish the AR etiology. Central AR is more common with root dilatation, eccentric AR is found in bicuspid AV and cusp prolapse. Shown here are a posteriorly directed AR jet from right cusp prolapse (**A**) and an anteriorly directed jet from a left cusp prolapse (**B**). **C,** Commissural AR between the left and the right cusps is shown in a 3D full-volume color view rotated to the ME AV SAX orientation.

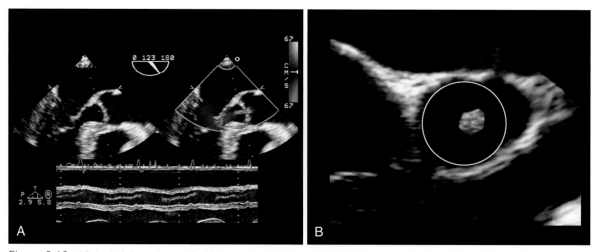

Figure 3-19. AR jet height and area. **A,** Measure the minimum AR jet height at its origin and compare it with LVOT width (jet height/LVOT width) to grade AR severity. Color M-mode assesses the duration of the AR jet and may not represent an optimal site for measurement of jet height and LVOT width. **B,** Comparison of the planimetered LVOT area and AR jet area in SAX should be preformed below the AV in the LVOT, ideally without the AV cusps visible.

TABLE 3-4   GRADING AORTIC REGURGITATION SEVERITY

Method	Mild	Moderate	Severe
Jet width/LVOT width* (%)	<25	25-64	≥65
Jet CSA/LVOT CSA* (%)	<5	5-59	≥60
CW density	Faint	Dense	Dense
Decay slope (m/s)	<2	2-3.5	>3
PHT (ms)	>500	200-500	<200
Descending aorta reversal (PW)	Brief, early	Intermediate	Holodiastolic
Vena contracta* (mm)	<3.0	3.0-6.0	>6.0
ERO area (cm²)	<0.10	0.1-0.3	>0.30
Regurgitant volume (cc/beat)	<30	30-60	>60
Regurgitant fraction (%)	<30	30-49	>50

*Nyquist limit 50-60 cm/s.
CSA, cross-sectional area; CW, continuous wave; ERO, effective regurgitant orifice; LVOT, left ventricular outflow tract; PHT, pressure half-time; PW, pulsed wave.
From Zoghbi WA, Enriquez-Sarano M, Foster E, et al. Recommendations for evaluation of the severity of native valvular regurgitation with two-dimensional and Doppler echocardiography. *J Am Soc Echocardiogr.* 2003;16:777-802.

although small jets reliably reflect mild AR and a larger area may indicate more significant AR.

- Numerous technical, physiologic, and anatomic factors affect the jet area size and alter its accuracy as an index of AR severity.
- Jet area may appear larger by increasing the driving pressure across the valve (flow momentum = flow rate × velocity); hence, the importance of measuring blood pressure.
- Eccentric jets occupy a small portion of the proximal LVOT appearing narrow, thus, underestimating AR severity, whereas central jets tend to expand fully in the LVOT and may overestimate AR.
- AR severity is poorly evaluated in diffuse jets that arise from the entire coaptation line as seen in AV SAX view.
- The maximal proximal jet width and its ratio to the LVOT diameter from the AV LAX and the ratio of cross-sectional jet to LVOT area from the AV SAX are measured within 1 cm of the AV. The criteria to define severe AR are ratios of 65% or greater for jet width and 60% or greater for jet area (Table 3-4).

Vena Contracta

- The vena contracta is the narrowest portion of a regurgitant jet that is slightly smaller than the anatomic regurgitant orifice and is characterized by high-velocity laminar flow.
- Vena contracta width is significantly smaller than jet width in the LVOT described previously because the jet expands immediately after the vena contracta (Figure 3-20).

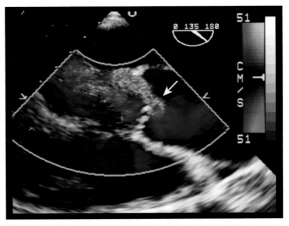

Figure 3-20. Vena contracta. To optimize visualization of the VC use a zoom of the ME AV LAX view and a small color sector. Measure the VC just below the area of proximal flow acceleration *(arrow)*, which may be difficult to determine in some central AR jets. The VC is smaller than the jet height. This linear measurement at a Nyquist of 50 to 60 cm/s grades AR severity (severe > 6 mm) and is also an estimate of the EROA.

- The vena contracta CSA represents a measure of the effective regurgitant orifice area (EROA), which is the narrowest area of actual flow.
- Vena contracta size is independent of flow rate and driving pressure for a fixed orifice but may change with a dynamic orifice and is less sensitive to technical factors.
- Vena contracta limitations occur with multiple or irregularly shaped jets, in which one diameter may not reflect AR severity; a SAX view may provide a better appreciation of the AR.

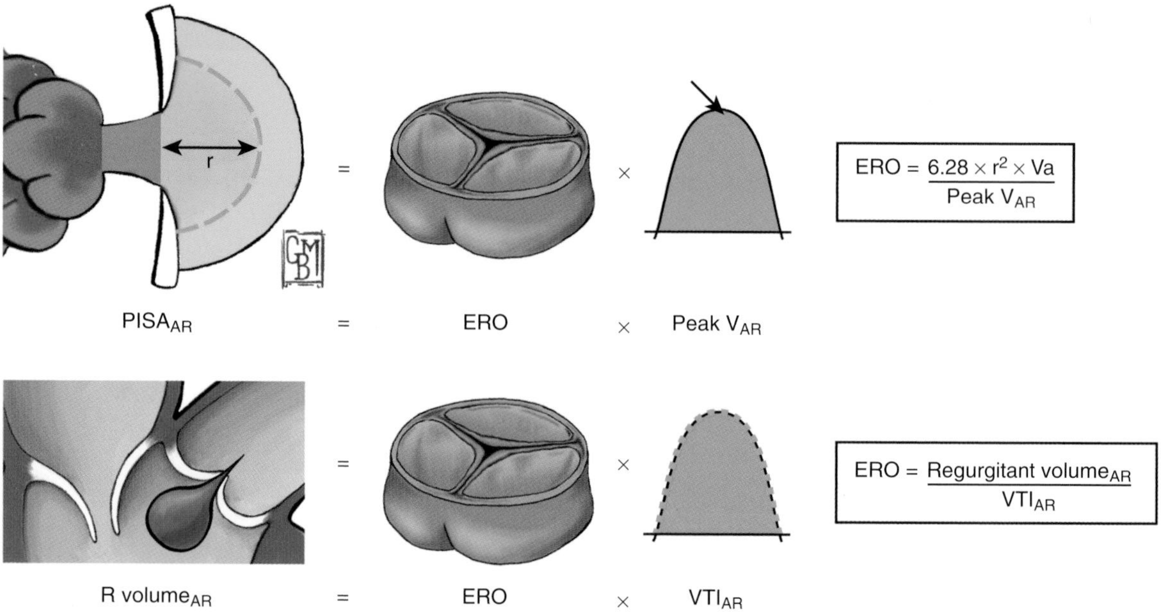

Figure 3-21. Effective regurgitant orifice (ERO). The ERO is the derived area of hemodynamic regurgitation calculated using regurgitant volume or PISA with the formulas as indicated. ERO greater than 0.3 cm² is severe.

- Minute errors measuring the small vena contracta values (usually < 1 cm) may result in a large error and misclassification of AR severity.
- Thresholds of vena contracta width associated with severe AR are 0.5 cm (highly sensitive), 0.7 cm (highly specific) and 0.6 cm (best combination of specificity and sensitivity).

Proximal Isovelocity Surface Area or Flow Convergence
- Blood appears as concentric, hemispheric shells of increasing velocity and decreasing surface area as it approaches a regurgitant orifice. EROA can be calculated as (Figure 3-21):

$$EROA = (2\pi r^2 \times Va)/PkVreg$$

  - Hemispheric surface area ($2\pi r^2$)
  - Aliasing velocity (Va)
  - CW Doppler peak velocity AR jet (PkVreg)
- Because the PISA calculation provides an instantaneous peak flow rate, EROA by this approach is the maximal EROA and may be slightly larger than EROA calculated by other methods.
- Compared with MR, less experience exists using PISA for AR assessment. Thresholds for severe AR are an EROA of 0.30 cm² or greater and a regurgitant volume of 60 mL or greater.

- PISA is more accurate for central than for eccentric AR jets and for a circular orifice.
- Any error in PISA measurement is squared, which can markedly affect the EROA.

Regurgitant Volume and Fraction
- Flow through the regurgitant AV is larger than that through other competent valves; regurgitant volume is the difference between the two.

$$Regurgitant\ volume = SV\ RegValv - SV\ CompValv$$

- Regurgitant fraction is the regurgitant volume divided by the forward SV through the regurgitant valve.

$$Regurgitant\ fraction = (SV\ RegValv - SV\ CompValv)/SV\ RegValve$$

- EROA is calculated from the regurgitant SV and the CW Doppler AR jet VTI (see Figure 3-21):

$$EROA = Regurgitant\ volume/VTIRegJet$$

- As with the PISA method, a regurgitant volume of 60 mL or greater and EROA of .30 cm² or greater are consistent with severe AR.
- Aortic SV can be derived from quantitative 2D measurements of LV end-diastolic and end-systolic volumes or pulsed

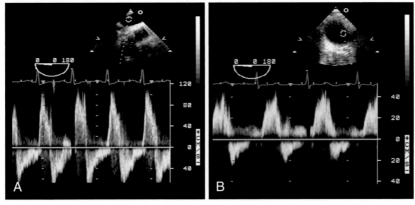

Figure 3-22. Aorta flow reversal. AR severity is indicated by diastolic flow reversal seen below the baseline with pulsed wave Doppler, in the distal arch upper esophageal (UE) arch LAX view (**A**) and descending aorta SAX view (**B**). More severe AR has holodiastolic flow with equivalent forward and reverse flow in a more distal portion of the descending aorta.

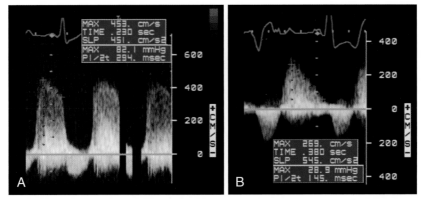

Figure 3-23. AR CW Doppler. CW Doppler density is a simple qualitative indicator of regurgitant volume, although with a lot of overlap between moderate and severe AR. The decay slope represents the rate of equalization of aortic and LV diastolic pressure with more rapid LV filling in severe AR. The slope can be expressed in cm/s (severe AR > 300 cm/s) or the time it takes for the pressure to fall by half ($PT_{1/2}$ or PHT, severe AR < 250 ms).

Doppler and compared with mitral or pulmonic SV.

- Quantitative Doppler method cannot be used if there is more than mild MR, unless the pulmonic site is used for systemic flow calculation.
- The most common errors encountered in determining these parameters are (1) inaccurate valve annulus measurement (error is squared), (2) failure to trace the modal velocity (brightest signal representing laminar flow) of the pulsed Doppler tracing, and (3) failure to position the sample volume correctly and with minimal angulation at the annular level.

Step 2b: Spectral Doppler
Aortic Diastolic Flow Reversal

- Brief diastolic flow reversal in the aorta is normal, which may be prolonged from reduced aorta compliance with aging.

- The duration and velocity of aortic flow reversal increase with worsening AR. The velocity, VTI, and VTI ratio of reversal to forward flow in the descending aorta have all been proposed as semiquantitative indices of AR severity.
- Prominent holodiastolic reversal indicates at least moderate AR. A similar diastolic VTI and systolic VTI is a reliable qualitative sign of severe AR (Figure 3-22).

Signal Density

- The density of the CW Doppler AR spectral display reflects the volume of regurgitation, especially in comparison with the antegrade spectral density (Figure 3-23).
- A faint spectral display is compatible with trace or mild AR. Significant overlap between moderate and severe AR exists in more dense recordings, making it an imperfect indicator of AR severity.

TABLE 3-5   LIMITATIONS AND IMPLICATIONS OF GRADING AORTIC REGURGITATION

Doppler	Limitations	Implications
Jet width (color Doppler)	Expands unpredictably Eccentric jets inaccurate	Simple screen
Vena contracta width (color Doppler)	Multiple jets invalid Small value, greater error	Simple quantitative Mild or severe AR
PISA method (color and CW)	AV calcifications Multiple jets invalid Less accurate eccentric jets Underestimate with aneurysms	Quantitative EROA (maximal) Regurgitant volume
Flow quantity (PW)	Invalid combined MR and AR	OK with multiple, eccentric jets EROA Regurgitant volume
Jet density (CW)	Overlap moderate and severe AR Incomplete trace	Simple Qualitative
PHT (CW)	Changes in LV pressure	Simple Qualitative
Aortic reversal (PW)	Age-related changes	Simple Qualitative

AR, aortic regurgitation; AV, aortic valve; CW, continuous wave; EROA, effective regurgitant orifice area; LV, left ventricular;
   MR, mitral regurgitation; PHT, pressure half-time; PISA, proximal isovelocity surface area; PW, pulsed wave.
From Zoghbi WA, Enriquez-Sarano M, Foster E, et al. Recommendations for evaluation of the severity of native valvular
   regurgitation with two-dimensional and Doppler echocardiography. *J Am Soc Echocardiogr.* 2003;16:777-802.

Diastolic Jet Deceleration

- The rate of deceleration of the diastolic regurgitant jet and the derived PHT reflect the rate of equalization of aortic and LV diastolic pressures (see Figure 3-23).
- With increasing AR severity, aortic diastolic pressure decreases more rapidly, the late diastolic jet velocity is lower, and hence, PHT is shorter. A value of 200 ms or less is consistent with severe AR.
- For a given AR severity, PHT is also determined by LV diastolic compliance and pressure; thus, it is further shortened by an elevated LV diastolic pressure or by vasodilators or lengthened with chronic LV adaptation to severe AR.

Grading Aortic Regurgitation

Integrative Approach to Aortic Regurgitation Assessment

- Grading of AR severity by Doppler echocardiography is an integrative and comprehensive process (see Table 3-4). It is made easier when the evidence from the different parameters is congruent.
- When different parameters are contradictory, closely examine for technical and physiologic reasons. Rely on best quality components

(regurgitant volume or fraction, EROA) to quantify AR severity.
- Limitations with clinical implications for grading AR are summarized in Table 3-5.

AORTIC VALVE ENDOCARDITIS

KEY POINTS

- Infective endocarditis affects normal and abnormal valves and is especially virulent when prosthetic valves are involved.
- Vegetations tend to occur on the low-pressure sides of valves.
- Vegetations are mobile, echodense structures similar in appearance to thrombus that must be viewed in clinical context.
- The development of abscesses and other perivalvular complications (pseudoaneurysm, fistulae, prosthetic valve dehiscence) significantly increases morbidity and mortality.

Etiology, Pathophysiology

- Infective endocarditis (IE) is caused by an infectious agent affecting normal (20%) or structurally abnormal (75%) valves with established risk factors of prior episodes of IE, invasive medical procedures and intravenous drug use.

- Native valve endocarditis (NVE) affects the left- more than the right-sided valves, in order of frequency: aortic > mitral > tricuspid > pulmonic.
- Prosthetic valve endocarditis (PVE) accounts for 7% to 25% of IE cases, 3% within the first year and 1% annual incidence thereafter, mechanical more than bioprosthetic valves in the first year, but that relationship reverses in later years after surgery.
- Early surgery will increase survival and is required in 40% to 45% of patients (similar rates for NVE and PVE). Surgery is more likely in younger age, congestive heart failure, abscess, coagulase-negative staphylococcal IE, and organisms resistant to medical management.

Echocardiography in Endocarditis

- The diagnosis of endocarditis is made with a combination of echocardiographic, clinical, and microbiologic data integrated in the Duke criteria.
- Based on AHA guidelines, the clinical scenario and patient probability of having endocarditis guide the use of transthoracic echocardiography (TTE) or TEE in the diagnosis of endocarditis. A negative TEE has a high negative predictive value (86-97%).
- Complications of endocarditis have a negative impact on clinical outcome so symptomatic patients with complicated left-sided NVE or PVE should undergo TEE to rule out valve ring abscess, valve perforation, or valvular dehiscence, which require immediate surgical intervention.
- Echocardiographic findings considered major criteria for the diagnosis of endocarditis are (1) vegetations, (2) abscesses, (3) new dehiscence of a valvular prosthesis, and/or (4) new valvular regurgitation.
- Abnormal echocardiographic findings not fulfilling those definitions are minor criteria: new nodular valve thickening, valve perforations and nonoscillating mass.

Vegetations
- Vegetative growth composed of platelets, fibrin, and microbes appears as irregular variable-sized vegetations on damaged endocardium exposed to turbulent flow.
- Typical vegetation locations are on valves and in the direction of blood flow: atrioventricular valves (atrial side), semilunar valves (ventricular side), VSD (orifice facing the right ventricle [RV]), AR (chordae tendinae of anterior mitral valve leaflet [AMVL]), MR (left atrial [LA] wall).
- Vegetation detection is better by TEE (90-100% sensitivity) than by TTE (60% sensitive, 98% specific). TTE is inadequate in 20% of cases because image resolution is limited to detecting vegetations greater than 3-mm size.
- Careful assessment by echocardiography documents the location, number, and size of vegetations that may involve multiple valves.
- Vegetations appear as irregular echodense independently mobile masses, although early small (<2 mm) vegetations may be difficult to detect using TEE (Figure 3-24).
- Both thrombus and pannus have a similar echogenic appearance and cannot be distinguished from vegetative material.
- Approximately 30% of IE patients have an embolic event. Emboli are most often cerebral with increased mortality, from large (>10 mm) and mobile vegetations on the MV. One embolic event increases the risk for a second event.

Abscess
- Abscess complicates up to 35% of endocarditis patients, worsening prognosis. There is a greater risk in patients with *Staphylococcus aureus* bacteremia, NVE (aortic > mitral > tricuspid) and PVE because the sewing ring is the primary site of infection.
- An *abscess* is defined as a region of necrosis or cavity containing purulent material that forms from perivalvular extension of microbes.
- AV abscesses are usually confined to the aortic valve plane but may extend into the weakest portion near the aortic-mitral intervalvular fibrosa or the base of the septum, causing a thickened posterior aortic root and heart block.
- Abscesses appear as an echodense or echolucent perivalvular area compared with the surrounding tissue, which may have color Doppler flow distinguishing it from pannus or thrombus (see Figure 3-24).
- TEE has superior sensitivity (87%) and specificity (96%) for perivalvular abscess, with aortic (86%) more easily detected than mitral (42%) and particularly in PVE.
- TEE evidence helpful in diagnosing abscesses includes (1) abnormal septal density (>14 mm), (2) greater than 15 degrees of prosthetic valve rocking (dehisced if > 40%), (3) mycotic aneurysm, and (4) aorta-ventricle discontinuity.
- Ring abscesses at the level of the aortic annulus may appear septated with either no

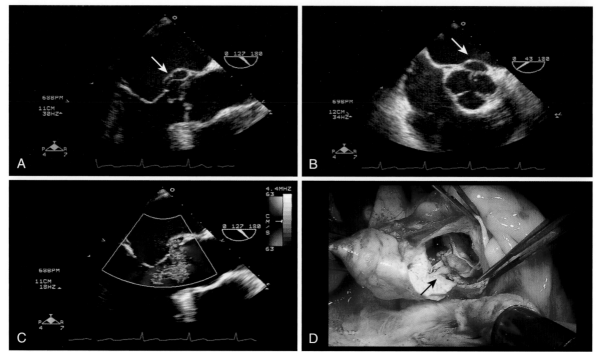

Figure 3-24. AV abscess and fistula. In the ME AV LAX view, (**A**) an echolucent septated cavity is clearly present and involves the noncoronary sinus as determined from the ME AV SAX view (**B**). The cavity is exposed to higher pressures throughout the cardiac cycle and does not collapse. **C,** Color Doppler shows flow into the cavity during early systole. **D,** The aortic vegetation and abscess are shown at the time of surgery. The abscess cavity was removed, the intervalvular fibrosa was reconstructed and an AVR was performed.

Doppler flow or systolic and diastolic flow from the higher aortic pressure, which minimizes collapse throughout the cardiac cycle.

Valve Regurgitation

- The presence of a new or worsening perivalvular regurgitation or valve dehiscence is a major criterion for endocarditis diagnosis.
- AR of varying severity is common (50% of cases) in aortic valve endocarditis is from cusp perforation or flail, perivalvular leak, or cusp malcoaptation from a vegetation.
- Cusp perforation is imaged as a discontinuity of the valve cusp at the site and an eccentric regurgitant AR jet with color flow Doppler.
- AMVL perforation represents a secondarily infected "jet lesion" that is associated with moderate AR from AV endocarditis.

Pseudoaneurysm

- Secondary involvement of the mitral-aortic intervalvular fibrosa and AMVL occurs as a result of direct extension of infection from an AV abscess or infected AR jet.
- A mitral-aortic intervalvular fibrosa pseudoaneurysm appears as a pulsatile echo-free space. The neck opens into the LVOT, bounded by the base of the AMVL, the medial wall of the LA, and the posterior aortic root (see Figure 3-24).
- Color Doppler distinguishes unruptured pseudoaneurysms that communicate only with the LVOT which show dynamic early systolic expansion and contraction during diastolic emptying.

Fistula

- Aortic root abscesses and pseudoaneurysms may rupture into adjacent chambers and create intravascular fistulous tracts.
- Fistulas may be single or multiple extending from the aorta to the RV, right atrium (RA), or LA and is easily imaged with color or CW Doppler (high-velocity flow).
- Abscess or pseudoaneurysm rupture can create a fistula tract between the LVOT, the pseudoaneurysm, and the LA, causing eccentric MR, or between the LVOT, the pseudoaneurysm, and the aorta with systolic fistula flow and diastolic AR flow (see Figure 3-24).
- Communication between the aortic root and the right ventricular outflow tract (RVOT) has been less commonly described.

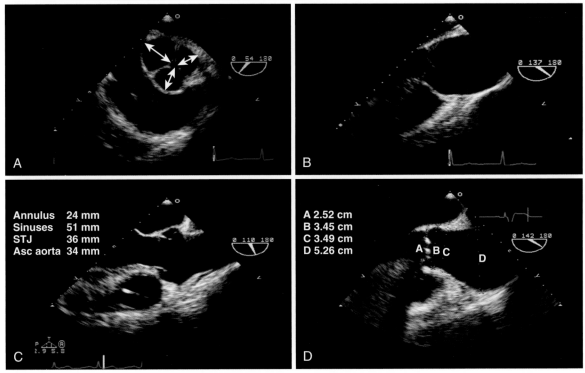

Figure 3-25. Aortic root disease. **A** and **B,** Annuloaortic ectasia in the ME AV SAX view appears as a prominent aortic root and central cusp malcoaptation with central AR. The noncoronary sinus is often stretched resulting in NCC distortion. The ME AV LAX view during diastole identifies poor cusp coaptation with a central gap. The dilated sinus may be the same size as the STJ, making it difficult to establish the exact STJ location. **C,** Sinus of Valsalva aneurysm with symmetrical sinus dilatation may result in central AR, although concurrent cusp prolapse may cause eccentric AR. **D,** Ascending aorta dilatation in a patient with a stenotic AV will require the aorta and valve to be replaced.

DISEASES OF THE AORTIC ROOT

Annuloaortic Ectasia

- Annuloaortic ectasia (Figure 3-25) describes annular, STJ, and ascending aorta dilatation associated with connective tissue (CT) disorders (e.g., Marfan, Ehlers-Danlos).
- Root replacement or valve-sparing root procedures aim to support the annulus to prevent recurrence of dilatation.

Sinus of Valsalva Aneurysms

- Isolated sinus of Valsalva aneurysms may be congenital (rare) or acquired defects from trauma, endocarditis, Marfan syndrome, or syphilis.
- A ruptured aneurysm is complex with fistula formation into an adjacent structure, whereas an unruptured aneurysm may cause RVOT obstruction, arrhythmias, or myocardial ischemia.

- Surgery (see Figure 3-25) is recommended when sinuses enlarge to greater than 50% (isolated) or greater than 40 mm (multiple). Surgery involves a tailored synthetic tube graft to replace the isolated diseased sinus and correct the AR.

Ascending Aorta Aneurysms

- Ascending aorta aneurysms (see Figure 3-25) from degenerative (aging, hypertension) or aortopathies (CT diseases, bicuspid AV) have a dilated STJ and ascending aorta that may involve the sinuses but not the annulus with central AR from outward displacement of the commissures.
- Surgery is indicated to prevent rupture in degenerative disease when the aortic diameter exceeds 60 mm or 55 mm (for AV sparing) and sooner in aortopathies at 50 mm or 48 mm (for AV sparing) or if there is a family history of acute type A aortic dissection.

Ascending Aorta Dissection

- Acute or chronic ascending aortic dissection dilates the STJ resulting in (1) acute distraction of the valve cusps (central AR) and (2) cusp unhinging and prolapse (eccentric AR).
- An aortic valve-sparing root procedure can be used for all aortic dissections limited to the ascending aorta above the STJ or involving the noncoronary cusp with AV prolapse.

INDICATIONS FOR AORTIC VALVE SURGERY

Native Aortic Valve Replacement

- Aortic valve surgery improves symptoms and survival with current indications as outlined in Table 3-6.
- The primary determinant for AVR with AS is symptoms and not the absolute AVA (or transvalvular pressure gradient); with AR, it is the presence of severe AR independent of symptoms.
- Class II indications for AVR may warrant further assessment using intraoperative TEE or visual inspection of the AV to decide whether intervention is needed.
- Age is not a contraindication to an open AVR but poor operative risk patients may be best treated with percutaneous balloon valvotomy or transcatheter AVR (see Case 3-2 on the companion website).

Prosthetic Valve Replacement

- Prosthetic valve failure from various causes (calcification or leaflet tears, pannus, thrombosis, infection) results in AR or AS, with the severity graded as previously described.
- Reoperation timing is based on symptoms, LV function, and the echocardiographic appearance of the valve. Elective early reoperation is safer and may improve the overall outcome.

TABLE 3-6   INDICATIONS FOR AORTIC VALVE REPLACEMENT

Aortic Stenosis	Aortic Regurgitation
Class I AVR Indicated	
1. Symptomatic severe AS* (B)	1. Symptomatic severe AR irrespective of LV (B)
2. Severe AS* + other cardiac surgery (C)	2. Asymptomatic chronic severe AR + LVEF < 0.50 at rest (B)
3. Severe AS* + LVEF < 0.50 (C)	3. Chronic severe AR + other cardiac surgery (C)
Class IIa AVR Reasonable	
Moderate AS* + other cardiac surgery (B)	Asymptomatic severe AR + normal LVEF but severe LV dilatation*† (B)
Class IIb AVR May Be Considered	
1. Asymptomatic severe AS* + abnormal exercise response or high risk for rapid progression or delayed surgery (C)	1. Moderate AR + other cardiac surgery (C)
2. Mild AS* undergoing CABG + rapidly progressive moderate to severe valve calcification (C)	2. Asymptomatic severe AR + normal LVEF > 0.50 + LV dilatation†, progressive LV dilatation, declining exercise tolerance, or abnormal hemodynamic responses to exercise* (C)
3. Asymptomatic extremely severe AS† + expected operative mortality ≤ 1.0% (C)	

(B) and *(C)* are current levels of evidence.
*Consider lower threshold values for patients of small stature of either gender.
†AVA < 0.6 cm², mean gradient > 60 mm Hg, and jet velocity > 5.0 m/s.
‡EDD > 75 mm or ESD > 55 mm.
AR, aortic regurgitation; AS, aortic stenosis; AVA, aortic valve area; AVR, aortic valve replacement; CABG, coronary artery bypass grafting; EDD, end-diastolic dimension; ESD, end-systolic dimension; LV, left ventricle; LV, left ventricular; LVEF, left ventricular ejection fraction.

From Bonow RO, Carabello BA, Chatterjee K, et al. 2008 focused update incorporated into the ACC/AHA 2006 guidelines for the management of patients with valvular heart disease: A report of the American College of Cardiology/American Heart Association Task Force on Practice Guidelines (Writing Committee to revise the 1998 guidelines for the management of patients with valvular heart disease). Endorsed by the Society of Cardiovascular Anesthesiologists, Society for Cardiovascular Angiography and Interventions, and Society of Thoracic Surgeons. *J Am Coll Cardiol.* 2008;52:e1-142.

Valve-Sparing Operations

- Aortic valve-sparing/-salvage reconstruction techniques are used to avoid prosthetic valves in patients with aortic root pathology and morphologically normal valve cusps with or without AR.
- The indications for AV sparing (Box 3-1) are as established for AVR for AR (see Table 3-6) with additional considerations of (1) aortic cusp quality, (2) surgeon's experience, and (3) inherent risk of reoperation.
- Salvage involves direct repair of the cusps to reestablish the plane of coaptation and consists of plicating the cusp-free margin for cusp prolapse or patch repairs for cusp perforations.
- Early repair failure can be prevented with the routine use of intraoperative TEE and adjustments of the reconstruction to achieve perfect valve function before leaving the OR.

- Abnormal AV cusps such as calcified, rheumatic, large fenestrations, severely overstretched, or multiple prolapsed cusps should not be spared (Figure 3-26).
- Valve-sparing operations require prolonged aortic cross-clamp times and, therefore, are

BOX 3-1 Indications for Valve-Sparing Aortic Root Procedures

- In age < 70 years
  - Acute type A aortic dissection
  - Degenerative aneurysm > 48 mm
  - Marfan syndrome or familial aneurysm/dissection > 45 mm
- In age < 60 years
  - Bicuspid aortic valve + ascending aneurysm > 45 mm
  - Repairable severe AR + dilated root > 40 mm

AR, aortic regurgitation.

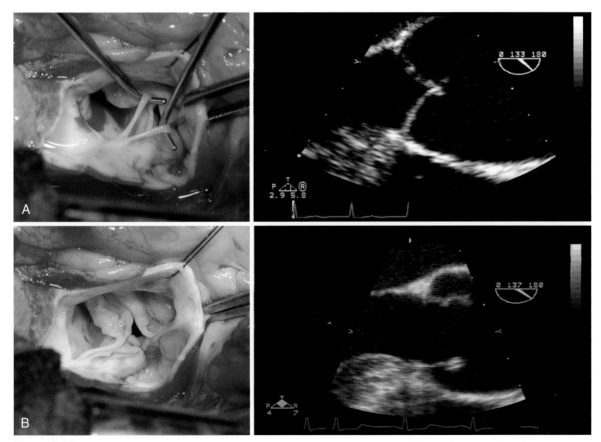

Figure 3-26. Cusp pathology. **A,** Fenestrations are tears at the cusp edge. In the ME AV LAX view, there is some cusp coaptation with AR appearing at the cusp edges. **B,** Chronic AR itself causes rolled up cusp edges. This appears as thickened cusp edges during systole in the ME AV LAX view. These cusp pathologies make AVs unsuitable for valve-sparing procedures.

TABLE 3-7   TYPES OF AORTIC VALVE PROSTHESIS

Valve Type	Mean Gradient	Advantages	Disadvantages
Mechanical	12.5 ± 6.4 mm Hg	Durability	Anticoagulation Hemodynamics
Stented bioprosthetic	14.4 ± 5.7 mm Hg	Good hemodynamics No anticoagulation	Durability
Stentless porcine		Increased EOA Low gradient	Complex procedure Long-term durability Difficult explantation
Homograft	7.8 ± 2.7 mm Hg	Low reinfection Favorable hemodynamics No anticoagulation	Valve failure (AR)

AR, aortic regurgitation; EOA, effective orifice area.

best avoided in patients with poor LV function or when other concomitant complex procedures are necessary.

Surgical Procedures

> **KEY POINTS**
>
> - Surgery in AS is guided by symptoms; with AR, it is determined by the severity of the AR.
> - Valve replacement may be with bioprosthetic or mechanical valves. The choice depends on the age of the patient, their suitability for anticoagulation, and the size of the aortic annulus.
> - Extensive involvement of the root and/or ascending aorta may dictate more complex operations.
> - Annular measurements guide the surgical valve sizing; if the prosthesis is too small for the patient's cardiac output, patient-prosthesis mismatch (PPM) may occur.
> - Specific patterns of intravalvular regurgitation are recognized for each valve. Periprosthetic leaks when small often disappear with heparin neutralization, but when large may underscore a persistent mechanical defect.
> - Damage to surrounding structures may occur and must be ruled out after aortic valve surgery is complete.
> - Aortic valve-sparing operations should be performed in centers where special expertise is present.

Aortic Valve Replacement

- Mechanical, bioprosthetic, stentless valves and homografts can be implanted in the aortic position, the choice depending on inherent advantages and disadvantages of each (Table 3-7).

> **KEY POINTS**
>
> - There are two types of stentless porcine prosthetic valves, the Freestyle aortic root prosthesis (Medtronic, Minneapolis, MN) and the Toronto SPV valve (St. Jude Medical, St. Paul, MN); both are glutaraldehyde-fixed porcine valves without a stent.
> - Human aortic and pulmonary valves from cadaveric human hearts are the valvular prostheses of choice for complex endocarditis because they have a low incidence of reinfection.

Bentall Procedure

- This traditional surgical approach has excellent reproducible results for patients with aortic root disease, particularly AS.
- The Bentall procedure involves replacement of the diseased aorta with a synthetic valved conduit, using either mechanical or biologic valve prostheses, along with coronary artery reimplantation.
- Any paravalvular leak will be visible in the surgical field, rather than with TEE.

Transcatheter Valvular Interventions

- Catheter-based interventions for AS are used in patients considered high operative risks.
- Two devices, the Edwards Sapien transcatheter heart valve (THV, Edwards Lifesciences Inc, Irvine, CA) and the Medtronic CoreValve System (Medtronic, Inc., Minneapolis, MN), have received commercial approval in Europe.
- The THV is a trileaflet bovine pericardial valve mounted on a balloon-expandable stainless steel stent and comes in two sizes, 23 mm (19-21 mm annulus) and 26 mm (22-24 mm annulus) for transfemoral (TF) or transapical (TA) deployment.

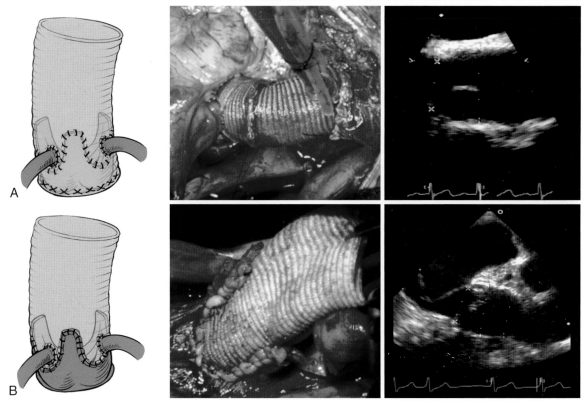

Figure 3-27. AV-sparing root techniques. **A,** In the reimplantation technique, the entire AV including the annulus is resuspended inside an appropriately sized (female 26-30 mm, male 28-34 mm) synthetic tube graft. There are two suture lines, one at the annulus and the other supporting the commissures. **B,** In the remodeling technique, each of the three native valve commissures is sewn with a single suture line to a synthetic tailored tripartite crown-shaped Dacron tube graft, creating neosinuses.

- The CoreValve has trileaflet porcine pericardial leaflets mounted in a self-expanding, nitinol frame. It comes in two sizes, 26 and 29 mm (23-27 mm annulus) and is only for TF insertion.
- Fluoroscopy and TEE are mandatory during the procedure for (1) AV annulus sizing, (2) valve positioning, (3) monitoring cardiac function, and (4) postdeployment valve function.
- TEE is the most reliable tool to measure the aortic annulus diameter at midsystole, taking multiple measurements, because AV calcification may make it challenging (see Case 3-2 on the companion website).
- For the retrograde TF approach, vascular access is the major limitation. Passage through the aortic arch may have stroke implications and retrograde crossing of a calcified stenotic AV is challenging.
- For the antegrade TA approach, the cardiac apex is accessed through a left minithoracotomy, sheaths are positioned across the stenotic AV; after a balloon valvuloplasty, the valve is positioned and deployed.

- The valve after deployment is assessed for position, stability, function and paravalvular leak.

Valve-Sparing Aortic Root Techniques

- Two basic types of valve-sparing operations, reimplantation and remodeling, have been designed for patients with aortic root dilatation and normal or near-normal AV (Figure 3-27).
- Both techniques involve excision of the dilated root tissue and use of a Dacron tube graft with re-attachment of the coronary arteries and distal ascending aorta.
  - In the reimplantation technique, pioneered by Dr. Tirone David,[9] the entire AV including the annulus is resuspended inside an appropriately sized synthetic tube graft, preventing future annular dilatation.
  - In the remodeling technique, created by Dr. Yacoub, each of the three native valve commissures is sewn to a synthetic tailored tripartite crown-shaped Dacron tube graft,

creating neosinuses without securing the aortic annulus.

- Modifications have been proposed to overcome limitations for both techniques (Table 3-8): the remodeling technique fails to secure the aortic annulus and prevent further dilatation and the reimplantation technique fails to provide neosinuses of Valsalva.

TABLE 3-8   MODIFICATIONS OF AORTIC VALVE-SPARING PROCEDURES

	Modifications	Implications
David 1	Graft attached to annulus, AV resuspended	Cylindrical sinus, annulus reinforced
David 2	Tailored graft attached to commissural posts	No reinforcement or reduction of the "annulus" and no STJ remodeling
David 3	David 2 + Annulus reinforced (Teflon felt)	Reinforces annulus, remodels STJ
David 4	David 1 using a 4-mm larger Dacron graft plicated at STJ	STJ remodeled
David 5	David 1 using a 8-mm larger Dacron graft plicated at annulus and STJ	Neosinuses created, STJ remodeled
Yacoub	Remodeling using a tripartite crown-shaped Dacron tube graft	Neosinuses without annular support or STJ remodeling

AV, aortic valve; STJ, sinotubular junction.

Intraoperative Echocardiography

- Intraoperative TEE is a Society of Cardiovascular Anesthesiologists (SCA)/AHA category 1 indication for aortic root-sparing procedures and a category 2 indication for patients undergoing AVR surgery.
- TEE is used to determine baseline valve function, detect any issues that require immediate reintervention, and monitor cardiac performance (Figure 3-28).

Aortic Valve Replacement (Figure 3-29) Pre-Cardiopulmonary Bypass

- Measurements of the annulus and aortic root size are obtained and, in conjunction with body surface area (BSA), help determine the prosthetic valve size.
- PPM implies the prosthesis EOA may be too small for the patient's cardiac output requirements. It occurs at an indexed EOA less than $0.85 \text{ cm}^2/\text{m}^2$ and may increase mortality in patients with impaired LV function.
- PPM has been used to describe an absolute small valve size (i.e., <21 mm), small valve size in a patient with a large BSA, excessive transvalvular gradient immediately postimplantation, increased transvalvular gradient with exercise, and various combinations of these variables.
- Implantation of an adequate-sized valve with a small aortic annulus may require

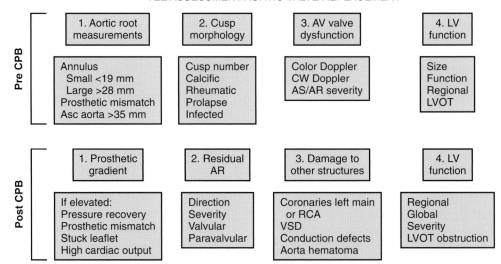

TEE ASSESSMENT AORTIC VALVE REPLACEMENT

Figure 3-28. TEE assessment for AVR. RCA, right coronary artery.

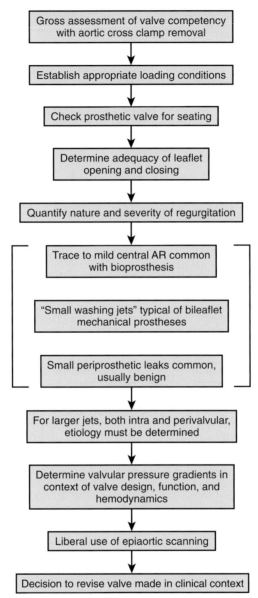

Figure 3-29. TEE assessment post AVR.

patch enlargement of the aortic annulus and aortic root, suprannular or slightly tilted orientation.

Post-Cardiopulmonary Bypass, Complications
Prosthetic Valve Gradients

- Most prosthetic valves have some degree of intrinsic stenosis (reference gradients in Table 3-7), although as a whole, as the prosthetic size increases, the transvalvular gradient decreases.
- The measured gradient is dependent upon current loading conditions, ventricular contractility, and the type and size of the implanted prosthesis (Figure 3-30).

- The same Doppler principles and formulas apply to native and prosthetic valves for evaluation of AR and AS.
- PR suggests the mean gradient obtained by CW Doppler may not be the spatial mean gradient, and care must be taken when comparing prostheses utilizing CW Doppler.
- Quantitative indices of valve function that are less dependent on flow include effective orifice area, Doppler velocity index (DVI), and valve resistance.
- DVI (Velocity$_{LVOT}$/Velocity$_{jet}$ = P$_K$V$_{LVOT}$/P$_K$Vjet) has no dimensions and incorporates the effect of flow on prosthetic valve velocity. A DVI

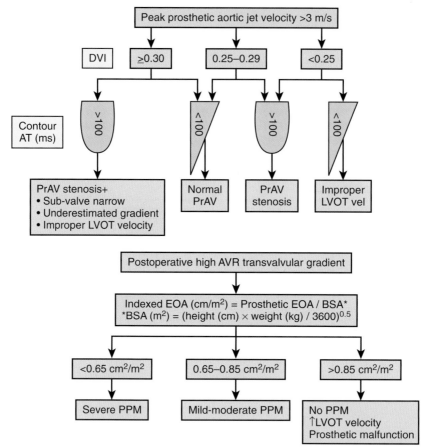

Figure 3-30. Elevated AVR gradient. The prosthesis EOA is too small for the patient's size, resulting in abnormally high pressure gradients and may be less relevant in obese patients. Avoidance of PPM in the aortic position may necessitate AVR implantation after patch root enlargement in the supravalvular or tilted rather than the intervalvular position. *From Zoghbi WA, Chambers JB, Dumesnil JG, et al. Recommendations for evaluation of prosthetic valves with echocardiography and Doppler ultrasound: A report from the American Society of Echocardiography's Guidelines and Standards Committee and the Task Force on Prosthetic Valves, developed in conjunction with the American College of Cardiology Cardiovascular Imaging Committee, Cardiac Imaging Committee of the American Heart Association, the European Association of Echocardiography, a registered branch of the European Society of Cardiology, the Japanese Society of Echocardiography and the Canadian Society of Echocardiography, endorsed by the American College of Cardiology Foundation, American Heart Association, European Association of Echocardiography, a registered branch of the European Society of Cardiology, the Japanese Society of Echocardiography, and Canadian Society of Echocardiography. J Am Soc Echocardiogr. 2009;22:975-1014.*

less than 0.27 is suspicious for significant valve obstruction.

- Valve resistance (dynes.s.cm⁵) is determined from the mean valve gradient (MG), ejection time (ET), and SV as

$$\text{Valve resistance} = (\text{MG} \times \text{ET/SV}) \times 1.33$$

Prosthetic Regurgitation

- Bioprosthetic valves may have a small jet located centrally or at a commissure (normal finding 10%). Abnormal significant AR results from a structural defect, leaflet damage, or strut deformation.
- Mechanical valves have specific patterns of washing jets within the sewing ring, which

occur early during valve closure and are of short duration and length.

- Paravalvular regurgitation results from an incomplete seal between the sewing ring and the annulus.
- Very small paravalvular jets often disappear after administration of protamine, but larger jets are unlikely to improve and usually require reintervention.

Damage to Other Structures

- Damage to surrounding structures may occur during access for AVR implantation.
- Sutures placed too deeply may injure or kink the left main coronary artery causing anterior and lateral wall motion abnormalities. A low

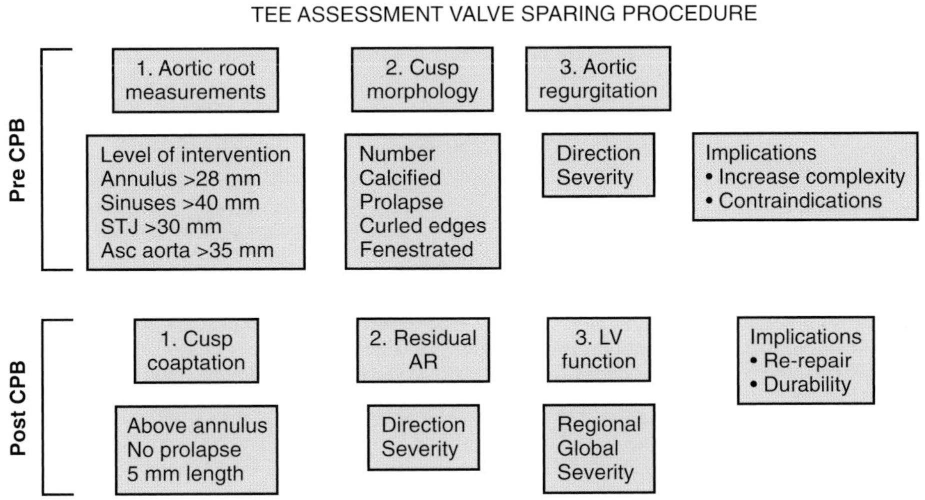

TEE ASSESSMENT VALVE SPARING PROCEDURE

Figure 3-31. TEE for AV-sparing root techniques.

aortotomy may compromise right coronary artery perfusion.

- It is common to see a hematoma at the base of the aortic root and dome of the LA when extensive dissection or patch enlargement has been required. This should not be confused with early prosthetic valve abscess formation.

Left Ventricular Outflow Tract Obstruction

- Dynamic LVOT obstruction by systolic motion of the AMVL (systolic anterior motion [SAM]) may occur after implantation of a small aortic prosthesis, particularly in the presence of septal hypertrophy.

Valve-Sparing Procedure

Pre Cardiopulmonary Bypass

- The presence of abnormal cusp morphology, eccentric AR, and a dilated aortic annulus (>28 mm) complicates valve-sparing procedures, reducing the outcome success (Figure 3-31).
- The single most important criterion in selecting patients for AV-sparing root procedures is the morphologic appearance of the aortic cusps during surgical inspection.

Post Cardiopulmonary Bypass

- Aortic cusps should coapt above the aortic annular plane in the sinuses of Valsalva, without evidence of residual cusp prolapse with at least a 5-mm coaptation length.

TABLE 3-9	FAILURE IN AORTIC VALVE-SPARING PROCEDURES	
	Cusp Coaptation	**AR presence**
Type A	2 mm above the annulus*	No AR
Type B	in the plane of the annulus	+ AR
Type C	below the plane of the annulus	+ AR

*Annulus base is the bottom of the Dacron graft.
AR, aortic regurgitation.
From Pethig K, Milz A, Hagl C, et al. Aortic valve reimplantation in ascending aortic aneurysm: Risk factors for early valve failure. Ann Thorac Surg. 2002;73:29-33.

- The presence of more than trace to mild AR will compromise the repair durability.
- Ventricular function is assessed to exclude regional wall motion abnormalities, which may signify inadequate coronary perfusion from problematic coronary reimplantation.

Failure of Valve-Sparing Operations

- Accelerated cusp degeneration can occur from systolic contact between the cusp and the wall or buckling of the cusps from lack of sinus expansion.
- Echocardiography defined a critical cause of failure results from sagging of the cusp with coaptation below the annulus (Table 3-9).
- This reemphasizes the importance of adequate resuspension of the pillars to reestablish the normal height of the cusp coaptation plane.

Suggested Readings

1. Baumgartner H, Hung J, Bermejo J, et al. Echocardiographic assessment of valve stenosis: EAE/ASE recommendations for clinical practice. *J Am Soc Echocardiogr*. 2009;22:1-23.
2. Bonow RO, Carabello BA, Chatterjee K, et al. 2008 focused update incorporated into the ACC/AHA 2006 guidelines for the management of patients with valvular heart disease: A report of the American College of Cardiology/American Heart Association Task Force on Practice Guidelines (Writing Committee to revise the 1998 guidelines for the management of patients with valvular heart disease). Endorsed by the Society of Cardiovascular Anesthesiologists, Society for Cardiovascular Angiography and Interventions, and Society of Thoracic Surgeons. *J Am Coll Cardiol*. 2008;52:e1-142.
3. Zoghbi WA, Enriquez-Sarano M, Foster E, et al. Recommendations for evaluation of the severity of native valvular regurgitation with two-dimensional and Doppler echocardiography. *J Am Soc Echocardiogr*. 2003;16:777-802.
4. Zoghbi WA, Chambers JB, Dumesnil JG, et al. Recommendations for evaluation of prosthetic valves with echocardiography and Doppler ultrasound: A report from the American Society of Echocardiography's Guidelines and Standards Committee and the Task Force on Prosthetic Valves, developed in conjunction with the American College of Cardiology Cardiovascular Imaging Committee, Cardiac Imaging Committee of the American Heart Association, the European Association of Echocardiography, a registered branch of the European Society of Cardiology, the Japanese Society of Echocardiography and the Canadian Society of Echocardiography, endorsed by the American College of Cardiology Foundation, American Heart Association, European Association of Echocardiography, a registered branch of the European Society of Cardiology, the Japanese Society of Echocardiography, and Canadian Society of Echocardiography. *J Am Soc Echocardiogr*. 2009;22:975-1014.

   The previous four references summarize the state of the art in the echocardiography and management of patients with valvular heart disease.
5. Evangelista A, Gonzalez-Alujas MT. Echocardiography in infective endocarditis. *Heart*. 2004;90:614-617.
6. Baddour LM, Wilson WR, Bayer AS, et al. Infective endocarditis: diagnosis, antimicrobial therapy, and management of complications: A statement for healthcare professionals from the Committee on Rheumatic Fever, Endocarditis, and Kawasaki Disease, Council on Cardiovascular Disease in the Young, and the Councils on Clinical Cardiology, Stroke, and Cardiovascular Surgery and Anesthesia, American Heart Association: Endorsed by the Infectious Diseases Society of America. *Circulation*. 2005;111:e394-e434.

   Excellent reviews of endocarditis from a clinical perspective and of the echocardiography findings.
7. Cohen GI, Duffy CI, Klein AL, et al. Color Doppler and two-dimensional echocardiographic determination of the mechanism of aortic regurgitation with surgical correlation. *J Am Soc Echocardiogr*. 1986;9:508-515.
8. Khoury G, Glineur D, Rubay J, et al. Functional classification of aortic root/valve abnormalities and their correlation with etiologies and surgical procedures. *Curr Opin Cardiol*. 2005;20:115-121.
9. Feindel CM, David TE. Aortic valve sparing operations: basic concepts. *Int J Cardiol Suppl*. 2004;1:61-66.
10. Van Dyck MJ, Watremez C, Boodhwani M, et al. Transesophageal echocardiography during aortic valve repair surgery. *Anesth Analg*. 2010;111:59-70.
11. Pethig K, Milz A, Hagl C, et al. Aortic value reimplantation in ascending aortic aneurysm: Risk factors for early valve failure. *Ann Thorac Surg*. 2002;73:29-33.

    Important references discussing the current management of aortic root abnormalities and valve sparing procedures. Citation 9 is from Toronto where much of the pioneering work in aortic valve-sparing surgery has been done.
12. Brinkman WT, Mack MJ. Transcatheter cardiac valve interventions. *Surg Clin North Am*. 2009;89:951-966, x.
13. Walther T, Dewey T, Borger MA, et al. Transapical aortic valve implantation: Step by step. *Ann Thorac Surg*. 2009;87:276-283.
14. Jayasuriya C, Moss RR, Munt B. Transcatheter aortic valve implantation in aortic stenosis: The role of echocardiography. *J Am Soc Echocardiogr*. 2011;24:15-27.
15. Moss RM, Ivens E, Pasupati S, et al. Role of echocardiography in percutaneous aortic valve implantation. *J Am Coll Cardiol Imaging*. 2008;1:15-24.

    Four important papers in the description of percutaneous aortic valve implantation. Citation 14 comes with superb illustrations. Citation 15 describes the TEE parameters that are used to guide the interventionalist.

Right-Sided Valvular Disease

4

Rebecca A. Schroeder, Jonathan B. Mark, and Atilio Barbeito

BACKGROUND

Tricuspid Valve Structure and Function

- The tricuspid valve (TV) is the largest cardiac valve (normal area 7-9 cm^2).
- It has a large anterior and smaller septal (medial) and posterior leaflets.
- There is great variability in leaflet and commissural morphology, chordal, and papillary muscle support.
- The anterior papillary muscle is the largest and arises from the moderator band in the right ventricle (RV).
- The tricuspid annulus is apically displaced relative to the mitral valve. It is supported medially by the right fibrous trigone and is thinner posteriorly and laterally.
- Tricuspid annular plane systolic excursion (TAPSE) toward the RV apex is reflective of right ventricular (RV) systolic function (normal 23 mm, range 15-31 mm).
- The tricuspid annulus shows horizontal, sphincter-like systolic motion during RV systole, reducing its area approximately 33%. Tricuspid annulus fractional shortening (TAFS) is indicative of RV systolic function.

Pulmonic Valve Structure and Function

- The pulmonic valve (PV) is similar to the aortic valve in its semilunar structure and area (normal area 2-4 cm^2), with lunula, nodulus of Arantii, and associated sinuses of Valsalva and sinotubular junction.
- Typically, the PV has thinner leaflets, which are termed *anterior*, *left posterior*, and *right posterior*.
- The PV annulus is thinner, less clearly defined, and more distensible than the aortic valve annulus, and it is attached to RV muscle.

OVERVIEW OF ECHOCARDIOGRAPHIC APPROACH

- Right-sided valvular assessment uses a similar echocardiographic approach to that used for assessment of the mitral and aortic valves.
- The echocardiographic modalities include
  - Two-dimensional (2D) imaging.
  - Color flow (CF) Doppler mapping.
  - Spectral Doppler imaging, including pulsed wave (PW) Doppler and continuous wave (CW) Doppler.
  - Three-dimensional (3D) imaging.
- The most efficient examination strategy begins with 2D imaging (structure), followed by CF Doppler mapping (flow, function), followed by PW or CW Doppler (quantitation).
- 3D data sets (including color flow) are easily acquired in real time, but best manipulated after examination or off-line.
  - 3D zoom mode is preferable for assessment of TV and PV leaflets.
  - 3D full-volume mode is probably better for assessment of tricuspid regurgitation (TR) and TV supporting structures.
- Structures to examine include
  - TV.
  - PV.
  - RV.
  - Right atrium (RA).
  - Interatrial septum (IAS) and interventricular septum (IVS)
  - Superior (SVC) and inferior (IVC) venae cavae.
  - Hepatic veins (HVs).
  - Pulmonary artery (PA).
- Compared with left-sided valvular assessment, imaging may be more difficult owing to more anterior (far-field) location of right-sided valves and acoustic shadowing from calcified or prosthetic aortic and mitral valves (Box 4-1).

BOX 4-1 Standard Scan Planes for Tricuspid and Pulmonic Valves

- ME four-chamber view
- ME RV inflow-outflow view
- Modified ME bicaval view
- TG RV midpapillary short axis view
- TG RV inflow view
- TG RV outflow view
- Deep TG four-chamber view
- TG hepatic vein view
- ME aortic valve short axis view
- ME ascending aortic short axis view
- UE aortic arch short axis view

ME, midesophageal; RV, right ventricular; TG, transgastric; UE, upper esophageal.

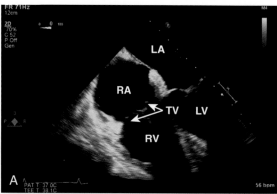

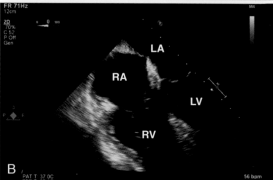

Figure 4-1. ME four-chamber view with the probe turned slightly clockwise to center the TV and display the RA, RV, LA, and left ventricle (LV) during systole (**A**) and diastole (**B**).

ANATOMIC IMAGING

Standard Scan Planes for Tricuspid and Pulmonic Valves

- *Midesophageal (ME) four-chamber view* allows assessment of TV and RA, RV, IAS, IVS, and adjacent left heart structures (Figure 4-1).

- The TV septal leaflet is seen medially, with either the anterior or the posterior leaflet seen laterally.
- Transesophageal echocardiography (TEE) probe insertion, which brings the coronary sinus into view, most likely displays the posterior TV leaflet.
- TEE probe withdrawal, which brings the RA appendage into view, most likely displays the anterior TV leaflet.
- Clockwise TEE probe rotation helps center the TV and right heart structures in the image display.
- The tricuspid annular dimension can be measured in this view (normal 28 mm, range 20-40 mm). TAFS and TAPSE can be measured to assess RV function.
- RA and RV size and function can be evaluated.
- CF Doppler allows assessment of a TR jet in the RA. However, the interrogation angle between the direction of the regurgitant jet and the ultrasound beam is often large, making this view suboptimal for spectral Doppler measurements.
- *ME RV inflow-outflow view* displays RA, TV, RV, PV, and PA, all "wrapping around" a centered aortic valve, seen in short axis (Figure 4-2).
  - The TV anterior leaflet appears medially and the TV posterior leaflet appears laterally, but there is some variability to this typical pattern.
  - The PV leaflets are seen between the RV and the proximal PA, generally in long axis, in the far right portion of the video display. The leaflets are often not distinctly seen.
  - CF Doppler allows assessment of a TR jet in the RA or a pulmonic regurgitation (PR) jet in the RV.
  - Spectral Doppler assessment of a TR jet is often better in this view, owing to a more parallel alignment with the ultrasound beam.
  - Spectral Doppler assessment of a PR jet and PV flow may be performed in this view, but the interrogation angle is often too large for accurate measurement.
- *Modified ME bicaval view* displays the TV in addition to the RA, LA, IAS, SVC, and coronary sinus (Figure 4-3).
  - This view is seen with slight counterclockwise probe rotation and a TEE probe angle greater than that needed for the bicaval view (typically 100-140 degrees).

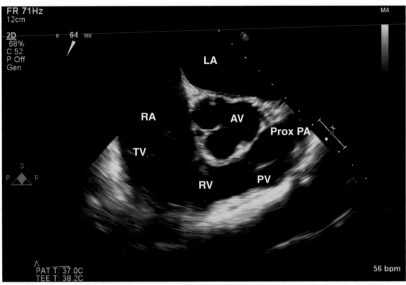

Figure 4-2. ME inflow-outflow view displays the aortic valve (AV) in the center of the image with the right-sided chambers wrapping around from left to right. Prox PA, proximal pulmonary artery.

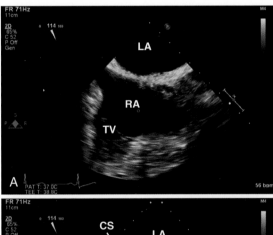

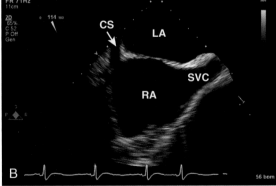

Figure 4-3. Modified bicaval view with the LA at the apex of the display, the RA near the center, and the TV appearing in the far left portion of the image. **A,** This view provides excellent alignment of the ultrasound beam with the direction of a regurgitant jet through the TV. **B,** Slight counterclockwise rotation brings the coronary sinus (CS) into view. SVC, superior vena cava.

- The SVC-RA junction is often seen, along with the origin of the coronary sinus in the RA.
- CF Doppler allows assessment of a TR jet in the RA.
- Spectral Doppler assessment of a TR jet and TV flow is often best in this view, owing to parallel alignment with the ultrasound beam.
- *Transgastric (TG) RV Midpapillary short axis view* is acquired with counterclockwise probe rotation beginning with a transgastric LV midpapillary short axis view. It often demonstrates the leaflets of the TV when the TEE probe is withdrawn or anteflexed slightly (Figure 4-4).
  - In this view, the large, redundant anterior TV leaflet appears to the left of the screen with the much smaller septal and posterior leaflets appearing to the right and in the near field, respectively.
- *TG RV inflow view* displays the TV in long axis as well as portions of the RA and the RV (Figure 4-5).
  - This view provides the best view of TV support structures.
  - The RV is seen to the left side of the display and the RA to the right.
  - This view is usually obtained with the probe turned slightly to the patient's right (clockwise) and a probe angle of 90 to 110 degrees.

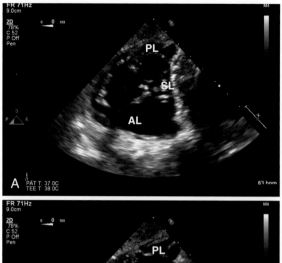

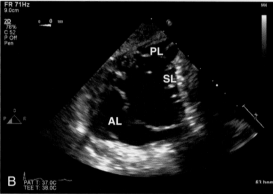

Figure 4-4. TG short axis view of the TV shows the leaflets approximated in systole (**A**) and open in diastole (**B**). Note the dominance of the large, redundant anterior leaflet (AL) compared with the small posterior (PL) and septal (SL) leaflets.

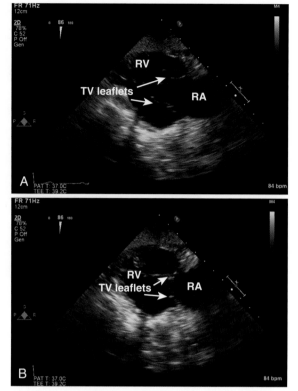

Figure 4-5. TG RV inflow view shows the RA and RV in long axis as well as the tricuspid leaflets in diastole (**A**) and systole (**B**). Given that flow across the TV is perpendicular to the ultrasound beam in this view, spectral Doppler measurements are not possible.

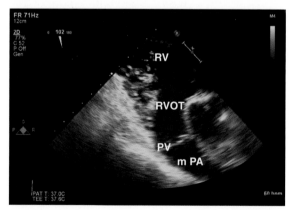

Figure 4-6. TG RV outflow view shows the RV and the RVOT, the PV, and the main pulmonary artery (mPA). This view is an excellent choice for Doppler interrogation of flow through the PV owing to alignment of the ultrasound beam and the direction of blood flow.

- The inferior free wall appears in the near field of the display and the anterior free wall is seen in the far field.
- Because TV flow is perpendicular to the ultrasound beam in this view, spectral Doppler measurements are generally impossible.
- *TG RV outflow view* displays the PV in long axis, with the TV, RV, RA, LA, and proximal PA in other orientations (Figure 4-6).
  - This view is acquired by slight counterclockwise probe rotation and using a probe angle of 130 to 145 degrees.
  - The right ventricular outflow tract (RVOT) and PV appear in the mid-far field, usually parallel to the ultrasound beam.
  - Measurements of PV annular dimensions in this view correlate best with intraoperative surgical measurements.
- *Deep TG four-chamber view* displays the RV and the other three cardiac chambers, much like the ME four-chamber view (Figure 4-7).
  - Beginning with a deep TG four-chamber view, clockwise probe rotation will often

show the RV, RA, and TV in the center of the image display.
- Alignment of a TR jet with the ultrasound beam is variable in this view.
- Clear images and alignment of the RV and TV make this view useful for measurement of TAPSE.

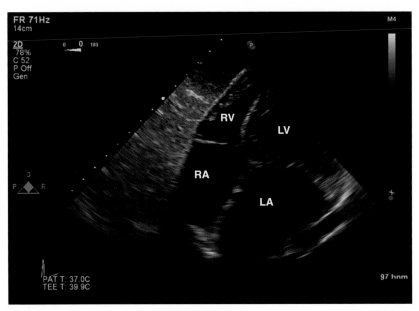

Figure 4-7. Deep TG four-chamber view shows the RA, LA, RV and LV. This view may be useful for Doppler analysis of a tricuspid regurgitant jet, especially in cases in which ME views are inadequate or poorly aligned.

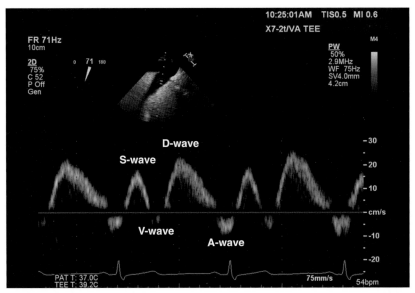

Figure 4-8. PW Doppler analysis of HV flow from the TG position with the probe turned slightly to the right (clockwise rotation). The antegrade S- and D-waves, as well as the retrograde A- and V-waves are labeled. The V-wave is not uniformly present.

- *TG HV view* can be acquired from a TG probe location and allows measurement of HV flow velocity with PW Doppler, which is useful for TR quantification (Figure 4-8).
  - Often best imaged from the RV short axis views by turning the probe to the right (clockwise), identifying an HV, and adjusting the multiplane angle to optimally align the direction of flow with the ultrasound beam.

- PW Doppler analysis yields patterns analogous to pulmonary venous flow patterns.
- *ME aortic valve short axis view* displays long axis views of the PV and proximal PA.
- *ME ascending aortic short axis view* is acquired with slight TEE probe withdrawal (Figure 4-9).
  - This view displays the proximal ascending aorta in short axis, the adjacent proximal PA, its bifurcation, and the right PA.

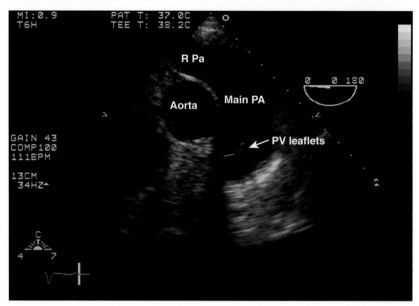

Figure 4-9. UE aortic short axis view demonstrates the main PA and its bifurcation into the right and left pulmonary arteries (R Pa). The PV leaflets are not uniformly seen as clearly as in this image.

- Alignment is ideal for spectral Doppler analysis of proximal PA flow or PV flow, especially when the valve is seen clearly.
- This is a useful view for assessment of pulmonary emboli in the main PA and its proximal branches.
- *Upper esophageal (UE) aortic arch short axis view* allows visualization of the PV in long axis as well as a significant portion of the main PA (Figure 4-10).
  - This view of the PV may be improved by turning the probe slightly to the left (counterclockwise) and retroflexing the tip.
  - This view also offers excellent alignment between flow and the ultrasound beam for accurate spectral Doppler assessment of flow across the PV.

TRICUSPID VALVE

Step-by-Step Examination

Step 1: 2D Examination
- Standard 2D views for TV examination include the ME four-chamber view (see Figure 4-1), the ME inflow-outflow view (see Figure 4-2), the modified ME bicaval view (see Figure 4-3), and the TG RV inflow view (see Figure 4-5). TG windows are very helpful for examination of the TV leaflets in short axis, although these are not uniformly obtainable. Other supplementary views

described previously may be helpful in difficult cases.
- Characteristics to examine include the general appearance of the TV annulus and leaflets, annular size (diameter), leaflet thickness and motion (restricted, excessive, coordinated, flail), leaflet coaptation, pathologic masses (e.g., vegetation or thrombus), and annular or leaflet calcification. In addition, RA, RV, and vena caval dimensions should be noted.
- Careful TEE 2D imaging is particularly important for the diagnosis of endocarditis. It is the most sensitive method to visualize vegetations, perivalvular abscesses, and leaflet perforations (Figure 4-11).

Step 2: CF Doppler
- CF Doppler examination of the TV should be performed in the ME four-chamber view (Figure 4-12A), the ME inflow-outflow view (see Figure 4-12B), and the modified ME bicaval view (see Figure 4-12C). The TG RV *inflow* view is not as useful for Doppler analysis owing to the large angle between the direction of flow and the direction of the ultrasound beam.
- The nature of flow (turbulent vs. laminar) as well as the magnitude and direction of antegrade and retrograde flow should be noted. In addition, eccentric CF Doppler signals that may indicate leaflet perforations or septal defects should also be noted.

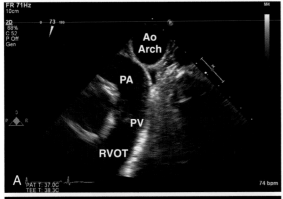

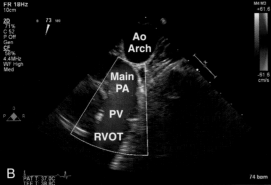

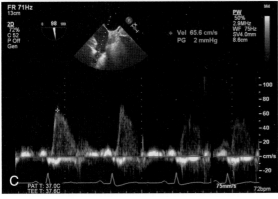

Figure 4-10. **A,** UE aortic arch short axis view shows the aortic arch (Ao Arch) in cross section and the RVOT, the PV, and the main PA in continuity. This image provides excellent positioning for CF (**B**) and spectral (**C**) Doppler analysis of RVOT or PV flow for estimation of pulmonary arterial mean or diastolic pressure, or assessment of severity of PS.

Step 3: Spectral PW Doppler and CW Doppler

- The choice of views in which to perform spectral Doppler analysis of the TV must be guided by which views yield adequate 2D and CF Doppler images of the valve. It is crucial that the direction of the flow be optimally aligned with the direction of the ultrasound beam.

- Estimation of peak RV pressure requires an adequate TR jet as well as alignment between the regurgitant jet and the interrogating beam. Inadequate alignment (>20-30 degrees) results in underestimation of peak velocity and errors in calculated pressure gradient.
- The modified ME bicaval view is often the best view in which to perform spectral Doppler analysis of a TR jet. Measurement of the pressure gradient across a stenotic TV may be best in the ME four-chamber view, the ME RV inflow-outflow view, or the modified ME bicaval view (Figure 4-13).
- **Pitfall to avoid:** The TV spectral Doppler trace may be contaminated by abnormal flow profiles across the aortic or mitral valves. CF Doppler mapping before spectral Doppler analysis should identify these other abnormal flow velocities.
- HV flow velocity (see Figure 4-8)
  - The HVs may be imaged from the TG TEE probe position. The probe angle is adjusted to identify a long axis view of a large HV and align the direction of flow with the direction of the ultrasound beam.
  - Normal HV flow velocity consists of an antegrade systolic (S) and diastolic (D) wave and a small retrograde atrial (A) wave resulting from end-diastolic atrial contraction. In patients with slow heart rates, another small retrograde wave (V) may be seen at end-systole.
- Survey for associated (secondary) clinical findings
  - The RV, RA, IVS, and IAS are important structures that may be affected by primary TV pathology or cause or exacerbate TR as a result of changes in normal chamber pressures and gradients.
- Alternative diagnostic techniques
  - The proximal isovelocity surface area (PISA) technique may be used to quantify TR severity but is not commonly used in the perioperative setting. A TR jet PISA radius greater than 9 mm indicates severe TR.
  - The pressure half-time (PHT) method may be used to quantify tricuspid stenosis (TS) severity (as with mitral stenosis), but it is not frequently performed with TEE or in the perioperative setting.
- 3D imaging may be used to obtain a more accurate assessment of the valve before possible repair or removal of a vegetation. However, 3D imaging of the TV is not as reliable as 3D imaging of the mitral valve.

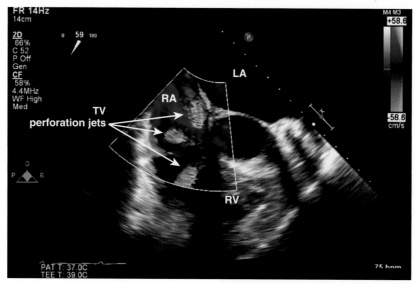

Figure 4-11. CF Doppler image demonstrates leaflet perforations of the TV secondary to infective endocarditis.

Tricuspid Regurgitation

- General Comments
  - "Normal" TR velocity **is 2 to 2.5 m/s** and is present in 65% of the general population and 93% of patients older than 70 years of age.
  - *Pitfall to avoid:* TR jet velocity is related to the pressure gradient between the RV and the RA and is NOT indicative of the severity of TR.
  - With more severe degrees of TR and resultant increases in baseline RA pressure, peak jet velocity may decrease due to decreasing pressure gradient between the RV and the RA.
  - The TR jet may be laminar (not turbulent) in cases of severe TR.
  - In cases of severe TR, there will be increased total flow through the TV. This may result in increases in peak antegrade velocities in the absence of valvular obstruction (≥1.0 m/s).
  - Other ancillary signs consistent with severe TR include
    - A large CF Doppler TR jet area (>10 cm^2) in the RA (Figure 4-14).
    - A TR jet with a large vena contracta width (>7 mm).
    - An HV flow velocity pattern showing S-wave reversal (Figure 4-15).
    - A TR CW Doppler spectral trace showing a low-velocity, dense, triangular, early peaking jet, with a spectral trace density equal to that of the antegrade TV flow velocity (Figure 4-16). The triangular shape of the CW Doppler trace indicates the "V-wave cutoff" resulting from the elevated systolic RA pressure.
  - Accompanying signs resulting from volume overload of the right heart chambers include enlargement of the RA, RV, and IVC. The IAS may show systolic displacement toward the left atrium (LA). The IVS will show diastolic flattening and abnormal systolic motion toward the RV.

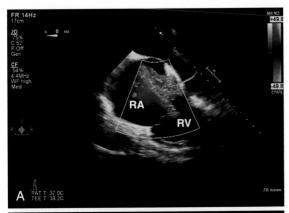

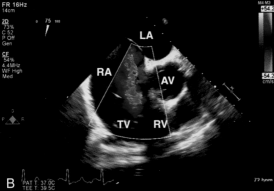

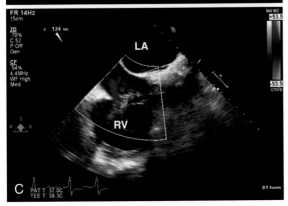

Figure 4-12. CF Doppler images demonstrate severe TR in the ME four-chamber (**A**), ME inflow-outflow (**B**) and modified bicaval (**C**) views. It is important to examine the extent of regurgitant flow in as many views as possible in order to completely assess the regurgitant jet and select the best view for spectral Doppler measurements.

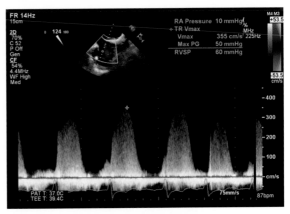

Figure 4-13. CW Doppler analysis of a TR jet in the modified bicaval view with calculation of peak right ventricular systolic pressure (RVSP) by the simplified Bernoulli equation. In this case, estimated RVSP is 60 mm Hg.

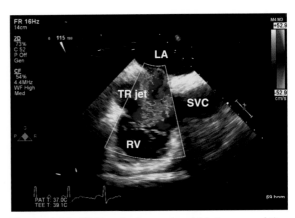

Figure 4-14. CF Doppler image, in which the area of the tricuspid regurgitant jet (TR jet) exceeds 10 cm², meeting criteria for severe TR.

- *Pitfall to avoid:* Catheters or wires that cross the TV do not generally cause significant regurgitation in the absence of preexisting valvular pathology.
- Specific diagnoses (Box 4-2)
  - Endocarditis.
    - Vegetations typically attach to the atrial side of the TV and are often larger than left-sided lesions.

- TEE has greater sensitivity than transthoracic echocardiography (TTE) for detection of vegetations and diagnosis of endocarditis.
- Large obstructing vegetations are more common on the TV than on other valves, with *Staphylococcus aureus* being one of the most common causative organisms.
- Intravenous drug abuse and presence of indwelling catheters and wires are significant risk factors for TV endocarditis (Figure 4-17).
- Ebstein's anomaly.
  - This congenital disorder involves apical displacement of the septal insertion of the TV leaflet (>8 mm/m² body surface

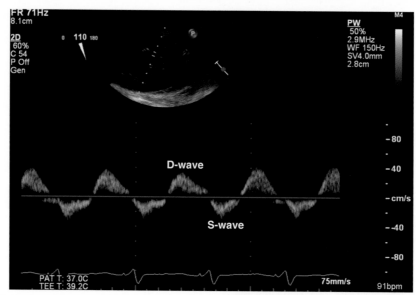

Figure 4-15. PW Doppler analysis of HV flow shows reversal of the S-wave in a patient with severe TR.

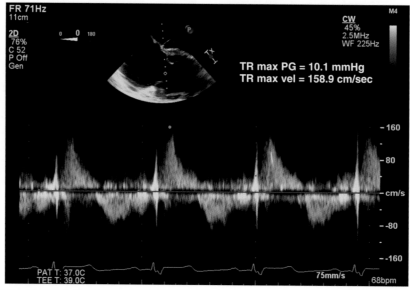

TR max PG = 10.1 mmHg
TR max vel = 158.9 cm/sec

Figure 4-16. CW Doppler analysis of a tricuspid regurgitant jet shows a low peak velocity, and a dense, triangular, early peaking jet, all consistent with severe TR.

BOX 4-2 Tricuspid Regurgitation: Etiology	
• Annular dilatation (secondary to pulmonary hypertension, constrictive pericarditis, pulmonic stenosis, RV ischemia or infarction) • Rheumatic heart disease • Endocarditis (infectious or noninfectious) • Carcinoid heart disease • Tumor (primary papillary fibroelastoma, secondary to obstructing atrial myxoma or renal cell carcinoma)	• Endomyocardial fibrosis • Trauma (blunt chest trauma, iatrogenic secondary catheters or wires) • Congenital anomalies (Ebstein's anomaly, tricuspid atresia) • Tricuspid valve prolapse (associated with Ehlers-Danlos or Marfan's syndromes, Ebstein's anomaly, or septum secundum ASD)

ASD, atrial septal defect; RV, right ventricle.

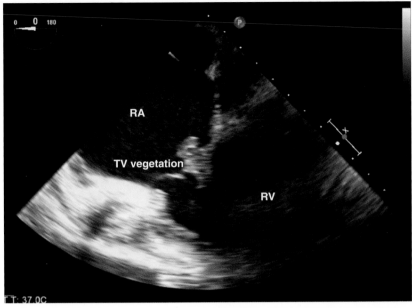

Figure 4-17. ME four-chamber view of the RA and RV shows a large vegetation arising from the leaflets of the TV.

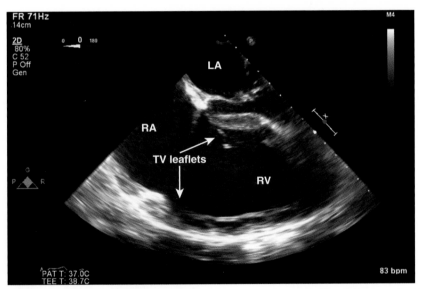

Figure 4-18. ME four-chamber view of the right-sided chambers in a patient with Ebstein's anomaly. Note that the TV annulus is in a more apical position than the mitral, separating the RV from its "atrialized" portion.

area) with associated RV dysfunction, severe TR, annular dilatation, and dilatation of an "atrialized" portion of the RV (Figure 4-18).
- The anterior TV leaflet is large, deformed, and described as "sail-shaped" or "curtain-like."
- There may be an associated large atrial septal defect in many cases.
- Although most patients with this disorder present in childhood, some with milder forms may not present until much later in life.
- Carcinoid heart disease. Circulating vasoactive amines in patients with carcinoid tumors lead to fibrosis and neovascularization of valve surfaces, with the right-sided valves almost exclusively affected (Figure 4-19).
  - Lesions occur on the ventricular side of the TV and affect up to 50% of patients with carcinoid tumors.

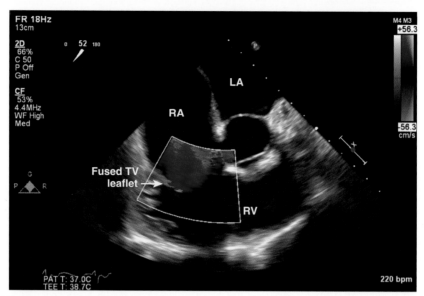

Figure 4-19. CF Doppler analysis of regurgitant flow through a deformed TV with leaflet fusion caused by carcinoid disease. Note that the regurgitant flow is laminar, indicating severe TR.

- Regurgitation is usually due to restricted leaflet closure, with short, thickened, and retracted valve leaflets that become immobile and often fixed in the open position.
- Surgical intervention for the valvular dysfunction is often indicated owing to the rapidly progressive nature of the valve involvement and the indolent nature of the primary tumors.
- Rheumatic heart disease.
  - Characteristic 2D findings include leaflet doming, thickening, and restricted motion. TR is a more common manifestation than TS.
  - Rheumatic involvement of the mitral and aortic valves is seen more often than TV disease and may result in secondary TR related to pulmonary hypertension.
  - Associated commissural fusion, calcification, and thickening of the subvalvular apparatus are often best seen in TG long and short axis views.
- Functional TR.
  - The most common cause of TR is annular dilatation secondary to pulmonary hypertension and RV dilatation from a variety of other primary processes.
  - Leaflet morphology is typically normal, and suture or ring annuloplasty is the standard treatment for severe functional TR (Figure 4-20).
- Assessment of severity (Table 4-1).

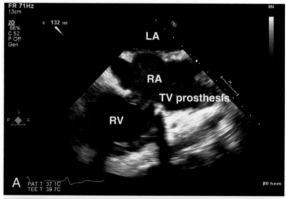

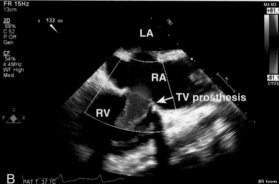

Figure 4-20. Modified bicaval view of the TV after bioprosthetic valve replacement. Note that the leaflets appear to open completely during diastole (**A**) and that flow through the prosthetic valve is laminar (**B**).

TABLE 4-1 TRICUSPID REGURGITATION: GRADING SEVERITY

	Trace (1+)	Mild (2+)	Moderate (3+)	Severe (4+)
2D and CF Doppler				Laminar TR jet appearance, ≥4 cm annulus diameter, poor leaflet coaptation
TR jet area in RA (%)		≤20	21-33	>33
TR jet area (cm²)	<2	2-4	4-10	>10
TR jet length (cm)	<1.5	1.5-3.0	3.0-4.5	>4.5
Vena contracta (mm)			<7	≥7.0
Hepatic vein flow velocity (PW Doppler)		Systolic dominance		Systolic flow reversal
Spectral Doppler		Soft, parabolic signal	More rounded signal	Dense triangular signal, early peaking

CF, color flow; PW, pulsed wave; RA, right atrium; TR, tricuspid regurgitation.

KEY POINTS

- The best views in which to perform spectral Doppler analysis of the TR jet are the modified ME bicaval view and the ME RV inflow-outflow view.
- The views that provide optimal alignment for spectral Doppler analysis of the PV are the TG RV outflow view, the UE aortic arch short axis view, and the ME ascending aortic short axis view.
- 3D zoom mode is preferable for valve leaflet examination whereas 3D full-volume is probably better for assessment of subvalvular structures and TR jet analysis.
- TR jet velocity is determined by the pressure gradient across the TV and compliance of the RA and RV. Laminar jets with low peak velocity may indicate severe TR of long standing.
- Increasing total flow across the valve in the setting of severe TR may result in increased antegrade peak velocity in the absence of valvular obstruction.
- Many pathologic processes that result in stenosis of the TV also result in significant TR.
- TEE has the greatest sensitivity and specificity for diagnosis of right-sided endocarditis, especially in the presence of indwelling lines or catheters (Figure 4-21).

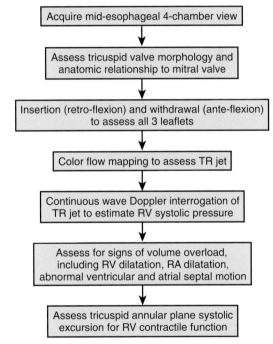

Figure 4-21. ME four-chamber view, the best single scan plane for assessment of TR.

Tricuspid Stenosis

- General Comments (Figure 4-22).
  - Because the TV has the greatest cross-sectional area, flow velocities across the valve are lowest (<0.7 m/s).
  - Significant TS is suggested when peak flow velocity exceeds 1.5 m/s.

- Many conditions that cause TS also result in significant TR (Box 4-3).
- Measurement of peak gradients with spectral Doppler is heavily dependent on loading conditions, the compliance of the RA and RV, and the correct alignment of the ultrasound beam with the direction of antegrade blood flow.
- TV leaflets affected by carcinoid disease are often fixed and retracted whereas those involved in rheumatic disease demonstrated characteristic

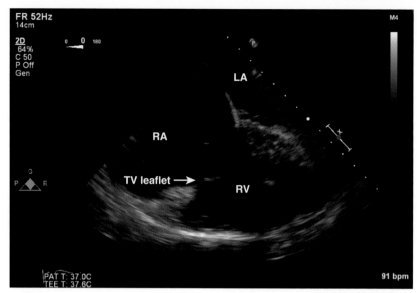

Figure 4-22. ME four-chamber view shows TV stenosis. Note the semiclosed position of the leaflet during diastole, as well as severe enlargement of the RA.

BOX 4-3 Tricuspid Stenosis: Etiology

- Rheumatic heart disease
- Congenital anomalies
- Endocarditis
- Methysergide toxicity
- Carcinoid heart disease
- Endomyocardial fibrosis

commissural fusion and doming during diastole.
- Assessment of severity (Table 4-2).

PULMONIC VALVE

Step-by-Step Examination

Step 1: 2D Examination
- Characteristics to examine include the general appearance of the annulus and the leaflets, annular size (diameter), leaflet thickness, and motion (restricted, excessive, coordinated, flail).
- Standard 2D views for PV examination include the UE ascending aortic short axis (see Figure 4-9), UE aortic arch short axis view (Figure 4-23A), ME inflow-outflow (Figure 4-24A), and TG RV outflow views (see Figure 4-6).
- Initial evaluation of the valve should focus on the structure (hypoplasia, dysplasia, absence),

leaflet motion (doming or prolapse), and the presence of masses. The diameter of the PA should also be noted.

Step 2: CF Doppler
- CF Doppler may be performed in any of the views mentioned previously (see Figures 4-23B and 4-24B).
- The CF Doppler jet characteristics, including length, width, duration, and turbulent or laminar pattern, should be assessed.

Step 3: Spectral PW Doppler and CW Doppler
- The UE aortic arch or TG RV outflow views usually provide the most favorable alignment of the ultrasound beam with the PV flow vector (see Figure 4-23C).
  - Indicators of PR severity include the density of the CW Doppler signal, the flow deceleration rate, and flow duration in relation to the electrocardiogram (ECG).
- When pressure gradients are derived from CW Doppler velocity measurements, mean gradients (as opposed to peak gradients) correlate best with catheter-based measurements.
- Survey for associated (secondary) clinical findings
  - Both the RV and the PA should be assessed. PV disease and dysfunction may be a consequence of or result in dilatation of proximate structures (PA and RV, respectively).

TABLE 4-2 TRICUSPID STENOSIS: GRADING SCALES

	Normal	Mild	Moderate	Severe
Valve area (cm²)	7-9			<2
Mean gradient (mm Hg)	<2	2-3	3-6	>7
Peak gradient (mm Hg)	<4			>25
Peak velocity (m/s)	<1	1-1.5	1.5-2.5	>2.5
CW Doppler signal		Steep deceleration		Delayed deceleration, dense signal

CW, continuous wave.

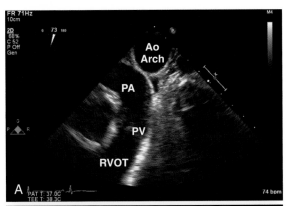

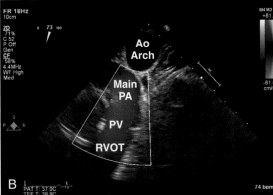

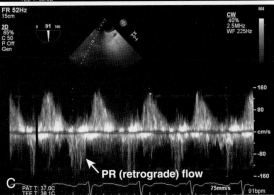

Figure 4-23. 2D (**A**), CF Doppler (**B**), and CW Doppler (**C**) recordings of a pulmonic regurgitation jet imaged from the UE aortic arch short axis position. The spectral Doppler trace shows antegrade flow (above the baseline) and retrograde flow (below the baseline), the latter resulting from PR. Ao Arch, aortic arch.

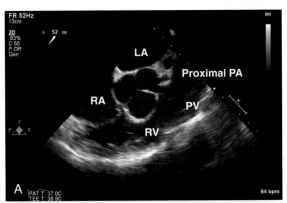

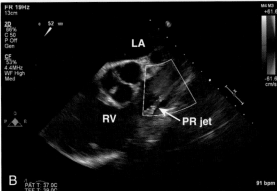

Figure 4-24. 2D (**A**) and CF Doppler (**B**) images of the PV in the ME inflow-outflow view. The regurgitant jet is consistent with moderate PR.

Pulmonic Regurgitation

- General comments
  - Trace or mild PR is very common in healthy individuals.
  - The most common cause of significant PR in the adult is primary or secondary pulmonary hypertension.
  - Initial evaluation of the valve should focus on cusp number (quadricuspid or bicuspid valves), structure (hypoplasia, dysplasia, absence), and leaflet motion (restriction, doming or prolapse).

TABLE 4-3   PULMONIC REGURGITATION: GRADING SEVERITY

Parameter	Mild	Moderate	Severe	Pitfalls
Pulmonic valve	Normal	Normal or abnormal	Abnormal	Not specific for PR
RV size	Normal	Normal or dilated	Dilated*	Enlargement seen in other conditions
Jet characteristics by color Doppler	Thin, usually <1 cm in length	Intermediate	Large, laminar, brief in duration	Poor correlation with severity of PR
Vena contracta width by color Doppler	Thin	Intermediate	Wide	Lacks published validation
Density and deceleration of PR signal by CW Doppler	Soft, slow deceleration	Dense, variable deceleration	Dense, steep deceleration, early termination of flow in diastole	Not specific for PR because it depends on pressure differential across the valve
Antegrade pulmonic flow velocity by CW Doppler*	Mildly elevated	Intermediate	Greatly elevated	Subject to errors due to difficulties with Doppler alignment
Pulmonic systolic flow compared with systemic flow by PW Doppler	Slightly increased	Intermediate	Greatly increased	Subject to errors due to difficulties with Doppler alignment and measurement of pulmonic annulus

*In the absence of pulmonic stenosis.
CW, continuous wave; PR, pulmonic regurgitation; PW, pulsed wave; RV, right ventricle.

- There are no validated, quantitative TEE methods for grading PR severity. As such, a qualitative approach that takes into account a variety of parameters is suggested (Table 4-3).
- Other ancillary signs consistent with severe PR include
  - Holodiastolic PA flow reversal.
  - Laminar, low-velocity PR flow detected by PW Doppler.
  - Premature opening of the PV (caused by atrial contraction at the end of diastole).
  - Premature closure if the TV (caused by rapid filling of the RV and equilibration of right atrial [RA] and RV pressures).
  - Low peak velocity of the PR jet by CW Doppler (<0.8 m/s).

KEY POINTS

- There is no validated grading schema for PR. Rather, a qualitative approach is recommended incorporating RV size, PV appearance, jet characteristics, vena contracta width, and spectral Doppler parameters.
- Although trace or mild PR is extremely common in older adults, pulmonary hypertension is the most likely cause of pathologic PR.
- Compression of the RVOT by extrinsic masses or dynamic obstruction in hypovolemic patients may mimic pulmonic stenosis (PS).

- Specific diagnoses
  - **Primary or secondary pulmonary hypertension** generally causes PA and PV annular dilatation, most frequently resulting in mild or moderate degrees of PR with a structurally normal PV.
  - **Endocarditis.** Isolated PV involvement is rare. Predisposing factors include a congenitally abnormal valve, the presence of intracardiac leads or catheters, and intravenous drug abuse (Figure 4-25).
  - **Rheumatic heart disease.** Echocardiographic features of rheumatic valvular disease include leaflet doming, thickening, and restriction. PV involvement in rheumatic disease usually accompanies TV pathology.
  - **Carcinoid heart disease.** Changes in carcinoid heart disease often result in PS with or without PR.
  - **Congenital abnormalities.** Previous PV or RVOT repair, as in tetralogy of Fallot or isolated congenital PS, may result in residual PR.
- Assessment of severity (see Table 4-3).

Pulmonic Stenosis

- General comments
  - Isolated PS is most commonly seen in neonates and infants and rarely presents in adulthood.

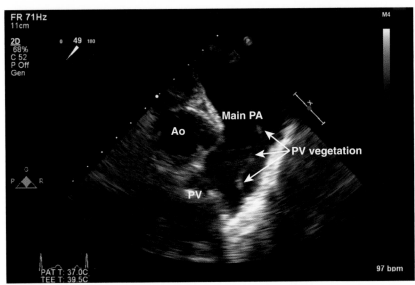

Figure 4-25. UE aortic short axis view demonstrates a long, filamentous vegetation in the main PA that arises from the PV. Ao, aorta.

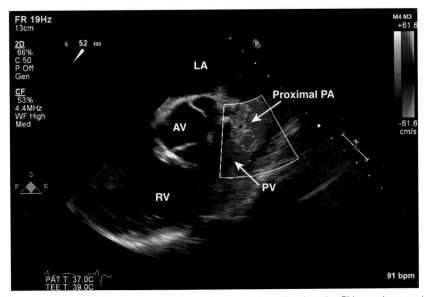

Figure 4-26. ME inflow-outflow CF Doppler image shows turbulent flow distal to the PV, consistent with PS. AV, aortic valve.

- It may be seen in carcinoid heart disease or recurrent bacterial endocarditis of the PV.
- 2D examination may reveal systolic doming of the valve, leaflet thickening, post-stenotic dilatation of the main PA and its branches, and signs of RV pressure overload (RV hypertrophy, paradoxical IVS motion in systole, varying degrees of TR).
- Subvalvular or supravalvular obstruction needs to be excluded. A variety of conditions, including extrinsic compression of the RVOT by postoperative hematoma, a pericardial cyst, or sarcoma, may mimic PS. Dynamic RVOT obstruction (analogous to dynamic left ventricular outflow tract obstruction) may be seen in hypovolemic postoperative patients treated with inotropic drugs.
- CF Doppler interrogation of the PV will demonstrate turbulent flow in the proximal PA when significant PS is present (Figure 4-26).

TABLE 4-4   PULMONIC STENOSIS: GRADING SEVERITY

Parameter	Mild	Moderate	Severe
Peak systolic jet velocity by CW Doppler (m/s)	<3	3-4	>4
Peak systolic gradient (mm Hg)	<36	36-60	>60

CW, continuous wave.

- CW Doppler is commonly used to determine the severity of the PS.
- Assessment of severity (Table 4-4).

Suggested Readings

1. Attenhofer Jost CH, Connolly HM, Dearani JA, et al. Ebstein's anomaly. *Circulation*. 2007;115:277-285.
   Detailed anatomic descriptions (with nice illustrations) of the pathophysiology of this disease as well as the echocardiographic findings and management guidelines.
2. Bonow RO, Carabello BA, Chatterjee K, et al. ACC/AHA 2006 guidelines for the management of patients with valvular heart disease. A report of the American College of Cardiology/American Heart Association Task Force on Practice Guidelines (Writing Committee to Revise the 1998 Guidelines for the Management of Patients with Valvular Heart Disease). *J Am Coll Cardiol.* 2006;48:e1-e148.
3. Maslow AD, Schwartz C, Singh AK. Assessment of the tricuspid valve: A comparison of four transesophageal echocardiographic windows. *J Cardiothorac Vasc Anesth.* 2004;18:719-724.
4. Bonow RO, Carabello BA, Chatterjee K, et al. ACC/AHA 2006 guidelines for the management of patients with valvular heart disease: Executive summary. A report of the American College of Cardiology/American Heart Association Task Force on Practice Guidelines (Writing Committee to Revise the 1998 Guidelines for the Management of Patients with Valvular Heart Disease). *J Am Coll Cardiol.* 2006;48:598-675.
   This practice guideline and the accompanying detailed executive summary provide up to date criteria for management, including many echocardiographic measures used to determine treatment.
5. Bruce CJ, Connolly HM. Right-sided valve disease deserves a little more RESPECT. *Circulation.* 2009;119:2726-2734.
   Recent summary of tricuspid and pulmonic valve diseases along with current practice guidelines for management and indications for surgical intervention.
6. David TE. Functional tricuspid regurgitation: A perplexing problem. *J Am Soc Echocardiogr.* 2009;22:904-906.
   Insights into the complexity of functional tricuspid regurgitation from the perspective of a renowned cardiac surgeon who specializes in valve repair.
7. Pellikka PA, Tajik AJ, Khandheria BK, et al: Carcinoid heart disease. Clinical and echocardiographic spectrum in 74 patients. *Circulation.* 1993;87:1188-1196.
   One of the most comprehensive reports of carcinoid heart disease, its many forms, and the echocardiographic findings.
8. Zoghbi WA, Enriquez-Sarano M, Foster E, et al. Recommendations for evaluation of the severity of native valvular regurgitation with two-dimensional and Doppler echocardiography. *J Am Soc Echocardiogr.* 2003;16:777-802.
   American Society of Echocardiography practice guideline for evaluation of valvular regurgitation, including all modes of echocardiography and criteria for assessing severity.

Echocardiographic Evaluation of Prosthetic Valves

5

Andrew D. Maslow and Arthur A. Bert

INTRODUCTION

> ### KEY POINTS
>
> - Echocardiography is the definitive technique for the noninvasive evaluation of prosthetic valve function, both bioprosthetic and mechanical.
> - On occasion, fluoroscopy is used as an adjunct in the evaluation of mechanical prostheses.
> - The echocardiographer should be most familiar with the prosthetic valves used at his or her institution; however, patients will present with different prostheses from other institutions, so that sources of reference (such as the tables in this chapter) must be readily available.
> - Acoustic shadowing from the prosthetic ring and leaflets may be critical; alternate windows and off-axis views become vital.

In patients with valvular (native or prosthetic) dysfunction, valve replacement remains a common definitive therapeutic intervention. Echocardiography is the method of choice for the noninvasive evaluation of prosthetic valve function.

Although many of the same principles and techniques utilized in the assessment of native valves are applied, echocardiography of prosthetic heart valves is much more demanding both to image and to interpret owing to imaging artifacts produced by the prosthetic materials. These artifacts vary depending on what type of valve is placed.

Although the evaluation of the prosthetic valve is primarily focused on the valve itself, the examiner must still perform a comprehensive examination of the surrounding cardiac tissues to assess for coexisting disease or secondary abnormalities and dysfunction.

Because there are so many available prosthetic valves, each with very distinctive two-dimensional (2D) and color flow (CF) Doppler acoustic profiles (Table 5-1), the echocardiographer should have access to the type and size of the in situ prosthetic valve and the reason the study has been ordered to focus the study and facilitate image interpretation.

This chapter describes and discusses the heart ultrasound examination using transesophageal (TE) and transgastric (TG) imaging and windows. It is accepted that epicardial and transthoracic examinations are complementary.

GENERAL CONSIDERATIONS WITH PROSTHETIC VALVES (Figure 5-1)

Types of Prosthetic Valves

Prosthetic valves are usually broadly grouped as biologic or mechanical.

Bioprosthetic Valves (Figure 5-2)
- Tissue valves are composed of three biologic cusps with an anatomic structure similar to that of the native aortic valve (AV). For imaging purposes, it is useful to know whether the valve is stented or stentless.
- All bioprosthetic valves are similar in that the trileaflet valve opens in a circular orifice.
- The normal flow pattern is similar to that of the native valve, specifically laminar flow with relatively low blood flow velocities.

Stented Bioprosthesis
- Commercially manufactured valves are composed of porcine AV cusps that are sewn into a fabric-covered metal support or cusps made from bovine pericardium using a template and sewn inside of stent supports.
- For stented and mechanical valves, the manufacturer's valve size refers to the external diameter of the sewing ring, not the actual diameter of the valve orifice.
- Stented bioprosthetic valves differ from the native valve in the presence of a metallic support, which limits imaging access and results in a reduced effective orifice area (EOA).

TABLE 5-1   REPORTED RANGES OF HEMODYNAMIC DATA FOR COMMONLY PLACED PROSTHETIC VALVES*

Diameter (mm)	Peak Gradient (mm Hg)	Mean Gradient (mm Hg)	Effective Orifice Area (cm²)
Bileaflet Mechanical Mitral Valve			
25	10	4	1.8-2.7
27	8-11	3-4	1.8-2.9
29	8-10	5	1.8-2.3
31	8-12	4-5	2.0-2.8
33	8-9	4-5	3.0
Stented Bioprosthetic Mitral Valve			
25	10-15	5-6.5	2.0-2.4
27	9-16	5-6.5	2.0-2.6
29	5-13	3-4.5	2.4-2.6
31	4-13	2-5	2.3-2.4
33	13	4	3.4
Bileaflet Mechanical Aortic Valve			
16	40-50	25-30	0.6
17	30-40	20-25	0.9-1.0
19	30-40	15-20	0.9-1.2
21	25-30	13-20	1.2-1.4
23	19-25	11-20	1.4-1.8
25	17-23	9-12	1.9-2.2
27	14-20	8-11	2.3-2.5
29	10-20	6-9	2.8-3.1
31	10-15	5-10	>3.1
Stented Bioprosthetic Aortic Valve			
19	32-44	24-26	0.8-1.2
21	25-28	17-20	1.1-1.5
23	21-29	12-16	1.3-1.7
25	16-24	9-13	1.9
27	19-22	6-12	2.2
29	18-22	10-12	2.8
Stentless Bioprosthetic Aortic Valve			
19	20-40	12-13	1.2-1.3
21	17-40	7.5-18	1.2-1.6
23	18-29	7-18	1.6-2.2
25	14-28	5-17	1.6-2.3
27	26	4.7-18	1.9-2.7
29	24	4	2.4

*Data are presented in ranges reflecting the variability reported in the literature.

Stentless Bioprosthesis

In this category, we take liberty by including all replacement tissues without a prosthetic stent. These include the better known stentless valves by St. Jude Medical and Medtronic (see Figure 5-2) as well as autograft and homograft tissues.

- Stentless valves differ based on their origin. They are considered xenografts consisting of either a preparation of porcine aorta or a sculpted bovine pericardium without any added strut support.
- Xenografts differ in method of preservation of valve cusps, anticalcification regimens, and

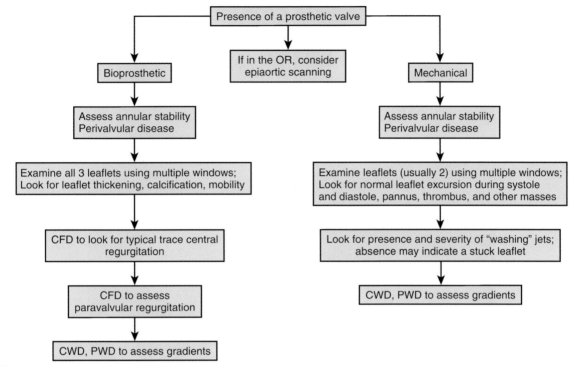

Figure 5-1. Flow chart of assessment of prosthetic valves in the operating room (OR). CFD, color flow Doppler; PWD, pulsed wave Doppler.

composition and designs of stents and sewing rings.

- Homografts are cadaveric human aortic or pulmonary valves (PVs) that are cryopreserved shortly after being harvested.
- Typically, the valve is harvested along with some of the respective ventricular outflow tract and great vessel, preserved as a block, and trimmed at surgery before implantation.
- Homografts are used in the aortic and pulmonary positions as well as in valved conduits.

Mechanical Valves (Figure 5-3)

- A wide variety of mechanical valves are currently available. Although this is the case, they all share commonalities.
- The most commonly implanted is a bileaflet valve in which two semicircular disks rotate around struts that are attached to the valve housing. These open to form two large lateral orifices and a smaller central orifice.
- The bileaflet valve forms the basis of all modern-day mechanical valve prostheses.
- Several other types of mechanical valves were implanted in the past and will be encountered in patients.
- The ball-cage valve houses a spherical occluder contained within a metallic cage. This occluder fills the cage orifice in the

closed position but rides above the orifice during antegrade flow.
- Single tilting-disk valves contain a single circular disk controlled by a metal strut that opens at an angle to the annulus plane.

BASIC PRINCIPLES OF THE ECHOCARDIOGRAPHIC EXAMINATION

Two-Dimensional

- Prosthetic valves should be imaged from multiple windows and angles to overcome the problem of acoustic shadowing that occurs owing to the highly reflective components inherent in many of these valves.
- Nonstandard windows and angles are often required to avoid imaging artifacts. Transesophageal echocardiography (TEE) becomes especially useful in evaluation of prosthetic valves in atrioventricular positions because it provides acoustic access from the atrial side of the valve.
- Prosthetic mitral valve (MV) assessment:
  - TE windows provide 2D and Doppler analyses.
  - TG windows offer a limited benefit in assessing the prosthetic MV.

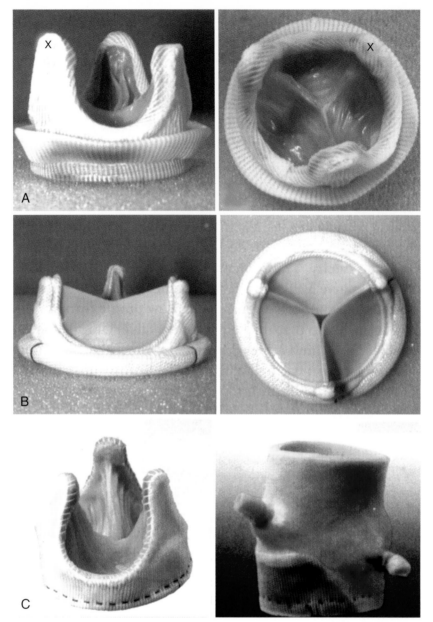

Figure 5-2. Bioprosthetic valves. Three examples of bioprosthetic/tissue valves that have been implanted. **A,** The Hancock Porcine Bioprosthesis with the cloth-covered stent. The "x" represents one of the three valve struts. This valve does not have a central opening as seen in the Carpentier Edwards Pericardial Valve (**B**). **C,** Examples of stentless valves are the Toronto Free-Style (left) and the Medtronic Freestyle Valve (right).

- Prosthetic AV assessment:
  - TE windows provide 2D and color Doppler imaging.
  - TG windows provide another view of the AV. Although farther from the transducer, these windows could be useful when TE imaging is limited possibly as a result of artifacts. Otherwise, TG imaging provides an opportunity to quantitatively interrogate the valve using pulsed wave (PW) and continuous wave (CW) Doppler.

- Prosthetic tricuspid valve (TV)
  - TE windows provide 2D and Doppler analysis, the latter including color, PW, and CW Doppler.
  - TG windows may provide imaging for 2D and color Doppler imaging more than PW or CW Doppler.
- Prosthetic PV
  - TE imaging is weaker than for other valves. Nonstandard windows may provide a more complete analysis.

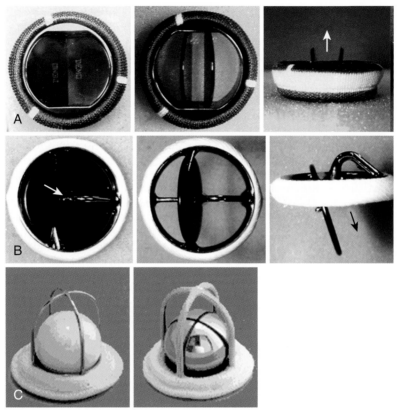

Figure 5-3. Mechanical valves. Three examples of mechanical valves. The *arrows* represent the direction of blood flow though the valve. **A,** Typical bileaflet valve in which forward flow moves through three orifices; two larger lateral and one small central. **B,** A single leaflet valve with flow moving through two orifices. **C,** A Starr-Edwards/Ball-in-cage valve for which flow occurs around the metal ball.

- TG windows can visualize the right ventricular outflow tract (RVOT) and PV.
- General points of 2D imaging of prosthetic valves
  - The opening and closing of the mechanical valve disks or bioprosthetic cusps must be evaluated.
  - Failure of a disk to open will significantly reduce the prosthetic valve's EOA and thus result in increased pressure gradients across that valve.
  - Failure to close properly will result in increased regurgitant flow.
  - Mechanisms of prosthetic valve dysfunction are both similar to and different from those of the native valves. Knowledge of these mechanisms is important to guide the echocardiographer during the assessment.
  - The presence of cusp thickening is usually an early sign of primary failure of a bioprosthetic valve.
  - Increased echo-dense lesions attached to a prosthetic valve sewing ring, stents, disks or occluder, and/or calcifications of

bioprosthetic leaflets are signs of possible prosthetic valve pathology and possible failure.
- Incomplete closure of prosthetic valve leaflets can be due to pannus growth, infection, thrombus, or suture materials around the sewing ring or the leaflets.
- Increased distance or separation of the prosthetic valve sewing ring from the native annulus is always pathologic and may appear as an echolucent space, a thickening, or a "rocking" motion of the valve during the cardiac cycle. These abnormal findings suggest a dehiscence of the prosthetic valve.
- "Focused" or magnified views are useful to assess the range of motion of individual disks or cusps as well as image and characterize abnormal perivalvular lesions.

Doppler Echocardiography

- The Doppler examination includes CF, PW, and CW Doppler examinations. Each method contributes toward qualifying and quantifying flow patterns of both normal and abnormally functioning prosthetic valves. The principles and rationale in utilizing Doppler techniques to qualify, measure, and quantify blood flow velocities, pressure gradients, and effective valve orifice areas of prosthetic valves are similar to that of native valves. However, the "normal" flow profiles of prosthetic valve are *NOT assumed to be equal* to that of normal functioning native valves.

- Given the variety of prosthetic valves available, different systolic and diastolic flow patterns across the valves exist. Although this is the case, assessment of severity of abnormal flows follow similar guidelines. For example, all perivalvular regurgitant leaks are considered abnormal. Those with a vena contracta width of greater than 3 mm have a greater potential to persist and/or worsen regardless of the prosthetic valve type.

Color Flow Doppler
Mechanical Valves

- All mechanical valves display "normal" regurgitant jets, sometimes referred to as "washing jets." These flows are thought to prevent the formation of thrombi at sites of blood flow stasis. These jets are typically small (vena contracta < 3 mm), have a low velocity and a uniform color pattern (minimal aliasing at most), and do not extend far from the valve plane.
- The "normal" degree of regurgitation of prosthetic valves, detected by CF Doppler, is greater than the trivial amounts seen in normal native valves. The patterns of regurgitation detected by CF Doppler are distinct ("signature patterns") for each mechanical valve type, corresponding to their fluid dynamics. While casting an identifiable "signature" pattern of regurgitant plumes, the associated regurgitant fraction is less than 10% to 15%.
- Valve types
  - Ball-cage valve
    - A ball-cage valve in the open position will demonstrate antegrade blood flow around all sides of the ball occluder and across the cage orifice. In the closed position, CF Doppler demonstrates a small regurgitant jet circumferentially around the ball as it seats in the cage orifice.
  - Single tilting disk valve
    - Antegrade blood flow across a single tilting disk prosthetic valve is characterized by a CF Doppler signal across a major and a minor orifice.

CF Doppler will indicate nonlaminar and asymmetrical flow as blood accelerates along the tilted surface of the open disk.
    - In the closed position, a single tilting disk normally demonstrates a regurgitation jet directed away from the sewing ring starting at the edge of the major orifice. Surgical preference on implantation determines the open disk position and, hence, the direction of the regurgitant jet normally seen on disk closure.
  - Bileaflet valve
    - This valve has a complex blood flow profile when interrogated by CF Doppler. In the open position, CF Doppler will demonstrate antegrade flow through two larger lateral orifices and a small central orifice.
    - When a bileaflet mechanical valve is imaged in the closed position, multiple "washing" jets of regurgitation are normally seen in the plane parallel to the leaflet-opening plane. All the regurgitant jets are located inside the sewing ring, with two jets originating from where the leaflets meet the housing and a third, central jet originating where the leaflets meet each other.

Bioprosthetic Valves

- Stented bioprosthetic valves display antegrade flow patterns closer to that of a normal native valve through a single orifice.
- "Normal" retrograde or regurgitant jets are centrally directed and do not extend far from the closed valve.
- Stentless valves including homografts and autografts usually demonstrate minor regurgitant jets that are central and limited in jet area and homogeneous in color.

General Points Regarding Color Doppler Assessment

- Pathologic regurgitant jets have higher velocities such that a color-mosaic pattern occurs from aliasing and create significant regurgitant momentum resulting in larger jet areas on CF Doppler imaging.
- The severity of prosthetic valve regurgitation is graded by criteria similar to that used for the native valve. The extent of the regurgitant jet into the receiving chamber as measured by CF Doppler (either the width of the vena contracta or the ratio of the CF Doppler jet area to the area of the atrium or the ratio of the width of the aortic insufficiency [AI] jet to

the width of the left ventricular outflow tract [LVOT]) is often utilized.

- CF Doppler-detected regurgitant jets that originate outside of the prosthetic sewing ring (paravalvular) are always pathologic.
- Although paravalvular regurgitation is always abnormal, small jets are often imaged on CF Doppler immediately after valve implantation in the operating room. To be clinically and hemodynamically insignificant, these jets should be small in comparison with the total circumference of the sewing ring they originate from. Many frequently resolve shortly after reversal of heparinization.
- Paravalvular regurgitation is not uncommon and results from a combination of surgical technique and the condition of the native annulus. A heavily calcified annulus complicates the placement of a prosthetic valve and may require extensive surgical débridement and repair before placement. These variables may increase the occurrence and severity of paravalvular regurgitation.
- For prosthetic valves in the mitral and tricuspid positions, it may be very difficult to detect pathologic regurgitation on transthoracic imaging. If suspected, it is an indication for TEE imaging. With TEE, CF Doppler imaging of a prosthetic valve in the mitral position is optimal because the ultrasound beam has access to the chamber receiving the regurgitant flow without intervening acoustic shadowing from crossing the prosthesis.
- For prosthetic valves in the atrioventricular position, a nondiagnostic transthoracic study for regurgitation does not exclude that possibility. Transthoracic echocardiography has a low negative predictive value for prosthetic valve regurgitation.

Pulsed Wave and Continuous Wave Doppler

- PW and CW Doppler modes provide quantitative evaluation of the prosthetic valve. Assessments regularly performed include peak transvalvular velocity (V_{max}), velocity time integral (VTI), peak and mean transvalvular pressure gradients, calculation of prosthetic valve area, and measurement of a dimensionless index in stenotic valves.
- These assessments are based on basic principles of physics including
  - **The simplified Bernoulli equation, $\Delta P = 4 \times (V_2)^2$,** forms the basis of much of the quantitative analysis including subvalvular and valvular velocities and gradients.

- For sites in which flow velocity proximal to the site of interest is high (>1.4 m/s), the simplified Bernoulli equation is not applicable and the proximal velocity must be included:

$$\Delta P = 4 \times (V_2^2 - V_1^2)$$

- The angle of interrogation (i.e., the angle between the Doppler beam and blood flow) should be less than 20 degrees to allow acceptable accuracy of blood flow velocities.
- For lower velocity flows (i.e., no aliasing), PW Doppler can be employed. The aliasing velocity is, in part, determined by the distance of the area of interest from the ultrasound probe. For higher velocity flows (i.e., exceeds the aliasing velocity), CW Doppler should be employed to allow assessment of high velocity flows.
- As a general practice, CW Doppler is most commonly used to assess prosthetic valve velocities and pressure gradients to allow measurement of a wide range of velocities and to ensure that the maximal velocities (i.e., vena contracta) is measured.
- **Conservation of mass/continuity equation**
  - This principle states that mass, flow, or volume (or stroke volume) measured at one site is equal to another provided that there are no intervening channels (inputs or outputs).
  - The basis of this assumes that volume can be measured by the equation VTI × Area (πr^2; r = radius of the site of interest). This equation assumes a circular and non-changing orifice.
  - If the volume or mass can be measured at a reference site, and the VTI across the valve can be obtained, then the **EOA** of the valve can be calculated using the **continuity equation:**

$$VTI_A \times Area_A = VTI_B \times Area_B$$
$$VTI_A \times \pi r^2_A = VTI_B \times \pi r^2_B$$

- The peak velocity (V) may be substituted for the VTI.
- Although the peak velocities of VTI for the reference are typically obtained using PW Doppler to target the same site at which the radius is measured, the respective Doppler values of the prosthetic valve are obtained using CW Doppler in order to measure flows across the vena contracta.
- Once three of the four values are obtained, the fourth can be solved for

$$VTI_A \times Area_A = VTI_B \times Area_B$$
$$Area_B = (VTI_A \times Area_A)/VTI_B$$

General Points

- Compared with a normal native valve, prosthetic valves have a smaller EOA. Antegrade velocities and pressure gradients across a normally functioning prosthetic valve are higher than a normal native valve.
- Smaller prosthetic valves may have hemodynamic profiles similar to that of mild stenosis for the given valve position (e.g., a 19 mm-prosthetic valve has an EOA ranging from 1.0-1.1 cm^2).
- Clinical application of Doppler-derived pressure gradients across mechanical valves may not be straightforward because a number of variables contribute to its value
  - Orifice area.
  - Cardiac output.
  - Viscosity.
  - Chamber pressures.
  - Chamber function.
  - Patient-prosthesis mismatch (PPM).
- Manufacturers publish data on the flow characteristics of each specific prosthetic valve and its various sizes. Published in vivo data vary more than in vitro data owing to variability in hemodynamic functions. Given the wide range of pressure gradients across any specific prosthetic valve, it may be best to determine the valve EOA or measure a dimensionless index across the valve and its outflow tract (described later).
- Doppler-derived peak and mean pressure gradients across *bioprosthetic valves* correlate closely with directly measured pressure gradients. For these valves, there is a single orifice.
- Doppler-derived pressure gradients across *mechanical valves* present a more complex clinical scenario. This has been best studied for the bileaflet valve where two hemicircular disks hinge open to form two larger semicircular lateral orifices and a smaller slitlike central orifice. Within the narrow central flow stream, higher blood velocities occur owing to local acceleration forces. Whether or not CW Doppler overestimates the transvalvular velocities by recording flow across the central smaller orifice is an issue. Theoretically, the pressure gradient across a narrower orifice of this valve will be identical to the peripheral ones because blood flow through the orifices is directly related to the orifice size.

- Utilizing pressure gradients across prosthetic valves as the sole indicator of functionality is limited because transvalvular gradients will vary directly with patient's cardiac output. Therefore, when valve patency is in question, it is important to determine the EOA of the prosthetic valve.
- *PPM* refers to an implanted prosthetic valve whose EOA is small relative to the patient's desired functional level. Implanted prosthetic valves have the unique possibility of functioning normally but still performing in a clinically detrimental manner through "PPM."
- This has been measured by comparing the EOA with the patient's body surface area (BSA) to obtain an indexed valve area: iEOA. The undersized valve's EOA results in
  - Excessive high-pressure gradients with the patient's blood flow requirements.
  - Decreased improvement of proximal chamber function or, in the case of aortic stenosis, a reduced regression of ventricular hypertrophy.
  - Decreased improvement of functional capacity.
  - Increased pressures, over time, in the chambers proximal to the prosthetic valve.
- Although indexing of EOA to a patient's BSA may not be appropriate in morbidly obese patients, it must still be considered because the patient will still need to function with the same body mass. For similar BSAs, obese patients have lower cardiac output requirements because fat is a vessel-poor tissue.
- A recent study found that PPM did not correlate with adverse clinical outcomes in patients with a body mass index greater than 30 kg/m^2. PPM may not have clinical importance in the elderly ($\geq$75 years old) or the smaller patient ($\leq$1.7 m^2).
- PPM can occur at any site at which prosthetic valves are implanted, but most clinical work has focused on prosthetic valves in the aortic position. Pressure gradients across prosthetic valves in the aortic position increase exponentially when the iEOA is 0.8 to 0.9 cm^2/m^2 or less. Based on these clinical data, PPM is considered to be hemodynamically insignificant if the EOA is 0.85 cm^2/m^2 or greater, moderate if the iEOA is between 0.65 and 0.85 cm^2/m^2, and severe if iEOA is less than 0.65 cm^2/m^2.
- The reported prevalence of moderate and severe PPM in aortic prosthetic valves varies considerably but should be deceasing as the

surgical community gains awareness of the impact of PPM on clinical outcomes.

- PPM results in reduced short- and long-term survival, especially when associated with preexisting left ventricular dysfunction. The severity of the PPM also correlates with reduced patient survival.
- PPM is best avoided by the preimplantation calculation of a valve's functional EOA against the patient's BSA and the choice of an appropriate sized valve.
- PPM has been reported for prosthetic valves implanted in the mitral position. Limited clinical data suggest that the iEOA on mitral prostheses should be greater than 1.2 to 1.3 cm^2/m^2 to avoid deleterious pressure gradients across the valve. PPM of mitral prosthetic valves has been reported to result in persistent pulmonary hypertension and reduced long-term survival.

PROSTHETIC MITRAL VALVE

KEY POINTS

- The severity of regurgitant flow is quantitated in a fashion similar to that of native valves. Special attention must be paid to the seating of the valve and the presence of pannus, thrombus, calcification or vegetation, and coexistent prosthetic stenosis.
- PPM for mitral prostheses may be considered to exist with iEOA less than 1.25 cm^2/m^2.
- The struts of bioprosthetic valves in the mitral position may rarely obstruct the LVOT. If the anterior mitral leaflet is redundant and preserved, outflow tract obstruction may occur with both mechanical and bioprosthetic valves.

Before evaluating the prosthetic MV, it is important to know what kind of valve was placed and to have some prior knowledge of how the images should appear. For all echocardiographic assessments, recording of the patient's hemodynamic status improves the perspective at the time of evaluation.

KEY POINTS

- The opening and closing of the mechanical valve disks or bioprosthetic cusps must be evaluated before decannulation so that abnormalities (see Cases on companion website) may be corrected before the patient leaves the operating room.
- Color Doppler in bioprosthetic valves often shows a small central jet of regurgitation; with mechanical prostheses, intravalvular washing jets are normally seen (see Cases on companion website).
- A small degree of paravalvular regurgitation, although abnormal, often resolves after the administration of protamine.
- PW and CF Doppler are used to assess transvalvular gradients. Although the accuracy in bioprosthetic valves seems intuitive, the complex flow characteristics of mechanical valves may be problematic.
- Evaluation of the functionality of a patient's particular valvular prosthesis must be made in light of the manufacturer's published data on the particular valves characteristics and, of course, on the patient's clinical context.
- Valve gradients are often higher than expected in the immediate post-bypass period and usually relate to the high flow state that exists; however, extremely high valvular gradients are unusual and should prompt close echocardiographic examination using TEE or alternative techniques such as epicardial echocardiography.

Step-by-Step Examination
(Figure 5-4)

- The 2D examination of the prosthetic MV is accomplished from a number of echocardiographic windows with particular emphasis on
  - Midesophageal (ME) windows from 0 to 150 degrees including but not limited to the standard ME windows.
  - TG views (0-30 degrees) are of limited value owing to its angle of interrogation; however, they may be useful to visualize the LVOT when shadowing artifact occurs during ME imaging (Figures 5-5 and 5-6)
- The CF, PW, and CW Doppler examinations of the prosthetic MV can be performed from the ME windows because the Doppler beam can be aligned with the direction of blood flow.
  - Imaging from multiple windows will improve the assessment and ability to differentiate between abnormal forward and regurgitant jets.

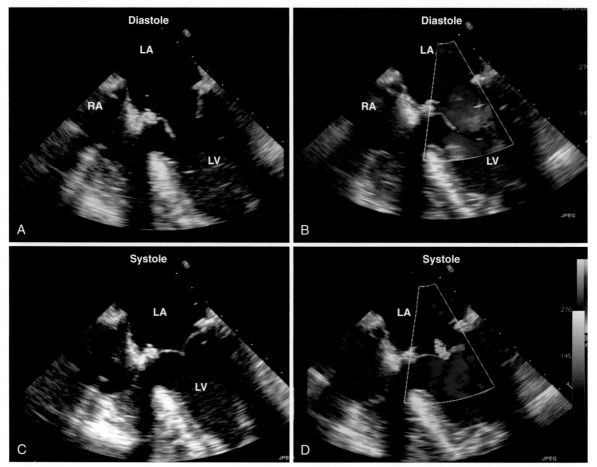

Figure 5-4. Normal functioning bioprosthetic valve in the mitral position. Four ME 0-degree images of a bioprosthetic valve in the mitral position. **A** and **C,** 2D images of valve opening and closing. **B** and **D,** The respective figures with CF Doppler demonstrating normal forward flow and a normal central regurgitation jet during ventricular systole. LA, left atrium; LV, left ventricle; RA, right atrium.

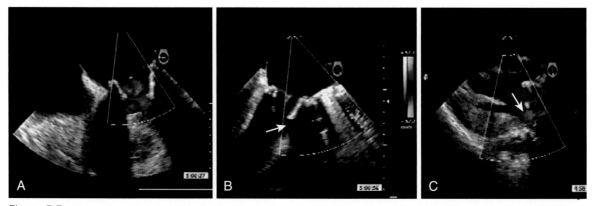

Figure 5-5. Normal functioning bioprosthetic valve in the mitral position using other echocardiographic windows. Three images of a normal functioning bioprosthetic valve in the mitral position. **A** and **B,** TE images. **C,** TG image. Images include both 2D and CF Doppler imaging. **B,** The *arrow* points to the LVOT. It is evident from TE imaging that prosthetic valve-related artifacts (e.g., shadowing) affects the ability to image the LVOT. **C,** This can be avoided by using TG imaging.

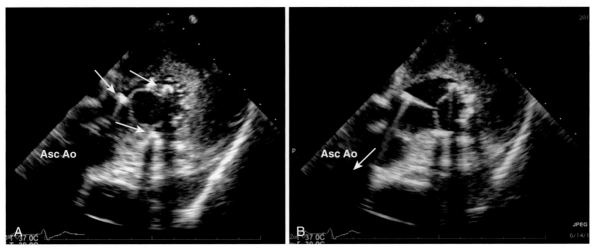

Figure 5-6. Bioprosthetic valve in the mitral position using TG imaging. Two images obtained during TG imaging (0-degree plane) of a bioprosthetic valve in the mitral position. The valve image is seen on cross section. The *arrows* in **A** point to the struts of the valve and the *arrow* in **B** points to the LVOT. Asc Ao, ascending aorta.

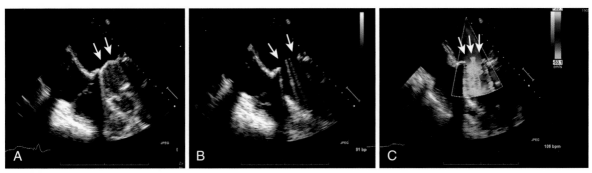

Figure 5-7. Normal functional mechanical valve in the mitral position. Three ME 0-degree images, perpendicular to the valve leaflets, of a normal functioning bileaflet mechanical valve in the mitral position. **A,** The valve in the closed position as demonstrated by the *arrows*. **B** and **C,** The leaflets in the open position, the latter with CF Doppler imaging. Three orifices each demonstrated by an *arrow* are seen with the central orifice appearing smaller and characterized by a higher velocity.

The Echocardiographer Should
- Have knowledge of imaging differences between prosthetic valves
- Attempt to identify the sewing ring, the leaflets, disks, or other occluder mechanism (i.e., ball-cage).

Step 1: Two-Dimensional Examination (Figure 5-7; see also Figure 5-4)
The 2D examination involves visualization of the prosthetic valve and its surrounding tissues. The assessment should evaluate valve stability, leaflet motion, and note any extraneous mobile structures, the latter of which may represent suture materials, fractured calcium deposits, native chordae, or leaflet components.

- Imaging includes primarily TE but may also include TG imaging.
- The stability of the valve should be determined and whether or not the prosthesis is rocking. As a rule, the prosthetic valve should sit firmly within its surrounding tissue.
- The valve leaflets should be visualized and their mobility noted.
- For mechanical valves, imaging perpendicular to the leaflets will allow one to see the opening and closing by noting the leaflet edges. Imaging parallel to the valve leaflets is not likely to visualize the leaflet edges opening and closing. If the valve is bileaflet and placed anatomically, optimal imaging is done at or close to a four-chamber orientation; if placed antianatomically, optimal imaging is done at approximately 50 to 80 degrees.

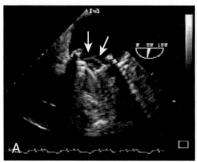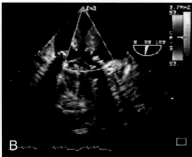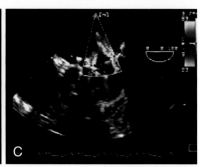

Figure 5-8. Normal functional mechanical valve in the mitral position. Three ME images of a normal functional bileaflet mechanical valve in the mitral position. **A** and **B,** ME two-chamber images. **C,** A four-chamber image. **A,** The valve leaflets *(arrows)* in the closed position. CF Doppler shows normal regurgitant jets in two nearly orthogonal views (**B** and **C**). The regurgitant jets are normal for this valve.

Step 2: Doppler Examination
(Figures 5-8 and 5-9)

The Doppler examination includes CF, PW, and CW examinations. The former allows both qualitative and quantitative evaluations including presence, direction, and width of normal and abnormal blood flows in and around the prosthetic valve.

- Both qualitative and quantitative imaging and assessments are achieved using TE windows.
- Although qualitative assessments may suggest high velocities (i.e., abnormal) based on the presence of aliasing (turbulence) during CF Doppler examination, this may or may not indicate abnormal flow. Further quantitative analysis should be performed to clarify the flow.

Regurgitant Flow: Normal versus Abnormal (Table 5-2; see also Figures 5-4, 5-8, and 5-9)

Prosthetic valves are association with "normal" or "expected" regurgitant jets. The former requires knowledge of normal regurgitant jets associated with each type of prosthesis. The assessment of abnormal prosthetic mitral regurgitation (MR) is similar to that of native valve assessment.

- Imaging includes both TE and TG windows.
- **Normal** regurgitant jets are less than 3 mm in width and do not extend far from the valve.
  - Bioprosthetic valves typically display a central regurgitant jet (see Figure 5-4).
  - Mechanical leaflets display a variety of regurgitant jets depending on the valve type (see Figures 5-8 and 5-9).
    - Imaging parallel to the valve leaflets will allow better visualization of the normal regurgitant jets.

- A bileaflet mechanical valve will usually have two regurgitant jets directed centrally.
- The normal regurgitant jet(s) of a single leaflet valve (tilting disk) may include 2 to 4 small jets with 1 larger central jet and 1 to 3 peripheral jets generating from the hinges of the valve.
- A ball-cage will have a surrounding series of small jets.
- **Abnormal** regurgitant jets can either be paravalvular or within the annular ring. Jets greater than 3 mm in width (vena contracta) are more concerning and are less likely to regress. Smaller jets may also be considered abnormal, but in the absence of obvious pathology (e.g., mobile materials; valve instability), these do not tend to progress over time. Abnormal regurgitant flows can result from a number of causes:
  - Paravalve (Figures 5-10 and 5-11)
    - Abscess.
    - Dehiscence.
  - Leaflet pathology
    - Abscess.
    - Tears.
    - Endocarditis (Figures 5-12 and 5-13)
      - Bioprosthetic valves: leaflet perforation/destruction.
      - Mechanical valves: interference with valve opening/closure.
  - Leaflet restriction/distortion (Figures 5-14 to 5-16)
    - Suture.
    - Thrombus.
    - Pannus.
    - Preserved valve apparatus interfering with closure of mechanical leaflets.
- **Assessing severity of regurgitant flow** is similar to that for native valve disease and includes

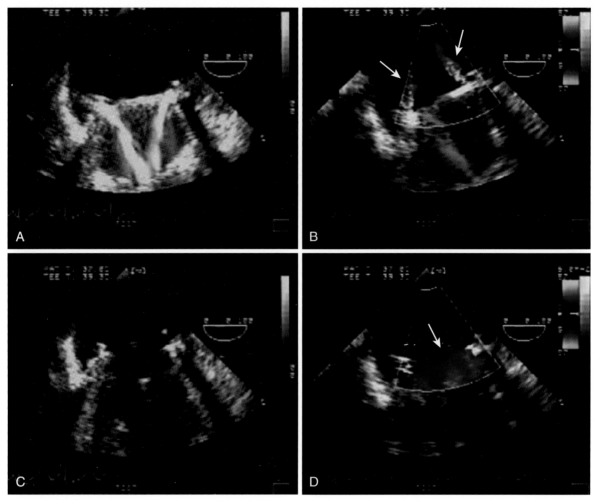

Figure 5-9. Normal functional mechanical valve in the mitral position. The four ME images, with the 2D imaging plane to be parallel to the valve leaflets, displays a normal functioning bileaflet mechanical valve in the mitral position. **A** and **B,** The valve in the closed position during ventricular systole demonstrates two regurgitant jets *(arrows)* directed toward each other. **C** and **D,** The valve in the open position during ventricular diastole. **D,** Three forward moving jets with one central *(arrow)* and two peripheral ones moving through the three orifices of the bileaflet mechanical valve.

TABLE 5-2 ASSESSING SEVERITY OF MITRAL REGURGITATION

Parameter	Mild	Moderate	Severe
Color flow jet area (CFD)	<4 cm² or <20% of LA area	Variable	>8 cm² or >40% of LA area
Jet density (CWD)	Incomplete/faint	Dense	Dense
Jet contour (CWD)	Parabolic	Parabolic	Early peaking, triangular
Pulmonary venous flow (PWD)	Systolic dominance	Systolic blunting	Systolic flow reversal
Vena contracta width (cm) (CFD)	<0.30	0.30-0.59	≥0.60
PISA			
Flow convergence (CFD)	None or minimal	Intermediate	Large
Regurgitant volume (mL/beat)	<30	30-59	≥60
Regurgitant fraction (%)	<30	30-49	≥50
Effective regurgitant orifice (cm²)	<0.20	0.20-0.49	≥0.50

CFD, color flow Doppler; CWD, continuous wave Doppler; LA, left atrium; PISA, proximal isovelocity surface area; PWD, pulsed wave Doppler.

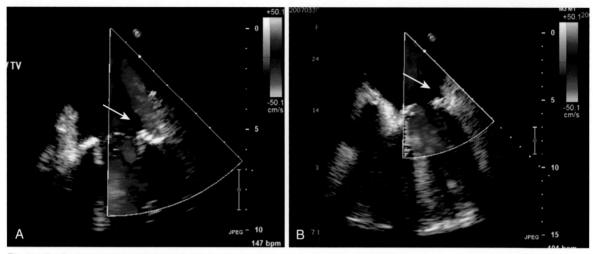

Figure 5-10. Post MV replacement with a paravalvular leak. Two images of a bioprosthetic valve with a decreasing paravalvular leak (left to right). **A,** The jet *(arrow)* appears to be nonturbulent or of lower velocity. **B,** After administration of protamine, the resulting image shows a significant reduction in the regurgitant CF Doppler jet area *(arrow)*.

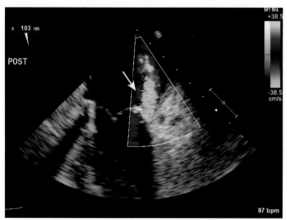

Figure 5-11. Post MV replacement with a significant paravalvular leak *(arrow)*. Large paravalvular turbulent jet directed toward the LA consistent with a paravalvular leak along the anterior aspect of the bioprosthetic valve.

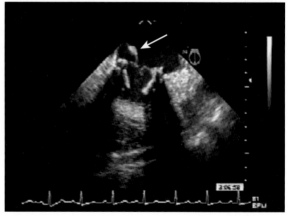

Figure 5-12. Endocarditis of a bioprosthetic valve in the mitral position. The image demonstrates an echodense mobile mass on the bioprosthetic valve *(arrow)*.

both assessments of the prosthetic valve and secondary effects on other cardiac functions, the latter including dilation of the left ventricle and atrium, elevation of the pulmonary artery pressures, right heart dysfunction, and tricuspid regurgitation (TR).

- Valve structure and motion.
  - Stable versus rocking.
- Extent or area of the regurgitant jet during CF Doppler.
  - Jet area less than 4 cm^2 is normal; greater than 8 cm^2 is abnormal.
  - Extent: Greater than 50% of the distance between valve and posterior atrial wall is significant.
- Eccentricity/centricity
  - Eccentric jets are one grade more severe than centrally directed jets.
- Pulmonary venous flows (PW)
  - Systolic dominance is normal; systolic blunting or reversal is abnormal.
- Flow convergence (proximal isovelocity surface area [PISA])
  - None is normal; convergence on the left ventricle side is abnormal.
- Jet density and contour
  - Faint/incomplete and parabolic are normal.
  - Dense/complete and early peaking are abnormal.

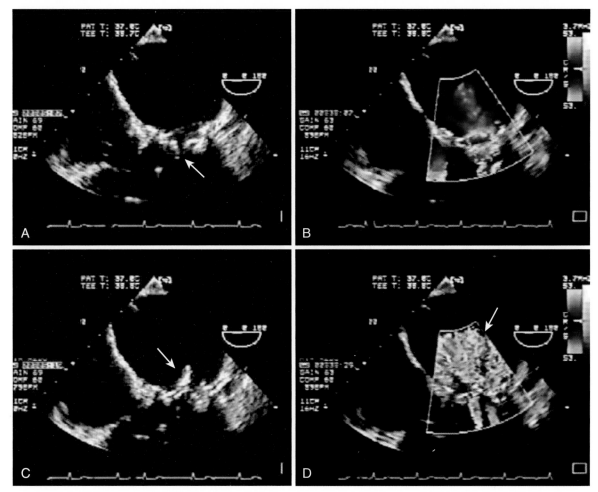

Figure 5-13. Endocarditis of a bioprosthetic valve in the mitral position with severe regurgitation. Four images demonstrate a mobile echodense mass attached to the prosthetic valve. **A** and **B,** The valve during diastole. **C** and **D,** Valve function during ventricular systole with severe MR *(arrow)*. The *arrows* in **A** and **C** point at the vegetation.

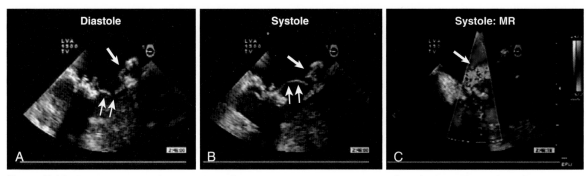

Figure 5-14. Stuck/restricted bioprosthetic leaflets due to suture between two of the leaflets. These three figures demonstrate the restriction of the lateral leaflet of a bioprosthetic valve, which on reevaluation, was due to suture. **A** and **B,** Restriction in forward motion of the medial leaflet *(two thinner arrows)* and immobility of the lateral leaflet *(thicker arrow)*. **C,** Mitral regurgitation during CF Doppler analysis.

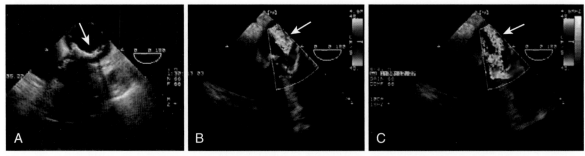

Figure 5-15. Distortion and dysfunction of a large mitral prosthesis in a relatively small annulus. These three images were obtained from a patient in whom a relatively large bioprosthetic valve was placed in the mitral position. **A,** The prosthetic valve appears to sit on top of the annulus *(arrow)*. **B** and **C,** Significant MR *(arrows)*.

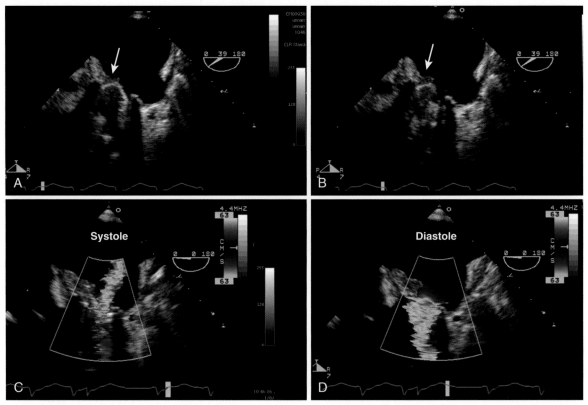

Figure 5-16. Thrombosis seen along the anterior medial leaflet of a mechanical MV. These four ME images demonstrate an echodense area on the mechanical valve consistent with thrombus. The stuck leaflet *(arrow)* during ventricular systole (**A**) and diastole (**B**). Ventricular systole (**C**) and ventricular diastole (**D**) show, with CF Doppler, that flow across the valve occurs only across the mobile mechanical leaflet.

- Doppler—quantitative
  - Vena contracta width (cm²)
    - Less than 0.3 cm² is acceptable as it is not likely to increase over time; greater than 0.6 is definitely abnormal.
  - Regurgitant volume (mL/beat; PISA or continuity equation).
    - Less than 30 is mild; 30 to 59 is moderate; greater than 60 is severe.
- Regurgitant fraction (%; PISA or continuity equation)
  - Less than 30 is mild; 30 to 50 is moderate; greater than 50 is severe.
- Regurgitant orifice (cm²; PISA or continuity equation)
  - Less than 0.2 is mild; 0.2 to 0.49 is moderate; greater than 0.5 is severe.

TABLE 5-3 ASSESSING SEVERITY OF MITRAL STENOSIS

Parameter	Mild	Moderate	Severe
Peak velocity (m/s) (CWD vs. HPRF)	<1.9	1.9-2.5	≥2.5
Mean gradient (mm Hg) (CW vs. HPRF)	≤5	6-10	>10
VTI_{MV}/VTI_{LVOT} (CWD and PWD)	<2.2	2.2-2.5	>2.5
Pressure half time (ms) (CWD)	<130	130-200	>200

Effective orifice area (cm^2)
  Pressure half time
  Continuity equation
  Planimetry (bioprosthesis)
	≥2.0	1-2	<1.0

CWD, continuous wave Doppler; HPRF, high pulse repetition frequency; LVOT, left ventricular outflow tract; MV, mitral valve; PWD, pulsed wave Doppler; VTI, velocity time integral.

Forward Flow: Normal vs. Abnormal (Table 5-3; see also Figures 5-4, 5-5, and 5-7 to 5-9)

Depending on the type of prosthesis, forward blood flow projects in different ways. Whereas bioprosthetic valves have a single forward flow, mechanical valves will have two (single leaflet) or three (bileaflet) forward projecting jets. The evaluation of forward flow consists of both qualitative (CF Doppler) and quantitative assessments (PW and CW Doppler), the latter consisting of transvalvular pressure gradients and calculation of prosthetic valve area.

- Doppler assessment is performed primarily from the TE windows (see Figures 5-5 and 5-7 to 5-9).
- **Normal flows** for prosthetic valves have been described and involve transvalvular velocities, pressure gradients, and valve areas. These data are largely determined during follow-up postoperative examination and may not be easily applied to intraoperative data, in which cardiac loading conditions and blood viscosity are significantly altered. Nevertheless, these data are often referred to and applied to the intraoperative examination.
- Normal EOA (or range) for each size and type of prosthesis has been reported. Suffice it to say, there are significant variations compared with that measured by the manufacturer.
- Although pressure gradients are a simpler measure, they are dependent on variables including valve area, cardiac output, blood viscosity, chamber pressures and compliances, and the angle of interrogation.
- **PPM** has been described for prosthetic MVs. PPM, for the MV, has been categorized as present or not, based on the iEOA (cm^2/BSA [m^2]). PPM for the MV may be considered present when the iEOA is less than 1.25 cm^2/m^2.

- Degrees of mitral stenosis follow similar charts for native valve assessment. Significant mitral stenosis is considered when the mean transvalvular gradient is greater than 6 mm Hg, a peak gradient 12 mm Hg or greater, and/or a mitral valve area (MVA) less than 1.8 cm^2.

Qualitative Assessment
Initial suspicion of obstruction to forward flow is seen during 2D and CF Doppler examination. Causes may include
- Thrombus (see Figure 5-16).
- Stuck leaflet (Figure 5-17; see also Figure 5-14).
- Distortion.
- Calcification.

Left Ventricular Outflow Obstruction after Mitral Surgery
An unusual type of obstruction is obstruction of the LVOT. This can result from attempts to retain native mitral tissues (leaflets or chordae) between the mitral annulus and the prosthetic ring. This is done to preserve ventricular geometry and reduce future negative remodeling. As an unusual consequence, these native tissues may become loose and lie in the LVOT, causing a dynamic and/or fixed obstruction to systolic outflow (Figure 5-18). Another cause of obstruction can result from placement of the struts of the bioprosthetic valve in the LVOT in a relatively small ventricle. Assessment of this complication may be difficult using ME imaging as a result of shadowing; therefore, TG imaging may be necessary (see Figures 5-5 and 5-6).

Quantitative Assessment
Doppler assessment of forward flow across the prosthetic MV is the standard to evaluate valve patency. A host of variables affect the Doppler data. These include changes in cardiac loading

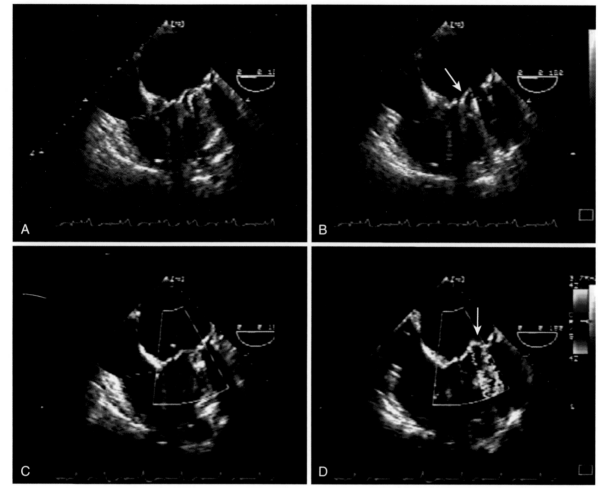

Figure 5-17. Stuck mechanical leaflet in the mitral position. These four ME 0-degree images demonstrate a stuck mechanical leaflet *(arrow)*. Images include 2D (**A** and **B**) and their respective CF Doppler (**C** and **D**) images during both ventricular systole (**A** and **C**) and ventricular diastole (**B** and **D**). **D,** During CF Doppler examination, ventricular inflow is seen across the one normally mobile leaflet *(arrow)*.

conditions and coexisting lesions that affect the forward flow across the MV or the pressure gradient between the left atrium and the left ventricle. These include, but are not limited to, AI (lowers pressure half time [PHT]), the presence of an interatrial septal defect (left to right flow lowers PHT), changes in atrial and/or ventricular compliances, and changes in heart rhythm.

- Peak velocity/gradient (CW). Although the presence of MR can affect the upper limit of normal, the following can be used as a general guide:
  - Less than 1.8 m/s or less than 12 mm Hg is considered normal.
  - 1.8 to 2.2 or 12 to 18 mm Hg is intermediate.
  - 2.2 m/s or greater than 18 mm Hg is considered abnormal.
- Mean transvalvular gradient (CW)
  - Less than 6 mm Hg is considered normal.
  - 6 to 10 is an intermediate range that deserves further clarification.
  - 10 mm Hg is considered abnormal.
- EOA
  - Planimetry (not widely studied for bioprosthetic valves and not feasible for mechanical valves)
  - PHT: $MVA = 220/PHT_{MV}$
    - Greater than 200 ms is abnormal.
    - 130 to 200 ms is intermediate.
    - Less than 130 ms is normal ($MVA > 1.7$ cm^2)

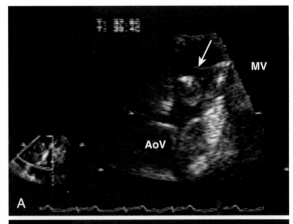

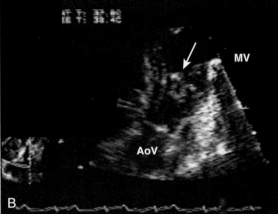

Figure 5-18. Example of a retained native anterior leaflet after valve replacement. Two TG images of the LVOT after MV replacement. During the prosthetic valve implantation, the anterior mitral leaflet was retained along the prosthetic valve annulus to prevent adverse ventricular remodeling. In both figures, the retained leaflet is identified by an *arrow* in the LVOT proximal to the aortic valve (AoV).

- Continuity equation
  - Deceleration time: EOA = 759/ Deceleration time
  - EOA_{MV} = stroke volume/VTI_{MV}
  - The stroke volume is measured from a reference area (LVOT, AV, or pulmonary artery)
    - Thermodilution stroke volume.
    - Doppler stroke volume (e.g., pulmonary artery; LVOT).
  - PISA. EOA = $(2\pi r^2 \times V_{NL})/(V_{MAX})$ corrected by the angle in inflow.
- Doppler velocity index (DVI) may also be used for the MV
  - VTI_{MV}/VTI_{LVOT}.
    - Greater than 2.2 is considered abnormal.
    - Less affected by changes in loading conditions.

PROSTHETIC AORTIC VALVE

KEY POINTS
<ul><li>Imaging of the AV must also include an assessment of the supra- and subvalvular tissues as well as the prosthetic valve.</li><li>TG imaging may be necessary to detect abnormal pressure gradients, because it is difficult to achieve an adequate angle of insonation from the esophagus. Movement of mechanical leaflets may be best appreciated from this window. Always remember to consider epiaortic scanning.</li><li>PPM may be most clinically relevant with valves in the aortic position. In general, mechanical valves give a larger EOA for a given ring diameter. If necessary, an aortic root enlargement procedure may be necessary.</li></ul>

Before evaluating a prosthetic AV, it is important to know the type of valve implanted and to have knowledge of how the characteristic 2D and CF Doppler images should appear. For all echocardiographic assessments, recording of the patient's hemodynamic status improves the perspective at the time of evaluation.

Step-by-Step Examination

- Imaging of the prosthetic valve includes assessment of the supra- and subvalvular tissues as well as the prosthetic valve.
- The 2D examination of the prosthetic AV is accomplished from a number of echocardiographic windows with particular emphasis on
  - ME four- or five-chamber view (0 degrees).
  - ME short axis view (40-60 degrees) (Figures 5-19 and 5-20).
  - ME long axis view (110-145 degrees) (Figure 5-21).
  - Trans-gastric views (0-155 degrees) (Figures 5-22 and 5-23)
- The CF Doppler examination of the prosthetic aortic can be performed from each of the same windows as the 2D examination (Figure 5-24).
  - Imaging from multiple windows will improve the assessment and ability to differentiate between abnormal forward and regurgitant jets.
- The PW and CW Doppler interrogation of the valve should be performed using TG imaging because the Doppler beam can be most easily aligned with the direction of blood flow.

• It is important to examine the LVOT and AV from multiple TG windows to obtain the maximum blood flow velocity. This would reduce the chance of underestimating peak subvalvular and transvalvular velocities.

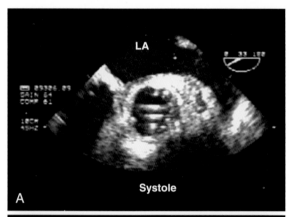

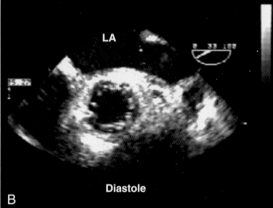

Figure 5-19. Normal mechanical valve in the aortic position. Two TE images show a short axis image of the bileaflet mechanical valve in the aortic position during ventricular systole and diastole. During systole, the medial edges of each mechanical leaflet are seen. During diastole, the leaflets are closed and not seen because of the angle of interrogation (i.e., the leaflets are not in the imaging plane).

The Echocardiographer Should
• Have knowledge of differences between prosthetic valves with (stented) or without (stentless) sewing rings. The latter (homografts, stentless valves) may not be distinguishable from native valves.
• Attempt to identify the sewing ring, the leaflets, disks, or other occluder mechanism (i.e., ball-cage).
• Recognize and appreciate the presence of perivalvular edema or hematoma that may be present immediately after valve surgery (Figures 5-25 and 5-26). This typically resolves over the first 24 to 48 hours after separation from cardiopulmonary bypass.
  • For patients with stentless valves, this may result in a smaller EOA in the immediate postoperative period. For stentless valves, data show a significant increase in EOA over the first 3 to 6 months after placement.
• Recognize changes in prosthetic valves over time. This is more of an issue with stentless AVs during which the cloth edges are sutured to the native aortic annulus. If the edges are not sutured completely, they may appear in the outflow tract. Over time, these edges will flatten out and any obstruction will resolve or reduce significantly over time.

Step 1: Two-Dimensional Examination
The 2D examination involves visualization of the prosthetic valve and its surrounding tissues. The assessment should evaluate valve stability, leaflet motion, and note any extraneous mobile structures, the latter of which may represent suture materials or fractured calcium deposits.
• Imaging includes both TE and TG imaging (see Figures 5-19 and 5-24).
• The stability of the valve should be determined and whether or not the prosthesis is rocking. As a rule, the prosthetic valve should sit firmly within its surrounding

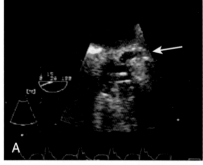

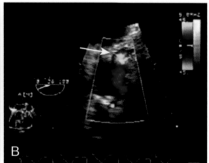

Figure 5-20. Normal mechanical aortic valve prosthesis with coronary flow in the left main coronary artery. Two TE images of the prosthetic AV in cross section show the left main coronary artery (**A**) with CF Doppler (**B**) as shown by the *arrows*.

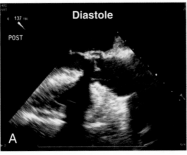
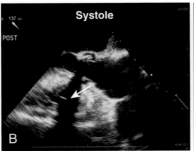
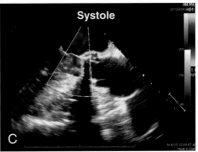

Figure 5-21. Normal bioprosthetic valve in the aortic position. Three TE images of a normal functioning bioprosthetic valve in diastole (**A**), and systole (**B** and **C**). **B,** Note the shadowing *(arrow)* caused by the prosthetic valve.

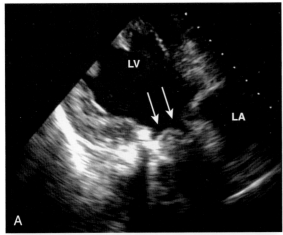

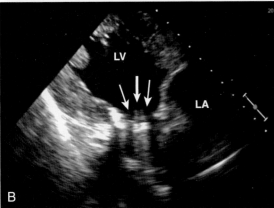

Figure 5-22. Normal aortic valve prosthesis seen during TG imaging. Two TG images of the LVOT *(arrows)*, LV, and LA. **A,** The *arrows* point toward the two closed mechanical leaflets. **B,** The *arrows* point toward the two leaflet edges/central orifice and the two lateral orifices in the open valve. These images were obtained with the transducer rotated to 100 degrees.

tissue without any qualitative evidence of rocking.
- The valve leaflets should be visualized and the mobility noted.
- Measurement of the LVOT diameter should be performed, from the ME long axis window,

to allow assessment of valve area using the continuity equation.
- Supra- and subvalvular areas should also be interrogated.
  - This is important for cases in which the LVOT was enlarged and/or when a homograft was placed.
  - Subvalvular imaging is needed to assess for evidence of LVOT obstruction.

Step 2: Doppler Examination

The Doppler examination includes CF, PW, and CW examinations. The former allows both qualitative and quantitative evaluations including presence, direction, and width of normal and abnormal blood flows in and around the prosthetic valve.
- Although qualitative imaging includes both TE and TG windows, most of the quantitative assessment is best achieved from the TG windows where blood flow and the Doppler beam can be best aligned (Figure 5-27).
- Although qualitative assessments may suggest high velocities (i.e., abnormal) based on the presence of aliasing (turbulence) during CF Doppler examination, this may or may not indicate abnormal flow. Further quantitative analysis should be performed to clarify the flow. As a rule, prosthetic valves in the aortic position are associated with higher flow velocities than a normal native valve in the aortic position.

Regurgitant Flow: Normal versus Abnormal (Table 5-4)

Prosthetic valves are associated with "normal" or "expected" regurgitant jets. The former requires knowledge of normal regurgitant jets associated with each type of prosthesis. The assessment of abnormal prosthetic AV regurgitation parallels that of native valve assessment.

TABLE 5-4	ASSESSING SEVERITY OF AORTIC VALVE REGURGITATION		
Parameter	**Mild**	**Moderate**	**Severe**
AI jet width (% LVOT diameter) (CFD)	Narrow (≤25%)	Intermediate (26-64%)	Large (≥65%)
AI jet density (CWD)	Incomplete or faint	Dense	Dense
AI jet pressure half time (CWD)	Slow (>500 ms)	Variable (200-500)	Steep (<200 ms)
Diastolic flow reversal in descending aorta (PWD)	Absent or brief	Intermediate	Prominent, holodiastolic
Regurgitant volume (ml/beat) (continuity equation)	<30	30-59	>60
Regurgitant fraction (%) (continuity equation)	<30	30-50	>50

AI, aortic insufficiency; CFD, color flow Doppler; CWD, continuous wave Doppler; LVOT, left ventricular outflow tract; PWD, pulsed wave Doppler.

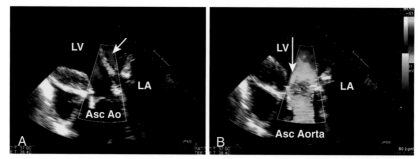

Figure 5-23. Normal bioprosthetic valve in the aortic position during TG imaging. Two TG images of a normal functioning bioprosthetic valve during diastole (**A**) and systole (**B**), the former showing ventricular inflow *(arrow)* and the latter showing ventricular outflow.

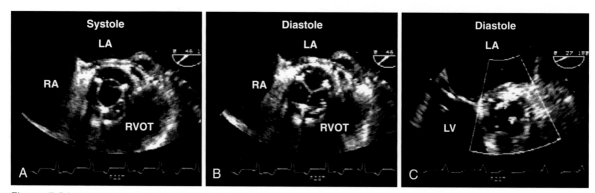

Figure 5-24. Normal aortic valve bioprosthesis with a normal regurgitant jet. Three TE images of the bioprosthetic valve during systole (**A**), diastole (**B**), and with CF Doppler demonstrate a small normal central jet of insufficiency in diastole. RA, right atrium.

- Imaging includes both TE and TG windows.
- **Normal** regurgitant jets, assessed with vena contracta, are less than 3 mm in width.
  - Bioprosthetic valves typically display a central regurgitant jet.
  - Mechanical leaflets display a variety of regurgitant jets depending on the valve type.
- A bileaflet mechanical valve will usually have two regurgitant jets directed centrally.
- A single leaflet valve (or tilting disk valve) will have a regurgitant jet directed away from the sewing ring from the edge of the major orifice.
- A ball-cage valve will have small circumferential jets around the occluder.

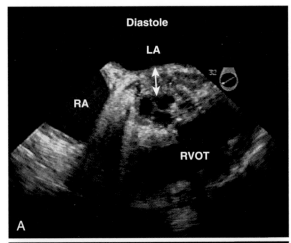

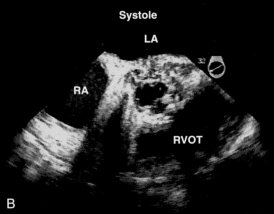

Figure 5-25. Normal homograft seen in the aortic position. Two TE images show a short axis view of the homograft valve in the aortic position during both ventricular diastole (**A**) and systole (**B**). Note the thickness of the paravalvular tissues (*double arrow* in **A**). This is the result of either edema or hematoma; it resolves over the following 24 hours to 3 to 6 months.

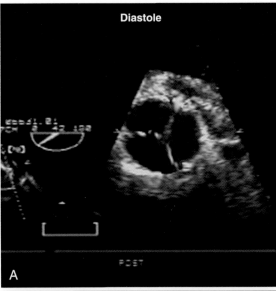

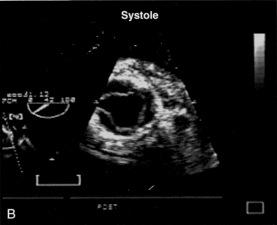

Figure 5-26. Normal homograft seen in the aortic position. Two TE images of a stentless AV in the short axis view seen during ventricular diastole (**A**) and systole (**B**).

- Homografts should NOT have any regurgitant jets; however, some may be seen depending on the native valve function before excision and preparation.
- **Abnormal** regurgitant jets, assessed using the vena contracta, are greater than 3 mm in width, however. Smaller jets may also be considered abnormal, but in the absence of obvious pathology (e.g., mobile materials; valve instability), these either do not progress or reduce in significance over time. Eccentrically directed jets (i.e., away from the middle) are considered abnormal. These abnormal flows can result from a number of causes:
  - Paravalve.
    - Calcification.
    - Abscess.
    - Dehiscence.
    - Retained native tissues.
  - Leaflet pathology (Figures 5-28 to 5-30).
    - Tears/Trauma.
    - Endocarditis.
  - Leaflet restriction/distortion.
    - Thrombus (Figure 5-31).
    - Stuck leaflet (Figure 5-32).
    - Suture.
    - Pannus.
- **Assessing severity of regurgitant flow** is similar to that for native valve disease
  - Valve structure and motion.
  - Left ventricular size (depends on acuity)
  - Doppler—qualitative to semiquantitative.
  - Jet width (% of LVOT diameter)
    - Less than 25% is mild; 25% to 50% is moderate; greater than 50% is severe.

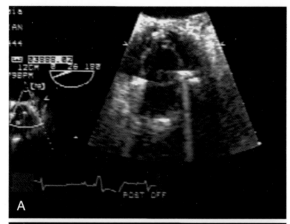

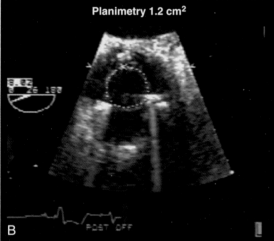

Planimetry 1.2 cm²

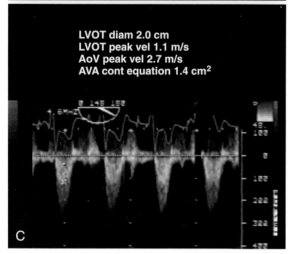

LVOT diam 2.0 cm
LVOT peak vel 1.1 m/s
AoV peak vel 2.7 m/s
AVA cont equation 1.4 cm²

Figure 5-27. Quantitative assessment of the prosthetic aortic valve (AoV). Two ME images (**A** and **B**) and one obtained during TG imaging (**C**). **A** and **B,** Short axis views allow 2D planimetry to be performed (**B**). **C,** CW Doppler profile during TG imaging. This can be performed on either mechanical or bioprosthetic valves to allow quantitative assessment of flow velocities, pressure gradients, and calculation of the aortic valve area (AVA) using the continuity equation.

- Jet density
  - Faint/incomplete is within normal limits.
  - Dense/complete is considered abnormal.
- PHT (ms)
  - Greater than 500 ms is mild; 200 to 500 is intermediate; less than 200 is severe.
- Diastolic flow reversal in descending aorta.
  - Absent is mild; intermediate is moderate; prominent is severe.
- Doppler—quantitative (continuity equation or PISA)
  - Regurgitant volume (mL/beat)
  - Less than 30 is mild; 30 to 59 is moderate; greater than 60 is severe.
  - Regurgitant fraction (%)
  - Less than 30 is mild; 30 to 50 is moderate; greater than 50 is severe.

Forward Flow: Normal versus Abnormal (Table 5-5)

Depending on the type of prosthesis, forward blood flow projects in different ways. Whereas bioprosthetic valves have a single forward flow, mechanical valves will have two (single leaflet valve) or three (bileaflet valve) forward projecting jets. The evaluation of forward flow consists of both qualitative (CF Doppler) and quantitative assessments (PW and CW Doppler), the latter consisting of transvalvular flow velocities and gradients, and calculation of the effective orifice area of the prosthetic valve.
- Although Doppler imaging from ME windows could add to the qualitative assessment,

TABLE 5-5	ASSESSING SEVERITY OF AORTIC VALVE STENOSIS		
Parameter	**Mild**	**Moderate**	**Severe**
Peak velocity (m/s) (CWD)	<3	3-4	>4
Mean gradient (mm Hg) (CWD)	<20-30	25-40	>40
Doppler velocity index (LVOT velocity/AV velocity)	0.35-0.30	0.30-0.25	<0.25
Effective orifice area (cm²) Continuity equation Planimetry (bioprosthetic valve)	>1.2	1.2-0.8	<0.8

AV, aortic valve; CWD, continuous wave Doppler; LVOT, left ventricular outflow tract.

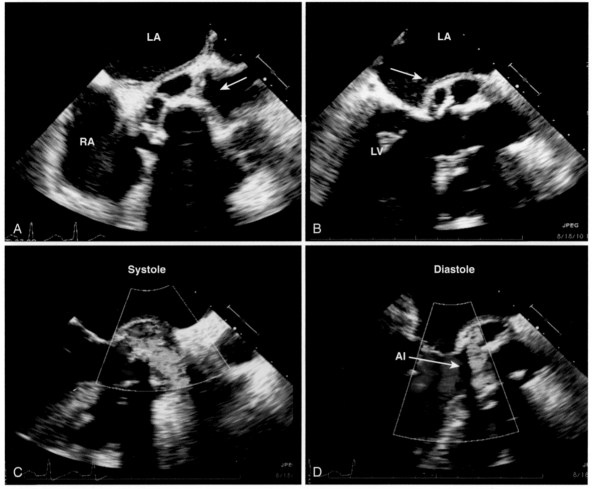

Figure 5-28. Paravalvular abscess after AV replacement. Four TE views of a paravalvular abscess surrounding a previously placed bioprosthesis. Short axis (**A**) and long axis (**B**) views of the valve and abscess *(arrow)*. **C** and **D**, CF Doppler images of the valve apparatus during systole and diastole, the latter demonstrating an eccentric jet of AI *(arrow)*.

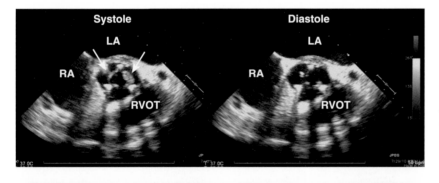

Figure 5-29. Endocarditis of a bioprosthetic AV. Two TE images of a bioprosthetic valve in the short axis window during systole and diastole. **Left,** The *arrows* point toward a small mass on the noncoronary cusp and a thickening of the left coronary cusp.

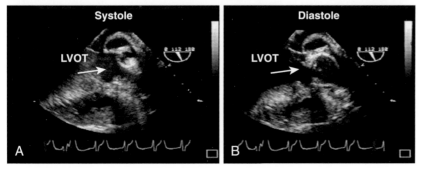

Figure 5-30. Dehiscence of an aortic homograft. Two TE long axis 2D views the LVOT and a dehisced homograft *(arrows)* seen during systole (**A**) and diastole (**B**).

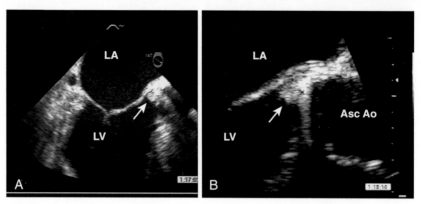

Figure 5-31. Thrombosis of a mechanical valve in the aortic position. Two TE images long axis view of the LVOT (**A**) and AV (**B**) show a mass along the posterior area of the prosthesis *(arrow)*. This was associated with an immobile leaflet and AV stenosis. The calculated AVA was 0.7 cm² with a mean gradient of approximately 50 mm Hg.

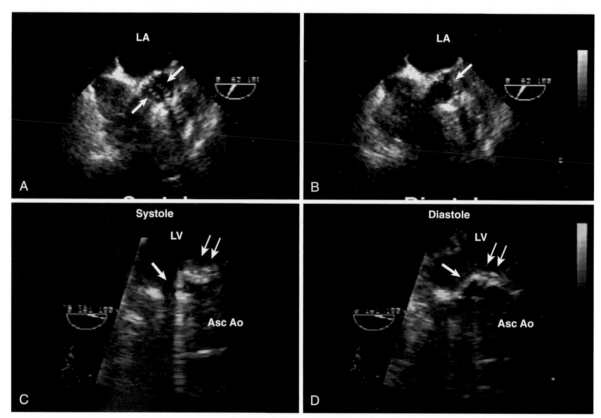

Figure 5-32. Stuck mechanical leaflet in the aortic position. Four images demonstrate restricted motion of one mechanical leaflet of the prosthetic AV. **A** and **B,** Short axis images of the mechanical valve. **A,** The two leaflet edges *(arrows)* are seen as also noted in Figure 5-19. However, in **B,** a leaflet edge *(arrow)* is still seen during diastole. **C** and **D,** TG imaging with the transducer rotated to 160 degrees. **C,** A single leaflet open *(single arrow)* while the other leaflet *(double arrow)* is stuck in an intermediate position. **D,** The mobile leaflet is shown to be closed and the stuck leaflet to be unchanged.

quantitative analysis primarily involves TG imaging.

- **Normal forward flows** for prosthetic valves have been described and the data include transvalvular velocities, pressure gradients, and valve areas.
- The normal **contour** of the flow velocity profile is an early peaking and triangular shape. With increasing narrowing/stenosis, the **contour** peaks later and the shape becomes more round. Along with this change in shape is a respective change in the **acceleration time** from a relatively short period to the peak velocity (≤80 ms) to a more prolonged **acceleration phase** (>100 ms).
- Although pressure gradients are a simpler measure, they are dependent on variables including valve area, cardiac output, blood viscosity, chamber pressures and compliances, and the angle of interrogation.
- Normal EOA (or range) for each size and type of prosthesis has been reported. Suffice it to say, there are significant variations compared with that measured by the manufacturer.
- These data are largely determined during follow-up postoperative examination and may not be easily applied to intraoperative data, in which cardiac loading conditions and blood viscosity are significantly altered. Nevertheless, data regarding expected EOA have been applied to the intraoperative examination.
- The **DVI** is a dimensionless index in which the peak subvalvular velocity (LVOT) is divided by the peak transvalvular velocity. Alternatively VTI may be used instead of peak velocities.
- **PPM** is a term used to describe the mismatch between the EOA of the prosthetic valve and the patient's BSA (m^2). The EOA is indexed to the patient's BSA to calculate the iEOA.
  - PPM has been categorized as mild, moderate, and severe based on the iEOA (cm^2/BSA [m^2]). For these divisions, the iEOA is 0.85 to 1.00 cm^2/m^2; 0.65 to 0.85 cm^2/m^2; and less than 0.65 cm^2/m^2, respectively.
  - PPM is associated with reduced short- and long-term survival, especially when associated with preexisting left ventricular dysfunction.
  - The clinical impact is more consistently reported for severe PPM (i.e., <0.65 cm^2/m^2).
  - PPM is best avoided by the pre-implantation calculation of a valve's functional EOA against the patient's BSA and the choice of an appropriate sized valve.

- PPM has less clinical impact on the elderly (>75 yr) and/or for smaller BSA (<1.75 m^2).
- Degrees of aortic stenosis follow similar charts for native valve assessment. A peak gradient greater than 4 m/s is considered significant whereas less than 2 m/s is considered clinically insignificant. The exception to the latter would be in the presence of reduced forward flow as seen in settings of severe ventricular dysfunction.
  - Causes of abnormal forward flow include
    - Leaflet pathology
      - Thrombus (see Figure 5-31).
    - Leaflet restriction
      - Stuck leaflet (see Figure 5-32).
    - Outflow obstruction
      - Dehiscence (see Figure 5-30).
      - Prosthetic valve materials (Figure 5-33).

Quantitative Assessment

Doppler assessment of forward flow across the prosthetic AV is the standard to evaluate valve patency. However, a host of variables affect the Doppler data. These include changes in cardiac loading conditions, coexisting lesions that affect forward flow across the valve, or the pressure gradient between the left ventricle and ascending aorta. These include, but are not limited to, left ventricular failure (decreased forward flow), AI (increased forward flow), MR (decrease forward flow), and atrial arrhythmias (reduced LV preload) (Figures 5-34 and 5-35; see also Figure 5-27).

- Peak velocity/gradient
  - Greater than 4 m/s is consistent with significant stenosis.
  - Less than 2 m/s is consistent with insignificant stenosis in absence of low cardiac output (forward flow across the AV).
- Acceleration time is the time from onset of outflow to peak velocity
  - The greater this value the more significant the stenosis
    - Normally less than 100 ms.
- DVI
  - VTI (or V)$_{LVOT}$/VTI (or V)$_{AV}$.
  - A DVI less than 0.3 is considered significant stenosis.
- EOA—continuity equation
  - EOA$_{AV}$ = cross-sectional area (CSA)$_{LVOT}$ × VTI$_{LVOT}$/VTI$_{AV}$.
  - Severity of stenosis may follow definitions put forth for native valve stenosis.
  - Valve areas may be reported directly (EOA) or after being indexed for BSA (iEOA).

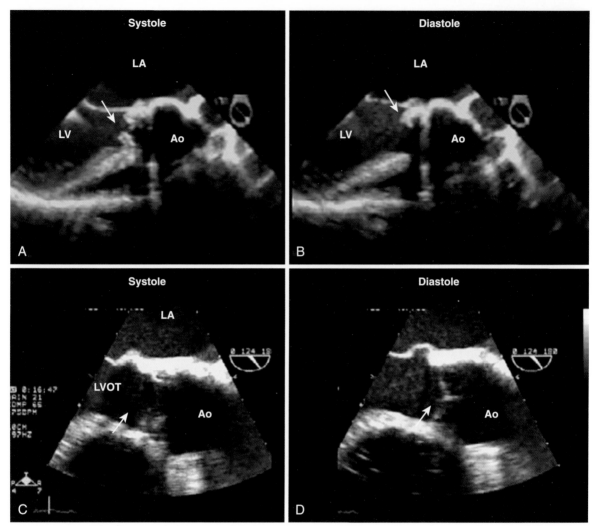

Figure 5-33. Before and after imaging of a stentless valve in the aortic position. Four TE images from the long axis view show a complication of the stentless AV. **A** and **B,** The *arrows* point to the cloth edges, which lay in the outflow tract causing functional stenosis. **C** and **D,** Follow-up at 6 months shows the cloth edges *(arrows)* to have flattened into the LVOT tissues and associated with a reduction in transvalvular pressures and an increase in the calculated EOA. Ao, aorta.

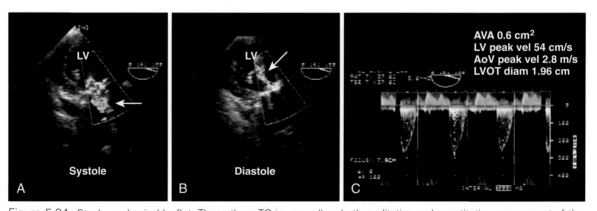

Figure 5-34. Stuck mechanical leaflet. These three TG images allow both qualitative and quantitative assessment of the same patient in Figure 5-32. **A,** Forward flow *(arrow)* is seen across the mobile leaflet. **B,** An abnormal regurgitant jet *(arrow)* coming from the stuck leaflet in the intermediate position. **C,** Significant AV stenosis with an AVA of 0.6 cm^2.

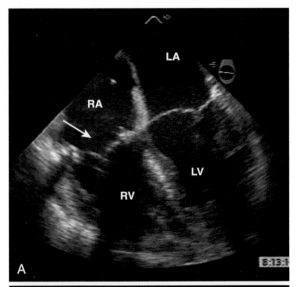

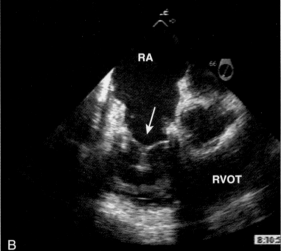

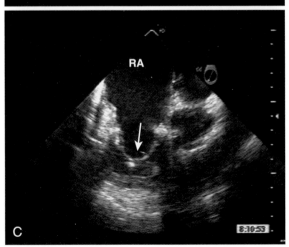

Figure 5-35. Normal bioprosthetic valve in the tricuspid position. Three ME images show a normal-appearing bioprosthetic valve *(arrow)* in the tricuspid position. **A,** The ME window. **B** and **C,** The right ventricular inflow view.

PROSTHETIC TRICUSPID VALVE

KEY POINTS

- Right-sided valve prostheses are less common than left-sided valve prostheses.
- Bioprosthetic valves are more commonly placed.
- Abnormalities of the TV necessitating valve replacement are most commonly the result of left-sided disease.
- Pulmonic valve replacement is most often done in the setting of congenital heart disease.

Before evaluating the prosthetic TV, it is important to know what kind of valve was placed and to have some prior knowledge of how the images should appear.

Step-by-Step Examination

- The 2D examination of the prosthetic TV can be most easily visualized from a number of echocardiographic windows:
  - ME windows from 0 to 150 degrees (Figures 5-35 and 5-36).
    - ME 0-degree window.
    - ME right ventricular inflow-outflow view (60-90 degrees).
    - ME coronary sinus view (100-120 degrees).
  - TG views (0-150 degrees) (Figure 5-37).
    - The lower-degree windows may allow either an apical view of the TV or a short axis view.
    - The higher-degree windows will allow a perpendicular view of the TV as well as views of the cavae.
- The CF, PW, and CW Doppler examinations of the prosthetic TV can be performed from primarily the ME windows because the Doppler beam can be most easily aligned with the direction of blood flow.
  - Imaging from multiple windows will increase the likelihood of detecting abnormal forward and regurgitant jets.

The Echocardiographer Should

- Attempt to identify the sewing ring, the leaflets, and disks.
- Have knowledge and imaging differences between prosthetic valves.

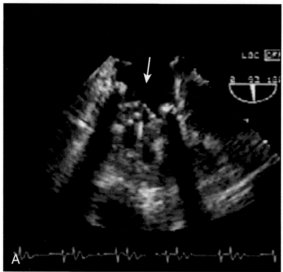

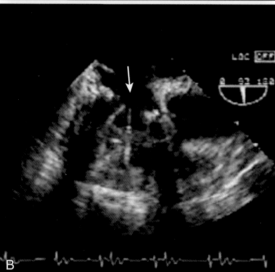

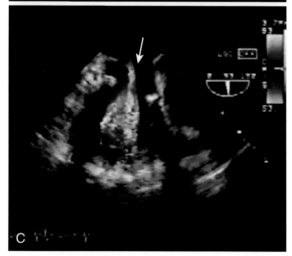

Figure 5-36. Normal mechanical valve in the tricuspid position. Three ME right ventricular inflow images show a normal-appearing mechanical valve *(arrows)* in the tricuspid position. **A,** During systole. **B,** During diastole. **C,** A normal CD flow pattern.

Step 1: Two-Dimensional Examination

The 2D examination involves visualization of the prosthetic valve and its surrounding tissues. The assessment should evaluate valve stability, leaflet motion, and any extraneous mobile structures that may represent suture materials.

- Imaging includes TE and TG imaging.
- The stability of the valve should be determined and whether or not the prosthesis is rocking. As a rule, the prosthetic valve should sit firmly within its surrounding tissue.
- Assessments of the right atrium and ventricle should make note of function and size. In considering the impact of the left heart on the right, assessment of the left heart structures should also be done.

Step 2: Doppler Examination

The Doppler examination includes CF, PW, and CW examinations. The former allows both qualitative and quantitative evaluations including occurrence, direction, and width of normal and abnormal blood flows in and around the prosthetic valve.

- Whereas qualitative imaging includes both TE and TG windows, most of the quantitative assessment is best achieved from the TE windows in which blood flow and the Doppler beam can be best aligned.
- Although qualitative assessments may be turbulent based on CF Doppler aliasing, this may or may not indicate abnormal flow. Further quantitative analysis should be performed to clarify the flow.
- Additional quantitative Doppler may include PW analysis of the caval flows looking for systolic blunting and/or reversal of flow. Assessment of the peak velocity of the tricuspid regurgitant jet allows one to estimate the right ventricular systolic pressure using the Bernoulli equation. This can be used to estimate the pulmonary artery systolic pressure.

Regurgitant Flow: Normal versus Abnormal (Table 5-6)

Prosthetic valves are associated with "normal" or "expected" regurgitant jets. Differentiating between normal and abnormal jets includes both echocardiographic and clinical assessments. The former requires knowledge of normal regurgitant jets associated with each type of prosthesis. The assessment of abnormal prosthetic TR parallels that of native valve assessment and should be distinct from normal regurgitant flows. On the whole, eccentric jets are considered abnormal.

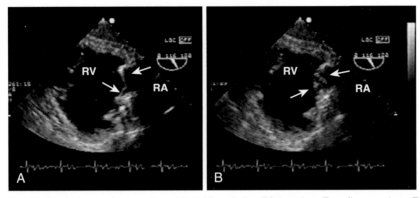

Figure 5-37. Normal mechanical valve in the tricuspid position during TG imaging. Two figures show TG imaging of a normal functional mechanical valve in the tricuspid position. **A,** The *arrows* show the mechanical leaflets during ventricular systole (i.e., closed). **B,** The *arrows* show the valve during ventricular diastole (i.e., open).

TABLE 5-6   ASSESSING PROSTHETIC TRICUSPID VALVE REGURGITATION

Parameter	Normal to Mild	Moderate	Severe
Jet area by color Doppler (cm²)	<5	5-10	>10
Vena contracta width (cm)		<0.7	>0.7
Jet density and contour (CWD)	Incomplete/faint and parabolic	Dense, variable contour	Dense with early peaking
Size of vena cava (cm)	≤1.5 with respiratory variation		>2.0 without respiratory variation
Cava and/or hepatic vein flow (PWD)	Systolic prominence ≥ diastole	Systolic blunting	Systolic blunting or reversal

CWD, continuous wave Doppler; PWD, pulsed wave Doppler.

- Imaging includes both TE and TG windows.
- **Acceptable** regurgitant jets are less than 3 mm.
  - Bioprosthetic valves typically display a central regurgitant jet.
  - Mechanical leaflets display a variety of regurgitant jets depending on the valve type.
  - A bileaflet mechanical valve will usually have two regurgitant jets directed centrally.
  - A single leaflet mechanical valve (or tilting disk valve) will have normal washing jets moving away from the major axis of the disk.
- **Abnormal** regurgitant jets can be either paravalvular or within the prosthetic ring. Paravalvular jets greater than 3 mm are associated with a greater chance of becoming more severe. As a rule, eccentrically directed regurgitant jets are considered abnormal. These abnormal flows can result from a number of causes that affect either the paravalvular space or the mobility of the leaflets:
  - Paravalve.
    - Calcification.
    - Abscess.
    - Dehiscence.
    - Retained native tissues.

- Leaflet pathology.
  - Tears/Trauma.
  - Endocarditis.
- Leaflet restriction/distortion.
  - Stuck leaflet (Figure 5-38).
  - Suture.
  - Thrombus.
  - Pannus.
- **Assessing severity of regurgitant flow** is similar to that for native valve disease and includes assessments of both the prosthetic valve and secondary effects on other cardiac functions, the latter including the left ventricle, atrium, tricuspid artery pressures, and secondary right heart dysfunctions.
  - Valve structure and motion.
    - Stable versus rocking.
  - Right atrium and ventricle.
    - Whereas dilation and dysfunction are consistent with significant TR, it is possible that the chamber adaptations have not yet occurred.
  - Inferior (or superior) vena cava size.
    - Inferior vena cava (IVC) diameter less than 1.5 cm with respiratory variation is considered normal.

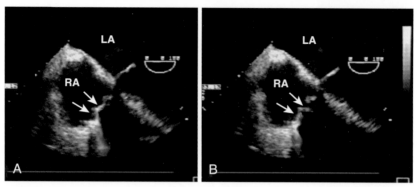

Figure 5-38. Stuck mechanical leaflet in the tricuspid position. These two ME 0-degree images show a stuck mechanical leaflet during both ventricular systole (**A**) and diastole (**B**). The mechanical leaflet closer to the septum appears to be moving. The *arrows* point to each mechanical leaflet. **A** shows both leaflets in the closed position, and **B** shows only one leaflet in the open position.

TABLE 5-7 ASSESSING PROSTHETIC TRICUSPID VALVE STENOSIS		
Parameter	**Normal**	**Abnormal**
Peak velocity (m/s) (CWD)	≤1.7	>1.7
Mean gradient (mm Hg) (CWD)	<5-6	>7
Pressure half time (ms) (CWD)	<200	>230
Size of vena cava (cm)	≤1.5 with respiratory variation	>2.0 without respiratory variation

CWD, continuous wave Doppler.

- IVC diameter between 1.5 and 2.5 is intermediate.
- IVC diameter greater than 2.5 cm with and without respiratory variation is abnormal.
- Extent of regurgitant jet
  - Jet area less than 4 cm² is normal; greater than 8 cm² is abnormal.
- Hepatic or caval venous flows
  - Systolic dominance is normal; systolic blunting or reversal is abnormal.
- Flow convergence (PISA)
  - None is normal; convergence on the right ventricle side is abnormal.
- Jet density and contour
  - Faint/incomplete and parabolic is normal.
  - Dense/complete and early peaking is abnormal.
- Vena contracta (cm)
  - Less than 0.3 cm is considered mild.
  - 0.3 to 0.7 cm is moderate.
  - Greater than 0.7 is severe.

Forward Flow: Normal versus Abnormal (Table 5-7)

Depending on the type of prosthesis, forward blood flow projects in different ways. Whereas bioprosthetic valves have a single forward flow, mechanical valves will have two or three forward projecting jets. The evaluation of forward flow consists of both qualitative (CF Doppler) and quantitative assessments (PW and CW Doppler), the latter consisting of transvalvular pressure gradients and calculation of prosthetic valve area.

- Doppler assessment is performed primarily from the TE windows.

Normal Flows

Normal forward flows for prosthetic valves have been described and involve transvalvular velocities and pressure gradients. There are no validated methods to assess TV area.

- Use of the continuity equation is compromised by the existence of pulmonary valve insufficiency and/or AI depending on which is used as the reference site.
- Calculation of valve area using the PHT and the equation 220/PHT has not been studied for the TV. It is not known whether or not the correction factor of 220 is applicable to the right side of the heart.
- Although there may be a theoretical value in using a dimensionless index such as the VTI_{TV}/VTI_{RVOT}, this has not been validated to date.

Abnormal Flows

There are, however, a constellation of findings that suggest obstruction to flow across the TV. These data are taken from a series of patients with normal valve function.

- Peak E velocity
  - Normal is less than 1.7 m/s.
  - Abnormal is suspected when greater than 1.7 m/s.
- Mean gradient
  - Normal is less than 6 mm Hg.
  - Abnormal is suspected when greater than 6 mm Hg.
- PHT
  - Normal is less than 200 ms.
  - Abnormal is suspected when greater than 230 ms.
- Right atrial and/or right ventricular enlargement is consistent with significant TR.

PROSTHETIC PULMONARY VALVE

Before evaluating the prosthetic PV, it is important to know what kind of valve was placed, and to have some prior knowledge of how the images should appear. The majority of valves are either stented or stentless (xenografts) bioprosthetic valves. There is a lack of data regarding prosthetic valve function in the pulmonic position. Determination of what is normal and abnormal parallels that of normal native valve function (Figures 5-39 and 5-40).

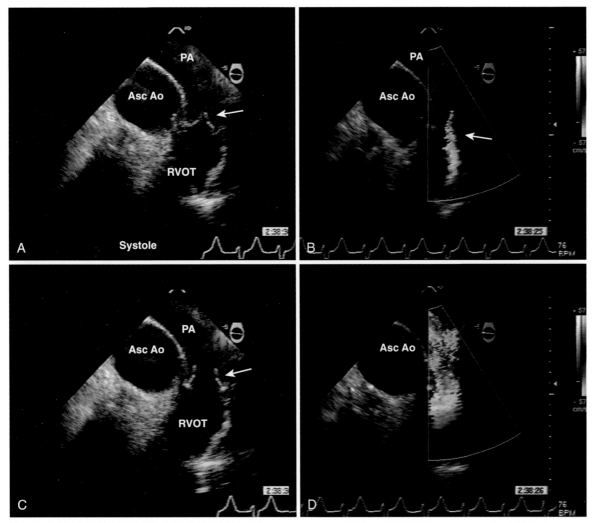

Figure 5-39. Normal bioprosthesis (stentless) in the pulmonary valve position. Four upper esophageal images of the RVOT, pulmonary artery (PA), and PV (*arrows* in **A** and **C**). **A** and **B,** During ventricular diastole. **B,** An acceptable amount of PV insufficiency *(arrow).* **C** and **D,** During ventricular systole, normal PV excursion and flow is demonstrated.

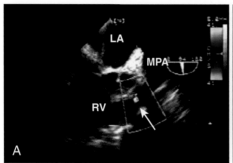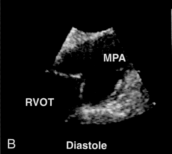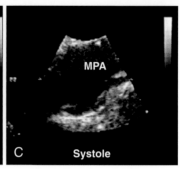

Figure 5-40. Example of epicardial imaging of the PV. These three images demonstrate the potential for imaging artifacts in assessing the PV leaflets during TE imaging (**A**) as well as the potential benefit of epicardial imaging (**B** and **C**), which show the PV during both ventricular systole and diastole. MPA, main pulmonary artery.

Step-by-Step Examination

- Because of its anterior location, and potential for artifact, the prosthetic PV may be difficult to image using TEE. Although not studied, epicardial imaging may prove to be the best modality for intraoperative evaluation.
- As is the case for other valves, assessment of the surrounding heart tissues and functions could suggest prosthetic valve dysfunction (e.g., right heart failure, elevated right ventricular pressures, and/or significant TR).
- Imaging, similar to the prosthetic AV, should include supra- and subvalvular areas.
- The 2D examination of the prosthetic PV can be most easily visualized from a number of echocardiographic windows:
  - ME right ventricular inflow-outflow window at approximately 70 to 100 degrees.
  - Starting from the same ME right ventricular outflow window at approximately 70 to 100 degrees, but with the TEE probe withdrawn from the esophagus and rotated toward the patient's right or the upper esophageal aortic arch short axis view.
  - TG views (100-145 degrees) with a rightward rotation of the TEE probe.
- The CF, PW, and CW Doppler examinations of the prosthetic PV can be performed from images described previously.

The Echocardiographer Should
- Attempt to identify the sewing ring, the leaflets, disks, or other occluder mechanism.
- Recognize limitations of imaging of the prosthetic PV during TEE examination.

- Assess the surrounding heart tissues and functions. These findings may allude to prosthetic valve dysfunction.

Step 1: Two-Dimensional Examination
The 2D examination involves visualization of the prosthetic valve and its surrounding tissues. The assessment should evaluate valve stability, leaflet motion, and note any extraneous mobile structures such as suture materials.
- Imaging includes both TE and TG imaging.
- The stability of the valve should be determined and whether or not the prosthesis is rocking. As a rule, the prosthetic valve should sit firmly within its surrounding tissue.
- The valve leaflets should be visualized and mobility noted.
- Supra- and subvalvular areas should also be interrogated. This is important for cases in which the RVOT was enlarged and/or when a homograft was placed.

Step 2: Doppler Examination
The Doppler examination includes CF, PW, and CW Doppler examinations. The former allows both qualitative and quantitative evaluations including occurrence, direction, and width of normal and abnormal blood flows in and around the prosthetic valve.
- Qualitative and quantitative imaging includes both TE and TG windows as described previously. It is important to view the PV from multiple windows to increase the chance of aligning the ultrasound beam with the direction of blood flow.
- Because right heart flows have lower velocity than their left heart counterparts, it may be necessary to reduce the color scale to highlight turbulent jets that might suggest the presence of abnormal flows.

TABLE 5-8 ASSESSING SEVERITY OF PULMONARY VALVE REGURGITATION

Parameter	Mild	Moderate	Severe
Jet width (% RVOT diameter or annulus) (CFD)	Narrow (≤25%)	Intermediate (26-50%)	Large (>50%)
Jet density (CWD)	Incomplete or faint	Dense	Dense
Pressure half time (CWD)	Slow (>500 ms)	Variable (200-500)	Steep (<200 ms)
Diastolic flow reversal in pulmonary artery (PWD)	Absent or Brief	Present	Present, holodiastolic
Regurgitant fraction (%) (continuity equation)	<30	30-50	>50

CFD, color flow Doppler; CWD, continuous wave Doppler; PWD, pulsed wave Doppler.

Regurgitant Flow: Normal versus Abnormal (Table 5-8)

Prosthetic valves are associated with "normal" or "expected" regurgitant jets. Differentiating between normal and abnormal jets requires knowledge of normal regurgitant jets associated with each type of prosthesis. The assessment of abnormal prosthetic PV regurgitation parallels that of native valve assessment. Most often, a bioprosthetic valve is placed in the pulmonary position; therefore, a small central regurgitant jet should be expected.

- Imaging includes both TE and TG windows.
- **Normal** regurgitant jets for prosthetic valves are known. Vena contractas less than 0.3 cm (3 mm) or jet widths less than 25% of the RVOT width are considered mild and are acceptable.
- **Abnormal regurgitant jets**
  - A wider jet (i.e., >50%) would be considered severe.
  - A jet width of 25% to 50% is considered moderate.
  - As a rule, eccentrically directed regurgitant jets are considered abnormal.
  - Reversal of diastolic flow in the pulmonary artery suggests at least moderate PV insufficiency.
- Abnormal flows can result from a number of causes
  - Paravalve
    - Abscess.
    - Annular calcification.
  - Leaflet pathology
    - Abscess.
    - Tears.
    - Endocarditis.
  - Leaflet restriction. An uncommon cause of PV insufficiency
    - Suture.
    - Thrombus.
    - Pannus.

TABLE 5-9 ASSESSING SEVERITY OF PULMONARY VALVE STENOSIS

Parameter	Mild	Moderate	Severe
Peak velocity (m/s) (CWD)	<3 (<2.5 homograft)	3-4	>4
Mean gradient (mm Hg) (CWD)	<20 (<15 homograft)	20-35	>35

CWD, continuous wave Doppler.

Forward Flow: Normal versus Abnormal (Table 5-9)

The evaluation of forward flow consists of both qualitative (CF Doppler) and quantitative assessments (PW and CW Doppler), the latter consisting of transvalvular pressure gradients and calculation of prosthetic valve area.

Assessment and/or prevention of PV stenosis is important to prevent right ventricular dysfunction, because the right ventricle does not tolerate acute increases in afterload.

- Doppler assessment is performed from the TE and TG windows.
- Normal flows have been described and involve transvalvular velocities, pressure gradients, and valve areas. The latter are usually described as the EOA.
  - There are little data assessing PV area with the continuity equation; therefore, much of the assessment is based on pressure gradients.
- Normal **peak velocity** across the PV is less than 2.5 m/s
  - This may be as high as greater than 3.0 m/s for xenografts.
  - As is the case with other prosthetic valves, flow velocities are affected by variables in addition to the prosthetic valve EOA.

- Normal **mean gradient** across the prosthetic PV is less than 15 mm Hg.
  - This may be as high as 20 mm Hg for xenografts.
- Measurements can be obtained directly using direct needle sticks.
- Findings of right ventricular hypertension, failure, or significant TR may allude to an increase in afterload.

Suggested Readings

1. Zoghbi WA, Enriquez-Sarano M, Foster E, et al. American Society of Echocardiography. Recommendations for evaluation of the severity of native valvular regurgitation with two-dimensional and Doppler echocardiography. *J Am Soc Echocardiogr.* 2003;16: 777-802.
2. Baumgartner H, Jung J, Bermejo J, et al. Echocardiographic assessment of valve stenosis: EAE/ASE recommendation for clinical practice. *J Am Soc Echocardiogr.* 2009;22:1-23.
3. Zoghbi WA, Chambers JB, Dumesnil JG, et al. Recommendations for evaluation of prosthetic valves with echocardiography and Doppler ultrasound. *J Am Soc Echocardiogr.* 2009;22:975-1014.

Three invaluable references in the management of patients with valvular heart disease.

4. Rosenhek R, Binder T, Maurer G, Baumgartner H. Normal values for Doppler echocardiographic assessment of heart valve prostheses. *J Am Soc Echocardiogr.* 2003;16:1116-1127.
An important reference for Doppler values of commonly used prosthetic valves.
5. Goetze S, Brechtken J, Agler DA, et al. In vivo short-term Doppler hemodynamic profiles of 189 Carpentier-Edwards Perimount pericardial bioprosthetic valves in the mitral position. *J Am Soc Echocardiogr.* 2004;17: 981-987.
6. Maslow AD, Haering JM, Heindel S, et al. An evaluation of prosthetic aortic valves using transesophageal echocardiography: the double-envelope technique. *Anesth Analg.* 2000;91:509-516.
An important technique in the Doppler assessment of aortic prosthetic valves using intraoperative TEE.
7. Chafizadeh ER, Zoghbi WA. Doppler echocardiographic assessment of the St. Jude Medical prosthesis valve in the aortic position using the continuity equation. *Circulation.* 1991;83:213-223.
8. Wiseth R, Levang OW, Sande E, et al. Hemodynamic evaluation by Doppler echocardiography of small (less than or equal to 21 mm) prostheses and bioprostheses in the aortic valve position. *Am J Cardiol.* 1992;70:240-246.

Ventricular Function

Wendy L. Pabich, Alina Nicoara, and Madhav Swaminathan

6

OVERVIEW

- The pump performance of the left (LV) and right (RV) ventricles is defined by their ability to eject (systolic performance) and relax and fill (diastolic performance).
- Evaluation of cardiac function with transesophageal echocardiography (TEE) is strongly indicated in cardiac surgery and is also seeing expanded utility outside of the operating room in both the intensive care units and emergency departments.
- When evaluating ventricular function in the perioperative period, changes in preload, pacing, respirations, and performance are dynamic and are affected significantly by the physiologic changes seen in the operating room.

LEFT VENTRICULAR SYSTOLIC FUNCTION

Background

Coronary Anatomy and Left Ventricular Wall Segmentation

- The left anterior descending (LAD) artery arises from the left main coronary artery and supplies the anterior wall and anterior septum.
- The left circumflex (LCX) artery arises from the left main coronary artery and supplies the lateral wall (Figure 6-1).
- The LV is divided into 17 segments for better characterization of wall motion and thickening. There are 6 segments at the basal and midpapillary levels, 4 segments each at the apex and the apical cap (Figure 6-2).
- Normal wall motion is defined as greater than 30% excursion of the endocardial border and 30% to 50% thickening (see Video 6-1 on the Expert Consult website).

Left Ventricular Anatomy: Wall Thickness and Size

- Normal values for left ventricular (LV) wall thickness are 0.6 to 1.0 cm in men and 0.6 to 0.9 cm in women. Measurements are best made of the septum and inferior walls at end-diastole (Figure 6-3).
- LV size is dependent upon patient size, but typical LV diastolic diameter is 3.9 to 5.3 cm in women and 4.2 to 5.9 cm in men.
- The LV is bullet-shaped and contracts in a twisting motion with the base and apex rotating in opposite directions.

Left Ventricular Ejection Fraction

- Left ventricular ejection fraction (LVEF) is a measure of contractility and can be calculated using LV systolic and diastolic volumes.
- LVEF depends upon preload and afterload.
- Normal LVEF is equal to or greater than 55%.
- LV systolic dysfunction exists when the ejection fraction (EF) is less than 55% and can be graded as mild (45-54%), moderate (30-44%), or severe (<30%) impairment.

Pathophysiology

- Wall motion and thickening are graded as normal, hypokinetic, akinetic (negligible thickening), dyskinetic (paradoxical systolic motion), or aneurysmal (diastolic deformation).
- Wall motion abnormalities (WMAs) can be either segmental or global and are most often due to decreased perfusion in the corresponding arterial distribution.
- Ventricular pacing can cause abnormal septal motion and WMAs may be difficult to assess, particularly in the perioperative period (see Videos 6-2, 6-3, and 6-4 on the Expert Consult website).
- LV function can also be affected by the long-term effects of valvular disease, particularly lesions that result in LV volume or pressure overload, such as aortic stenosis, aortic regurgitation (AR), and mitral regurgitation (MR; Figure 6-4).

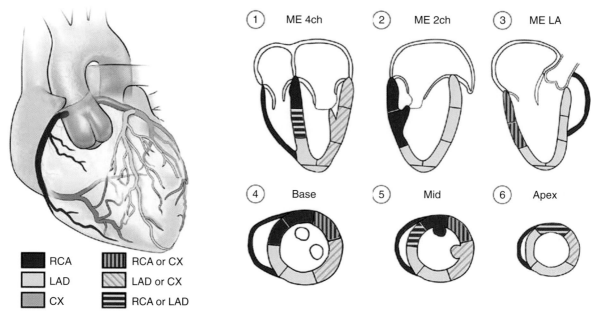

Figure 6-1. Typical distributions of the RCA, the LAD, and the LCX coronary arteries. *Modified with permission from Lang RM, Bierig M, Devereux RB, et al; Chamber Quantification Writing Group; American Society of Echocardiography's Guidelines and Standards Committee; European Association of Echocardiography. Recommendations for chamber quantification: A report from the American Society of Echocardiography's Guidelines and Standards Committee and the Chamber Quantification Writing Group, developed in conjunction with the European Association of Echocardiography, a branch of the European Society of Cardiology. J Am Soc Echocardiogr. 2005;18:1440-1463.*

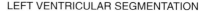

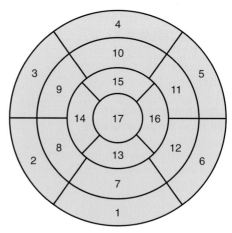

Figure 6-2. Display, on a circumferential polar plot, of the 17 myocardial segments and the recommended nomenclature for tomographic imaging of the heart. *Modified from American Society of Nuclear Cardiology. Imaging guidelines for nuclear cardiology procedures, part 2. J Nucl Cardiol. 1999;6:G47–G84.*

1. Basal anterior
2. Basal anteroseptal
3. Basal inferoseptal
4. Basal inferior
5. Basal inferolateral
6. Basal anterolateral

7. Mid anterior
8. Mid anteroseptal
9. Mid inferoseptal
10. Mid inferior
11. Mid inferolateral
12. Mid anterolateral

13. Apical anterior
14. Apical septal
15. Apical inferior
16. Apical lateral
17. Apex

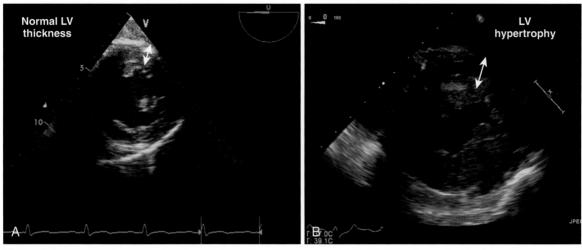

Figure 6-3. TG mid SAX views of the LV in a patient with normal LV thickness (**A**) and in a patient with LVH (**B**). Measurements of the inferoseptal wall of the LV are shown.

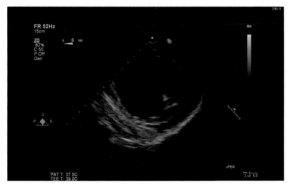

Figure 6-4. TG mid SAX view of the LV in a patient with severe aortic insufficiency and dilatation of the LV cavity. A reasonable estimate of LV cavity dimensions can be made in this view considering the depth of view (15 cm) and the 1-cm markings on the cursor to the *left* of the display.

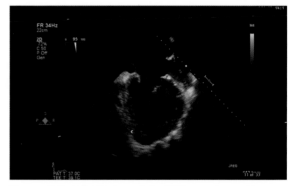

Figure 6-5. ME 2C view of the LV in a patient with dilatation of the LV cavity. A reasonable estimate of LV cavity dimensions can be made in this view considering the depth of view (22 cm) and the 1-cm markings on the cursor to the *right* of the display.

Left Ventricular Hypertrophy

- *Concentric* hypertrophy is ventricular wall thickening as a compensatory response to chronic LV pressure overload (e.g., hypertension and aortic stenosis).
  - Elevated intracavitary pressures.
  - Reduced compliance.
- *Eccentric* hypertrophy results from chronic volume overload (e.g., aortic insufficiency).

Cardiomyopathies

- Cardiomyopathies can affect ventricular function and can result from chronic ischemic, valvular, or intrinsic myocardial disease.
- Dilated cardiomyopathy may be ischemic or nonischemic in nature (Figure 6-5).
- Tako-Tsubo cardiomyopathy is associated with specific septal ballooning.
- Peripartum cardiomyopathy.

- Hypertrophic obstructive cardiomyopathy (HOCM)
  1. Familial inheritance with risk of sudden death.
  2. Characterized by dynamic obstruction.
  3. Worsened by hypovolemia or administration of inotropes and chronotropes.
  4. Septal hypertrophy results in left ventricular outflow tract (LVOT) obstruction and elevated LVOT gradients.
  5. Patients are at risk for systolic anterior motion (SAM) of the anterior leaflet of the mitral valve (MV) and MR (Figure 6-6; and see Video 6-5 on the Expert Consult website).
- Restrictive cardiomyopathy
  1. Restrictive cardiomyopathy can be difficult to distinguish from constrictive pericardial disease (see "Left Ventricular Diastolic Function").

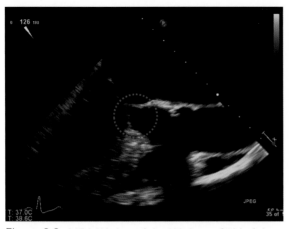

Figure 6-6. ME LAX view of the LV shows SAM of the anterior mitral leaflet *(circle)* in a patient with HOCM.

2. Infiltrative disorders such as amyloidosis, sarcoidosis, and carcinoid disease frequently lead to restrictive cardiomyopathy.

Overview of Echocardiographic Approach

Table 6-1 presents an evaluation of LV systolic function.

Anatomic Imaging

An orderly sequence of image acquisition ensures that all views will be obtained. A suggested approach is to start with the midesophageal (ME) views, progress to the transgastric (TG) views, and

TABLE 6-1   EVALUATION OF LEFT VENTRICULAR SYSTOLIC FUNCTION

TEE View	What to Look For	Imaging Modality	Measurements Possible
ME 4C	EF Segmental wall motion analysis Volume status LVH Septal hypertrophy	2D	Chamber dimensions Simpson's method of disks Systolic strain/strain rate
		Doppler	dP/dT (MR jet) Tissue Doppler MV annulus Doppler strain
ME 2C	EF Segmental wall motion analysis LVH	2D	Chamber dimensions Simpson's method of disks Systolic strain/strain rate
		Doppler	dP/dT (MR jet)
ME LAX	EF Segmental wall motion analysis LVOT obstruction/SAM LVH Septal hypertrophy	2D	Septal thickness Chamber dimensions Systolic strain/strain rate
		Doppler	dP/dT (MR jet)
TG SAX	EF Segmental wall motion analysis Volume status LVH	2D	Wall thickness Chamber dimensions Systolic strain/strain rate
		M-mode	Wall thickness Chamber dimensions
TG LAX	EF Segmental wall motion analysis	2D	Chamber dimensions
		M-mode	Chamber dimensions
DEEP TG LAX	EF	Doppler	CO (LVOT PW Doppler)
3D	Ejection fraction Segmental wall motion analysis	3D full-volume data set	Tissue velocity Timing strain/rate

EF, ejection fraction; 4C, four-chamber; LAX, long axis; LVH, left ventricular hypertrophy; LVOT, left ventricular outflow tract; ME, midesophageal; MR, mitral regurgitation; MV, mitral valve; PW, pulsed wave; SAM, systolic anterior motion; SAX, short axis; TEE, transesophageal echocardiography; TG, transgastric; 2C, two-chamber; 2D, two-dimensional; 3D, three-dimensional.

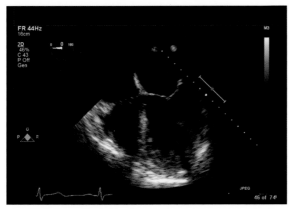

Figure 6-7. ME 4C view of the LV with the multiplane scan angle at 0 degrees.

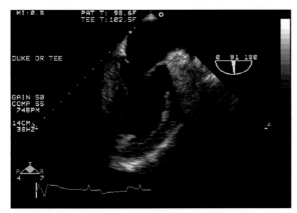

Figure 6-8. ME 2C view of the LV with the multiplane scan angle at approximately 90 degrees.

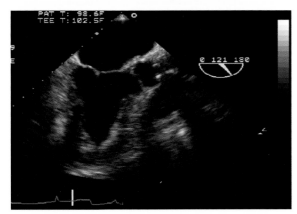

Figure 6-9. ME LAX view of the LV with the multiplane scan angle at approximately 120 degrees.

conclude with three-dimensional (3D) image acquisition.

Acquisition

- ME four-chamber (ME 4C) (Figure 6-7).
- ME two-chamber (ME 2C) (Figure 6-8).
- ME long axis (ME LAX) (Figure 6-9).

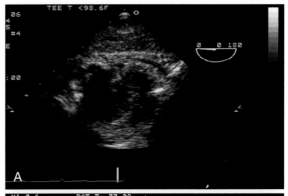

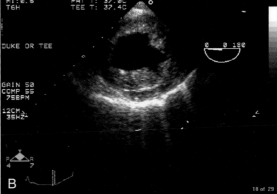

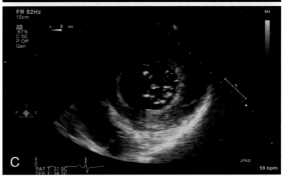

Figure 6-10. TG SAX views of the LV with the multiplane scan angle at 0 degrees at the apical (**A**), mid (**B**), and basal (**C**) levels.

- TG short axis (TG SAX) at the apex, midpapillary, and basal levels (Figure 6-10).
- TG long axis (TG LAX 2C) (Figure 6-11).
- Deep TG (TG DEEP) (Figure 6-12).
- 3D ME 4C, focusing on the left side (Figure 6-13).

Analysis
Dimensions
- Chamber dimensions
  - The LV chamber can be quantified by measuring the LV length (major diameter) in ME 2C and diameter (minor diameter) in ME 2C and TG LAX (Figure 6-14).

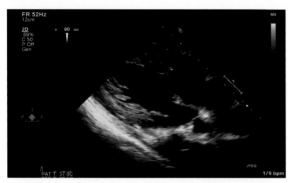

Figure 6-11. TG 2C view of the LV with the scan angle rotated to 90 degrees.

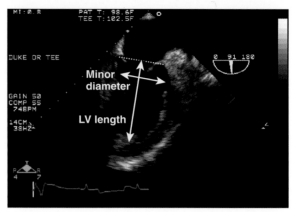

Figure 6-14. ME 2C view of the LV demonstrates the LV length (major) and the minor diameter measurements.

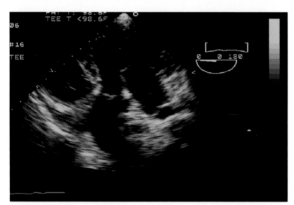

Figure 6-12. Deep TG LAX view of the LV with the scan angle at 0 degrees and the probe tip anteflexed.

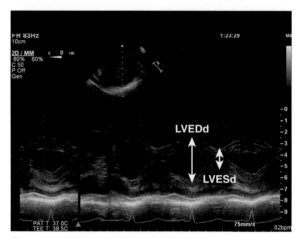

Figure 6-15. TG mid SAX of the LV with the M-mode cursor directed perpendicularly across the image. Measurements are shown of the LVEDd and LVESd, respectively, from one endocardial border to the other.

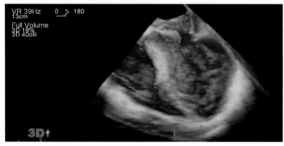

Figure 6-13. 3D image of the LV acquired using the ME 4C view as the reference 2D image.

- Wall thickness
  - Septal and inferior wall thicknesses are best measured in the midpapillary TG SAX view. Normal wall thickness is less than 1 cm (see Figure 6-3).

Ejection Fraction Linear Measurement
- Fractional shortening (FS) (%) = [(left ventricular end-diastolic dimension [LVEDd] − left ventricular end-systolic dimension [LVESd])/LVEDd] × 100.

- LV internal dimensions at end-diastole and end-systole are measured from endocardial border to endocardial border with M-mode at a TG SAX view just above the papillary muscles (Figure 6-15).
- Superior temporal resolution of M-mode allows for more accurate identification of endocardial borders.
- FS is not accurate in patients with marked regional differences such as WMA or aneurysms.
- Normal FS is defined as 27% to 45% in women and 25% to 43% in men.

Ejection Fraction Area Measurement
- Fractional area of change FAC (%) = [(left ventricular area in end-diastole [LVAd] − LV area in end-systole [LVAs])/LVAd] × 100

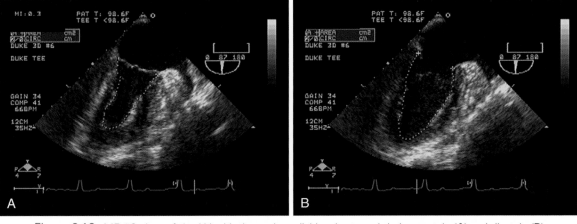

Figure 6-16. ME 2C view of the LV with the endocardial border traced during systole (**A**) and diastole (**B**).

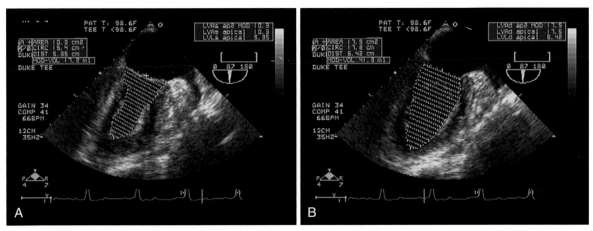

Figure 6-17. ME 2C view of the LV with internal volume measured using Simpson's method of disks during systole (**A**) and diastole (**B**).

- LV cavity area is measured via manual tracing of the endocardial border to assess area at end-diastole and end-systole in the TG SAX or TG LAX views.
- The papillary muscles should be ignored when estimating the chamber area.
- FAS provides an improved estimate over linear measurements, because information regarding septal and lateral ventricular walls is taken into account.
- Normal FAC is 59% to 65% in women and 56% to 62% in men.

Ejection Fraction Volumetric Measurements
- LVEF = [(left ventricular end-diastolic volume [LVEDV] – left ventricular end-systolic volume [LVESV])/LVEDV] × 100%
- Biplane: LV systolic and diastolic volume estimation utilizing the endocardial border.

- Volume is calculated from the manually traced endocardial border in the ME 4C and ME 2C views (Figure 6-16).
- Assumes a symmetrically shaped LV.
- Simpson's method of disks calculates diastolic and systolic volume from a summation of stacked elliptical disks.
  - Measured in the ME 4C and ME 2C views (Figure 6-17).
  - Endocardial border detection may be improved using automated software, enhanced tissue harmonics, or contrast-based LV opacification.

Ejection Fraction Three-Dimensional Measurement
- Involves construction of a ventricular model based upon endocardial border detection.
- Typically a 3D data set is best obtained from an ME 4C view (Figure 6-18).

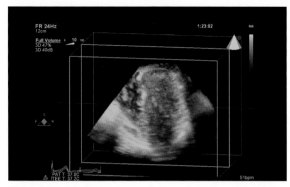

Figure 6-18. Image of a 3D full-volume data set of the LV acquired using the ME 4C view as the reference 2D image. The default setting ensures that the 3D image displayed reflects the reference 2D image.

- 3D modeling may be performed using specific 3D software at the time of acquisition or off-line when the images are reviewed (Figure 6-19).
- 3D imaging accounts for regional abnormalities, yielding more accurate stroke volumes (SVs) than two-dimensional (2D) analysis (see Videos 6-6 and 6-7 on the Expert Consult website).
- Problems associated with foreshortening in 2D can be avoided with 3D imaging.

KEY POINTS: PITFALLS

- Identification of the LV endocardial borders can be difficult, particularly with shadowing of the ventricular walls secondary to calcification, prosthetic valve artifact, air, and other factors. This can make estimates of LVEF inaccurate.
- Linear LV measurements may be inaccurate if there are regional WMAs because they evaluate only two opposing walls in one imaging plane.
- Volumetric calculations involve geometric assumptions of the shape of the LV. This may be inaccurate with regional WMAs and aneurysms.
- Foreshortening of the LV apex is common in 2D imaging, which may result in underestimations of LV dimensions, volume, and EF.
- High-quality 2D images are necessary to generate a usable 3D data set. Suboptimal 2D imaging can lead to inaccurate 3D calculations.
- Ventricular function may be more difficult to interpret in the patient with dysrhythmias that cause variability in SV, such as atrial fibrillation.
- Acquisition of full-volume 3D data sets requires minimal translational motion, electrocautery interference, or irregular rhythms. These can be difficult to avoid in the perioperative setting.

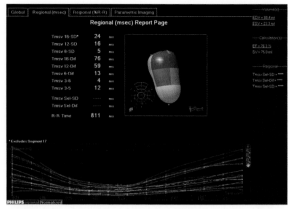

Figure 6-19. Image of a 3D full-volume analysis of the LV using 3D advanced quantification software. Detailed segmental analysis is obtained for wall motion, volume, and timing of contractility.

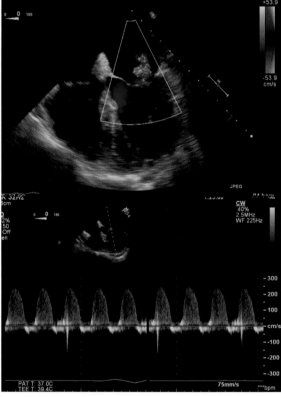

Figure 6-20. **Top,** ME 4C view with color flow Doppler across the MV shows a regurgitant jet. **Bottom,** CW spectral Doppler tracing across the MV shows high-velocity systolic waveforms consistent with MR.

Physiologic Data

Acquisition

- ME 4C continuous wave (CW) Doppler of MR jet for dP/dT. (Figure 6-20).
- TG DEEP or TG LAX pulsed wave (PW) Doppler of the LVOT velocity time

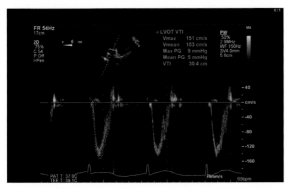

Figure 6-21. PW spectral Doppler across the LVOT shows a tracing (VTI) for calculating the LV SV.

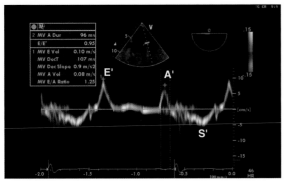

Figure 6-22. Spectral recording of tissue velocity of the lateral mitral annulus using TDI in the ME 4C view. Diastolic velocities (E' and A') and timings (deceleration time and slope) measurements are shown.

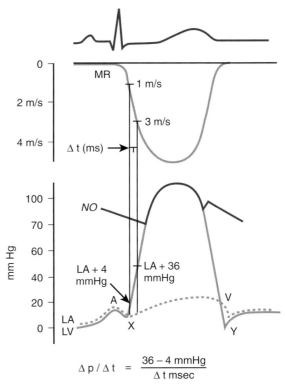

$$\Delta p / \Delta t = \frac{36 - 4 \text{ mmHg}}{\Delta t \text{ msec}}$$

Figure 6-23. Pressure tracing diagram. *From Pai RG, Bansal RC, Shah PM. Doppler-derived rate of left ventricular pressure rise. Its correlation with the postoperative left ventricular function in mitral regurgitation. Circulation. 1990;82:514-520.*

integral (VTI) for cardiac output (CO; Figure 6-21).

- ME 4C tissue Doppler imaging (TDI) PW Doppler of lateral mitral annulus peak systolic velocity (Figure 6-22).

Analysis
Rate of Rise in Left Ventricle Pressure (dP/dT)

- The rate of rise in LV pressure is well correlated with systolic function and can be measured using the rate of rise in velocity of the MR jet (Figure 6-23).
- The MR jet is interrogated using CW Doppler and the time interval between velocities of 1 and 3 m/s is measured (Figure 6-24).
- The pressure differential can be calculated by converting the measured velocities into pressures using the simplified Bernoulli equation.

dP = pressure gradient at 3 m/s – pressure gradient at 1 m/s

$$= 4(v_{3m/s})^2 - 4(v_{1m/s})^2$$

dT = time interval in seconds

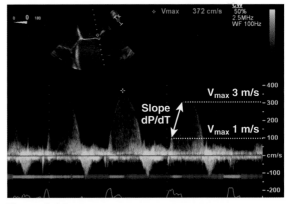

Figure 6-24. Spectral recording of CW Doppler interrogation of an MR jet in the ME 4C view shows the measurement of dP/dT on the MR jet waveform from 1 to 3 m/s.

- Normal dP/dT values are greater than 1000 mm Hg/s.

Cardiac Output

- SV (in mL or cm^3) can be calculated by measuring flow through a known cross-sectional area (CSA).
- Although SV can be theoretically measured anywhere, the most common site for

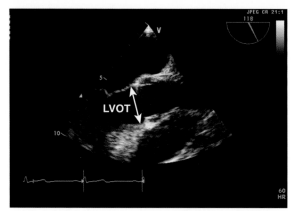

Figure 6-25. ME aortic LAX view shows the location of measurement of the LVOT.

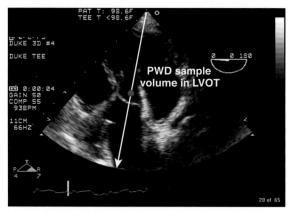

Figure 6-26. Deep TG LAX view with a PW Doppler sample volume shown located in the LVOT for measurement of the VTI at the level of the LVOT.

measurement is the relatively cylindrical LVOT, just below the aortic valve (Figure 6-25).

- CSA (in cm^2) is measured utilizing LVOT diameter obtained in the ME LAX view, assuming that the CSA is a circle.

$$CSA_{LVOT} = 3.14(d_{LVOT}/2)^2$$

- Flow through the LVOT is measured using range-specific PW Doppler, obtaining a sample velocity over time. The distance traveled by blood through the cylindrical LVOT in a single beat is measured in centimeters and known as the VTI (Figure 6-26):

$$SV\ (cm^3) = CSA\ (cm^2) \times VTI\ (cm)$$

- CO can be calculated by multiplying the SV by the heart rate (HR).

$$CO\ (L/min) = [SV\ (mL) \times HR\ (beats/min)]/1000$$

- Cardiac index (CI) can be calculated by factoring in the patient's body surface area (BSA in m^2). A normal cardiac index is greater than 2 L/min/m^2.

Tissue Doppler Imaging of the Mitral Annulus

- Lateral mitral annular motion is measured using PW Doppler.
- Myocardial velocities are much lower than the velocities of blood flow, and adjustments to the sector width may be necessary to achieve high frame rates.
- Measurement is less dependent of loading conditions.
- Velocities are measured in the ME 4C and ME 2C views (see Figure 6-22).
- Velocities are age- and gender-dependent, but globally normal LV systolic function is associated with velocities greater than 7.5 cm/s. Velocities less than 5.5 cm/s are seen in LV impairment.

Strain/Strain Rate and Speckle Tracking

- Strain (ε) is the change of length of an object divided by its original length.
- Positive strain indicates lengthening and negative strain indicates shortening.
- Myocardial strain occurs in three dimensions: longitudinal, circumferential, and radial.
- During systole, there is negative strain in the longitudinal and circumferential dimensions and positive strain in the radial dimension.
- Strain rate is the change of strain over time (Δε/Δt).
- TDI of the mitral annulus in the ME 4C view can be used to assess strain and strain rate. Specialized software is necessary to calculate strain and strain rate.
- 2D speckle tracking can be used in place of TDI as a means of assessing strain and is not dependent upon the angle of interrogation like tissue Doppler. Specialized software is necessary for speckle tracking and may not be available on all ultrasound machines.

KEY POINTS: PITFALLS

- CO and dP/dT are load-dependent and can vary widely as a result.
- Measurements of velocities will be underestimated if the angle of Doppler interrogation is not parallel to motion/flow, giving falsely low estimations of ventricular function.
- Inaccurate 2D measurements of LVOT diameter will grossly impair the ability to calculate an accurate CO, particularly because this measurement is squared.
- dP/dT can be performed only if there is MR.
- TDI of the mitral annulus is difficult in the presence of mitral annular calcification or prosthetic valve.

Alternate Approaches— When Transesophageal Echocardiography Is Insufficient

- Visual estimation of LVEF and WMA using 2D images can be a quick method to roughly assess ventricular function. The reliability of this method may improve with observer experience, although it is still subject to interobserver variability.
- Echocardiographic assessment of LV systolic function can always be correlated with other modalities (cardiac magnetic resonance imaging [MRI], cardiac catheterization, left ventriculogram, or pulmonary artery [PA] catheterization).

Figure 6-27 presents an LV assessment flow chart.

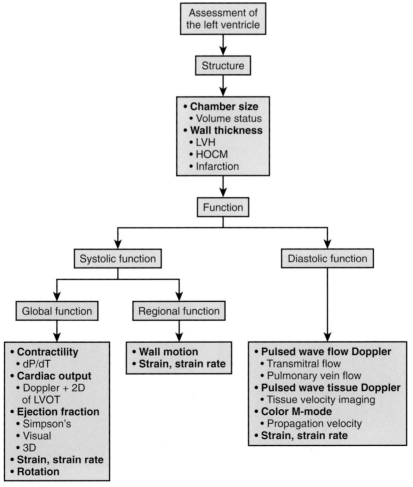

Figure 6-27. LV assessment flow chart.

RIGHT VENTRICULAR SYSTOLIC FUNCTION

Background

Coronary Anatomy and Right Ventricular Wall Motion

- The RV is primarily supplied by the right coronary artery (RCA). A small portion of the anterior free wall may be supplied by a branch of the LAD (see Figure 6-1).
- The posterior descending artery (PDA) supplies the RV, the inferior wall and the posterior third of the septum.
- In the majority of the population, the PDA arises from the RCA and the coronary circulation is termed *right dominant coronary circulation.*
- If the PDA extends off the LCX artery, the circulation is known as *left dominant coronary circulation.*
- The RV medial wall is composed of the ventricular septum, and its function is evaluated as part of the LV.
- The RV free wall can be divided into basal, mid, and apical segments.
- Systolic function is assessed solely by endocardial excursion. The typical RV wall is too thin to evaluate wall thickening.
- Normal wall motion is defined as greater than 30% excursion of the endocardial border (see Video 6-8 on the Expert Consult website).

Right Ventricular Anatomy

- The RV is asymmetrically crescent shaped. The chamber is composed of the ventricular septum and the RV free wall (Figure 6-28).
- Trabeculae carnae line most of the RV chamber.

- The moderator band is a prominent muscular trabeculation that divides the right ventricular (RV) inflow and outflow tracts and is often easily visible on TEE (Figure 6-29).
- Owing to its irregular shape, multiple views may be necessary to assess RV chamber size.

Right Ventricular Ejection Fraction

- Right ventricular ejection fraction (RVEF) is a measure of contractility and can be calculated using RV systolic and diastolic volumes.
- RVEF depends upon preload and afterload.
- RV systolic function is typically graded qualitatively as normal, mildly reduced, moderately reduced, or severely reduced.
- Typically, RV systolic function is graded in comparison with LV systolic function.
- Normal RVEF is equal to or greater than 55%.

Pathophysiology

Wall Motion

- WMAs can be either segmental or global and are most often caused by decreased perfusion in the corresponding arterial distribution.
- Wall motion is graded as normal, hypokinetic, akinetic, dyskinetic (paradoxical systolic motion), or aneurysmal (diastolic deformation) (see Video 6-9 on the Expert Consult website).
- RV wall motion is more afterload dependent than LV wall motion and prone to dysfunction with elevated PA pressures.
- The RV is particularly prone to perioperative ischemia for the following reasons:
  - Retrograde cardioplegia delivery intraoperatively may be inadequate to protect the RV.

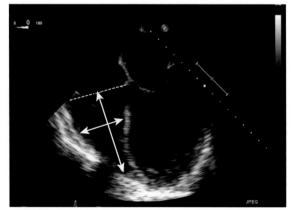

Figure 6-28. ME 4C view of the RV with the major *(vertical arrow)* and minor *(horizontal arrow)* axes indicated.

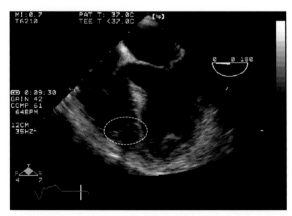

Figure 6-29. ME 4C view with a moderator band *(circle)* in the RV.

- Intracardiac air will preferentially enter the RCA given the anterior position of the right coronary ostium in the supine patient (see Video 6-4 on the companion website).
  - The anterior position of the RV makes it more susceptible to warming intraoperatively from surgical lights and ambient air.
- Significant RV infarction may be accompanied by inferior LV wall infarction as well, given the shared coronary perfusion.
- Other signs of RV infarction include right atrium (RA) enlargement, increased central venous pressure (CVP), RV dilation, tricuspid regurgitation (TR), paradoxical ventricular septal motion, and right-to-left shunting in the presence of a patent foramen ovale.
- RV function can also be affected by the long-term effects of pulmonary and valvular disease, particularly lesions that result in RV volume or pressure overload, such as pulmonic stenosis, pulmonary hypertension, pulmonary valve insufficiency, and TR.

Right Ventricular Dilatation
- The RV is a thin-walled volume-pumping chamber that is extremely sensitive to increases in afterload, which frequently result in systolic dysfunction.
- RV dilation typically is the result of volume overload but can also occur with pressure overload.
- RV CSA is typically 60% of LV cross-sectional area at end-diastole.
- RV dilation can be quantified as mild (60-100% LV size), moderate (equal to LV size), and severe (>LV size) (Figure 6-30).

- The LV typically forms the apex of the heart. However, with RV dilation, the apex includes the RV (Figure 6-31).

Right Ventricular Hypertrophy
- Right ventricular hypertrophy (RVH) may indicate pulmonic stenosis (PS) or elevated PA pressures. Trabeculae are more prominent when RVH is present.
- RV free wall hypertrophy occurs before septal hypertrophy (Figure 6-32).

Interventricular Septum
- Flattening of the septum is a characteristic feature of RV dysfunction. The septum normally functions as part of the LV and has a convex curvature in regards to the RV chamber.
- Septal flattening will occur at different times in the cardiac cycle, dependent upon whether the RV is volume or pressure overloaded (Figure 6-33; and see Video 6-10 on the Expert Consult website).
  - RV volume overload
    - Septal flattening in end-diastole during peak RV overfilling.
    - Septum resumes the normal convex shape during systole, and the neighboring LV appears circular.
  - RV pressure overload
    - Septal flattening in end-systole during peak RV afterloading and the neighboring LV chamber appears D-shaped rather than circular.
    - Septum may appear more normal during diastolic filling.
- Conduction abnormalities, ventricular pacing, previous surgery, and pericardial disease can also cause abnormal ventricular septal motion.

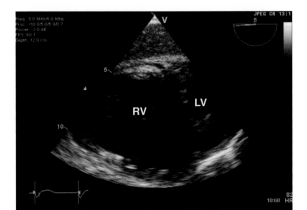

Figure 6-30. TG mid SAX view of a dilated and severely hypokinetic RV. The LV is seen to the right of the image and is smaller in comparison.

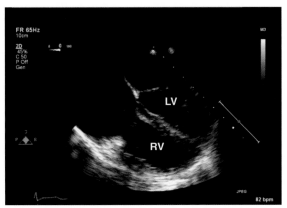

Figure 6-31. ME 4C view of a dilated RV that forms a part of the cardiac apex. The LV is seen to the right of the image.

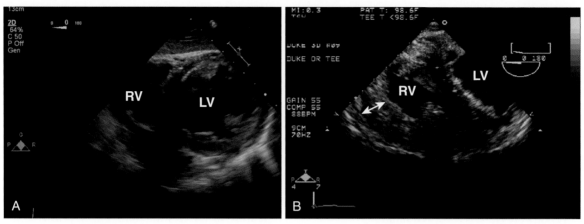

Figure 6-32. TG mid SAX view demonstrates a normal-sized RV (**A**) and a severely hypertrophied RV (**B**). The thickness of the RV is indicated by the *double-sided arrow*. The LV can be seen adjacent to the RV in each panel.

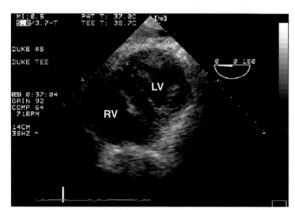

Figure 6-33. TG mid SAX view in a patient with high RV systolic pressures demonstrates flattening of the septum at systole.

Figure 6-34. ME 4C view obtained with the scan plane at 0 degrees.

Overview of Echocardiographic Approach

Table 6-2 presents an evaluation of RV systolic function.

Anatomic Imaging

As with the LV images, it is important to maintain an orderly acquisition sequence. A suggested approach is to start with the ME views, progress to the TG views, and conclude with 3D image acquisition.

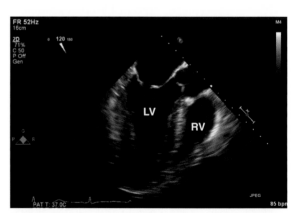

Figure 6-35. ME LAX view obtained with the scan angle rotated to 120 degrees.

Acquisition

- ME 4C (Figure 6-34).
- ME LAX (Figure 6-35).
- ME RV inflow-outflow (Figure 6-36).
- ME bicaval (Figure 6-37).
- TG SAX at the midpapillary and basal levels (Figure 6-38).

- TG LAX (Figure 6-39).
- TG DEEP (Figure 6-40).
- Upper esophageal aortic arch short axis (UE aortic arch SAX) (Figure 6-41).
- 3D ME 4C focusing on right side (Figure 6-42).

TABLE 6-2 EVALUATION OF RIGHT VENTRICULAR SYSTOLIC FUNCTION

TEE View	What to Look For	Imaging Modality	Measurements Possible
ME 4C	EF Wall motion analysis Chamber size Septal motion RVH TR	2D	Wall thickness Chamber dimensions TV annular plane excursion
		Doppler	Tissue Doppler TV annulus
ME LAX	Chamber size RVH	2D	RVOT dimension
Modified ME bicaval	EF Wall motion analysis TR	2D	Chamber dimensions
		Doppler	dP/dT (TR jet) RVSP (TR maximum velocity)
ME RV inflow-outflow	Wall motion analysis RVH TR	2D	RVOT dimension Wall thickness
		Doppler	dP/dT (TR jet) RVSP (TR maximum velocity) CO (RVOT PW Doppler)
TG SAX (RV outflow)	EF Wall motion analysis Chamber size Septal motion	2D	Wall thickness Chamber dimensions
		Doppler	CO (RVOT PW Doppler)
TG RV inflow	EF Wall motion analysis Chamber size	2D	Wall thickness Chamber dimensions
Deep TG LAX	EF	2D	Wall thickness Chamber dimensions
		Doppler	dP/dT (TR jet)
UE aortic arch SAX		2D	RVOT diameter
		Doppler	CO (RVOT PW Doppler)
3D	EF Segmental wall motion analysis	3D full-volume data set	EF

CO, cardiac output; EF, ejection fraction; 4C, four-chamber; LAX, long axis; ME, midesophageal; PW, pulsed wave; RV, right ventricular; RVH, right ventricular hypertrophy; RVOT, right ventricular outflow tract; RVSP, right ventricular systolic pressure; SAX, short axis; TEE, transesophageal echocardiography; TG, transgastric; TR, tricuspid regurgitation; TV, tricuspid valve; 2D, two-dimensional; 3D, three-dimensional; UE, upper esophageal.

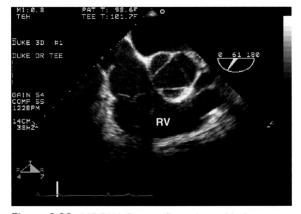

Figure 6-36. ME RV inflow-outflow view with the scan angle rotated to 61 degrees.

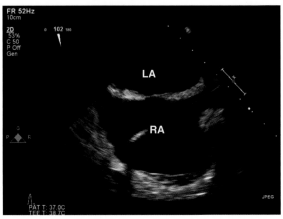

Figure 6-37. ME bicaval view with the scan plane rotated to 102 degrees.

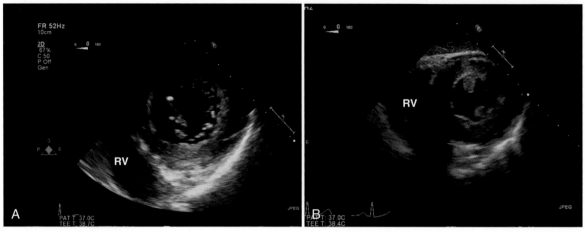

Figure 6-38. TG SAX views at the basal (**A**) and midpapillary (**B**) levels obtained with the probe in the stomach and the scan angle at 0 degrees.

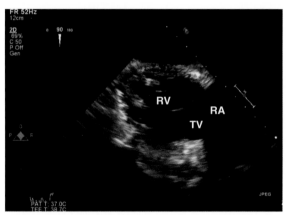

Figure 6-39. TG RV inflow view obtained with the probe in the stomach at the midpapillary level with the scan angle rotated to 90 degrees and manually turned to the right.

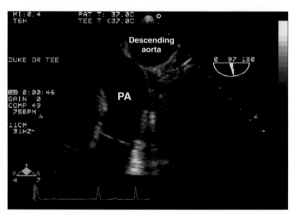

Figure 6-41. UE aortic arch SAX view with the scan angle rotated to 97 degrees.

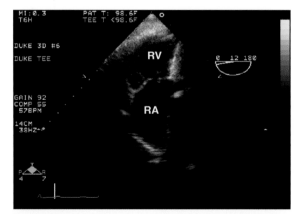

Figure 6-40. Deep TG view with the probe deep in the stomach at 12 degrees, anteflexed and manually turned to the right to obtain a view of the RV. The RA is seen in the lower part of the image.

Analysis
Chamber Dimensions

- The RV chamber can be quantified by measuring the RV major and minor diameters in ME 4C. Normal dimensions are 3.5 cm ± 0.2 and 2.8 cm ± 0.2, respectively (see Figure 6-28).
- Normal RV diastolic area ranges from 11 to 28 cm^3 and normal RV systolic area ranges from 7.5 to 16 cm^3.

Wall Thickness

- Normal RV wall thickness is less than 0.5 cm.
- Measurement is best made of the free wall at end diastole.
- Free wall thickness greater than 1 cm may be present with severe pulmonary hypertension.

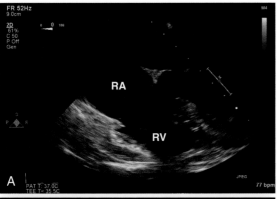

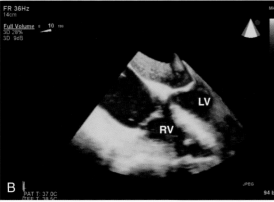

Figure 6-42. **A,** ME 4C view focusing on right side, obtained with the probe at the midesophagus at 0 degrees, manually turned toward the right. **B,** 3D acquisition data set in the ME 4C view, focusing on the right side.

- Trabeculae carnae will also be more prominent if RVH is present.

Ejection Fraction

- Area measurement

$$FAC\ (\%) = [(\text{right ventricle area in end-diastole [RVAd]} - \text{right ventricle area in end-systole [RVAs]})/RVAd] \times 100$$

  - RV cavity area is measured via manual tracing of the endocardial border to assess area at end-diastole and end-systole in the TG SAX or TG RV inflow views.
  - Papillary muscles should be ignored when estimating the chamber area.
- Volumetric measurements

$$RVEF = [(\text{right ventricular end-diastolic volume [RVEDV]} - \text{right ventricular end-systolic volume [RVESV]})/RVEDV] \times 100\%$$

  - Biplane
    - RV systolic and diastolic volume estimation utilizing the endocardial border. Volume is calculated from the manually traced endocardial border in the ME 4C view.

- Simpson's method of disks may be used, although this technique has not been validated.
  - As with the LV, endocardial border detection of the RV may be improved using automated software, tissue harmonic imaging, or contrast-based RV opacification.
- Tricuspid annular plane systolic excursion (TAPSE)
  - Apical to basal shortening of the lateral annulus of the tricuspid valve (TV) is measured as an assessment of global RV function (Figure 6-43; see Videos 6-11 and 6-12 on the Expert Consult website)
  - Normal TAPSE is 1.5 to 2 cm.
  - TDI may be used to quantify TAPSE.
- 3D estimation of EF
  - 3D EF analysis involves construction of a ventricular model based upon endocardial border detection. Typically, a 3D data set is best obtained from an ME 4C view (see Figure 6-42B).
  - 3D modeling may be performed using specific 3D software at the time of acquisition or off-line when the images are reviewed (see Videos 6-13 and 6-14 on the Expert Consult website).
  - 3D imaging accounts for regional abnormalities, yielding more accurate SVs than 2D analysis.
  - Problems associated with foreshortening in 2D can be avoided with 3D imaging.

KEY POINTS: PITFALLS

- The irregular shape of the RV makes quantification of RVEF difficult. Therefore, qualitative methods are more commonly used.
- Ventricular function may be more difficult to interpret in the patient with dysrhythmias that cause variability in SV, such as atrial fibrillation.
- Identification of the RV endocardial borders can be difficult, particularly with shadowing of the ventricular walls secondary to calcification, prosthetic valve artifact, intracardiac catheters, air, and other factors. This can make estimates of RVEF inaccurate.
- High-quality 2D images are necessary to generate a usable 3D data set. Suboptimal 2D imaging can lead to inaccurate 3D calculations.
- Acquisition of full-volume 3D data sets require minimal translational motion, electrocautery interference, or irregular rhythms. These can be difficult to avoid in the perioperative setting.

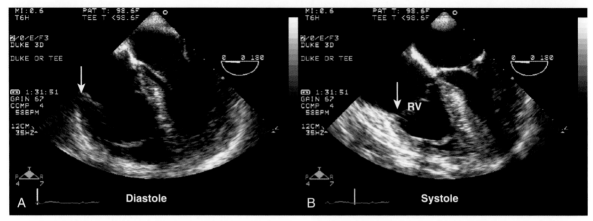

Figure 6-43. ME 4C view of the RV with the tricuspid annulus *(arrow)* indicated in diastole (**A**) and systole (**B**).

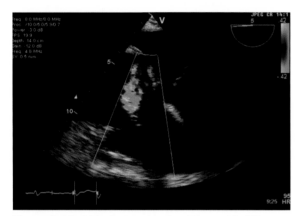

Figure 6-44. ME 4C view shows a TR jet with CW Doppler.

Physiologic Data
Acquisition
- ME 4C or ME RV inflow-outflow views for CW Doppler of TR jet for dP/dT (Figures 6-44 and 6-45).
- ME RV inflow-outflow or UE aortic arch SAX for PW Doppler of RVOT flow to calculate right-sided CO (Figure 6-46).
- TG of the liver for PW Doppler of hepatic venous flow (Figure 6-47).

Analysis
- Rate of rise in RV pressure (dP/dT)
  - The rate of rise in RV pressure is well correlated with systolic function and can be measured using the rate of rise in velocity of the TR jet.
  - The TR jet is interrogated using CW Doppler and the time interval between velocities of 1 and 2 m/s is measured (in contrast to the 1–3 m/s time interval used with LV dP/dT assessment from the MR jet).

- The pressure differential can be calculated by converting the measured velocities into pressures using the simplified Bernoulli equation.

  dP = pressure gradient at 2 m/s − pressure gradient at 1 m/s

  $$= 4(v_{2m/s})^2 - 4(v_{1m/s})^2$$

  dT = time interval in seconds

- Normal dP/dT values are greater than 1000 mm Hg/s.
- CO
  - As with the LV, SV (in mL or cm^3) of the RV can be calculated by measuring flow through a known CSA.
  - Although SV can be theoretically measured anywhere, the most common site for measurement is the relatively cylindrical RVOT.
  - CSA (in cm^2) can be measured utilizing RVOT diameter obtained in the ME RV inflow-outflow or the UE aortic arch SAX views, assuming that the CSA is circular.

  $$CSA_{RVOT} = 3.14(d_{RVOT}/2)^2 \text{ or } CSA_{PA}$$
  $$= 3.14(d_{PA}/2)^2$$

- Flow through the RVOT is measured using PW Doppler, obtaining a sample velocity over time. The distance traveled by blood in a single beat is measured in centimeters and known as the VTI (Figure 6-48).

  $$SV (cm^3) = CSA (cm^2) \times VTI (cm)$$

- Right-sided CO can be calculated by multiplying the SV by the HR:

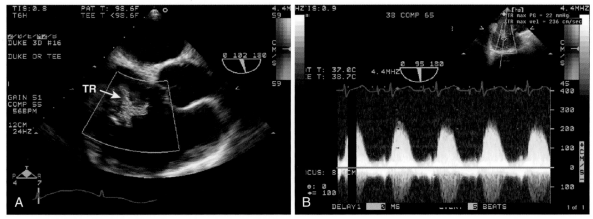

Figure 6-45. **A,** Modified ME bicaval view with color flow Doppler shows a TR jet. **B,** CW Doppler interrogation of the TR jet.

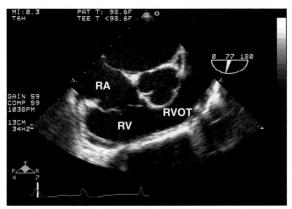

Figure 6-46. ME RV inflow-outflow view with the scan plane at 77 degrees shows RVOT.

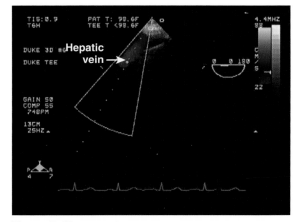

Figure 6-47. View of the hepatic vein adjacent to the IVC with the probe in the lower esophageal position, rotated toward the right, following the path of the IVC from the right atrial-IVC junction in the 4C view. The PW Doppler sample volume is shown placed in the hepatic vein. Color flow Doppler is helpful in identifying flow within the hepatic vein.

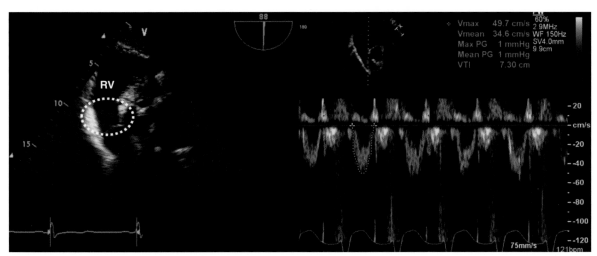

Figure 6-48. TG deep view with RVOT PW Doppler.

$$CO \ (L/min) = [SV \ (mL) \times HR \ (beats/min)]/1000$$

- Right-sided CI can be calculated by factoring in the patient's BSA (in m^2). A normal CI is greater than 2 $L/min/m^2$.
- Calculation of right-sided CO may be particularly beneficial when intracardiac shunts are present and pulmonary flow is greater than systemic flow (Qp/Qs > 1).
- Right ventricular systolic pressure (RVSP)
  - The pressure gradient between the RV and the RA is first calculated using the simplified Bernoulli equation and the maximum velocity of the TR jet (see Figure 6-45).

$$\Delta P_{RV-RA} = 4(TR \ jet)^2$$

  - The RSVP can be calculated if right atrial (RA) pressure is known.

$$RVSP = \Delta P_{RV-RA} + Ra \ pressure \ (CVP)$$

  - In absence of PS or RVOT obstruction, RVSP and PA systolic pressure are equivalent.
- Hepatic venous flow may be used to assess global RV function
  - Impaired RV systolic function can result in blunting of systolic inflow and augmentation of diastolic inflow, but this must be differentiated from elevated RA pressures for other reasons.
  - Severe TR results in reversal of systolic hepatic venous flow, and this may be seen with severe RV systolic dysfunction (Figure 6-49).

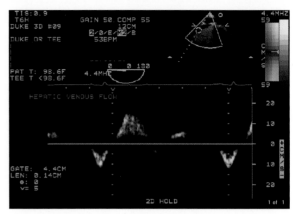

Figure 6-49. PW spectral Doppler image of hepatic venous flow shows systolic flow reversal.

---

method may improve with observer experience, although it is still subject to interobserver variability.
- Echocardiographic assessment of RV systolic function can always be correlated with other modalities, and this may be valuable when echocardiographic images are unavailable or of insufficient quality.
- Cardiac MRI estimation of RVEF and right-sided cardiac catheterization estimation of RVEF.
- RV function can also be assessed with central venous catheters and measured pressures.
- Filling pressures (right ventricular end-diastolic pressures [RVEDPs]) as measured with CVPs. Elevated filling pressures are indicative of impaired RV systolic function.

KEY POINTS: PITFALLS

- The RV is particularly load dependent, and wide variation in CO and dP/dT can be seen with differences in afterload.
- dP/dT and RVSP can be calculated only if there is TR.
- Measurements of velocities will be underestimated if the angle of Doppler interrogation is not parallel to motion/flow, giving falsely low estimations of ventricular function.
- Inaccurate 2D measurements of RVOT diameter will grossly impair the ability to calculate an accurate right-sided CO, particularly because this measurement is squared in the equation.

Alternate Approaches

- Visual estimation of RVEF and WMA using 2D images can be a quick method to roughly assess systolic function. The reliability of this

---

KEY POINTS

- RV dilatation is present when the apex is formed by the RV.
- The RV is more sensitive to increases in afterload than the LV.
- The RV is generally assessed qualitatively and compared with LV function.
- Abnormal ventricular septal motion can be seen with either volume or pressure overload, and the bowing of the septum during the cardiac cycle can offer clues to the etiology.
- TR may be an indicator of systolic RV dysfunction, particularly with hepatic venous flow reversal.

Figure 6-50 is a flow chart for the RV.

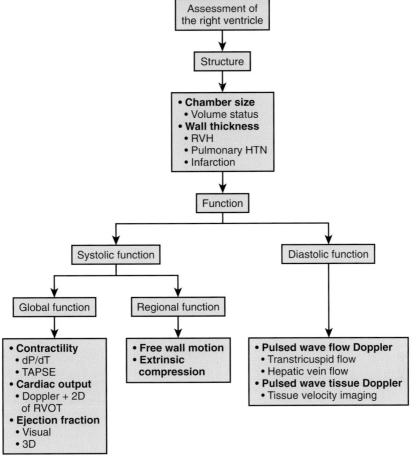

Figure 6-50. RV assessment flow chart. HTN, hypertension.

LEFT VENTRICULAR DIASTOLIC FUNCTION

Background

- The pump performance of the LV depends on its ability not only to eject and empty (systolic performance) but also to relax and fill (diastolic performance).
- Diastolic dysfunction is common and often severe, even when silent.
- When symptomatic, its clinical presentation may be attributed to other conditions; therefore, diastolic dysfunction may remain undiagnosed or ignored because symptoms may mimic other conditions.
- Diastolic heart failure may occur in isolation with a normal EF and is also known as heart failure with a normal ejection fraction (HFNEF).
- Concentric left ventricular hypertrophy (LVH) frequently coexists with diastolic dysfunction.

- Echocardiography has emerged over the past two decades as a reliable and relatively noninvasive method of evaluating LV diastolic function and filling pressures.
- The treatment of intraoperative diastolic heart failure per se is limited to rate reduction, which can be challenging in the immediate postoperative period.

Physiology of Diastole

- The classic approach is to divide diastole into four phases (Figure 6-51):
  - Isovolumetric relaxation extends from aortic valve (AV) closure to MV opening. During this phase, LV pressure steadily declines without a change in volume.
  - Early filling begins with the opening of the MV. Most of the diastolic filling occurs during this phase in healthy subjects and is the result of the pressure gradient between the left atrium (LA) and the LV at the opening of the MV.

TABLE 6-3   DIASTOLIC DETERMINANTS*

Diastolic Function Determinant	Intrinsic Factors	Extrinsic Factors
LV relaxation	Synchrony of cardiac contraction Velocity of cardiac contraction Duration of systole Stored energy during systole (elastic recoil) Calcium homeostasis Cytoskeleton alterations Neurohormonal activation (sympathetic nervous system, renin-angiotensin-aldosterone)	Arterial impedance Preload
LV compliance	Fibrillar collagen (amount, geometry, distribution, type) Myocardial fibrosis, scar, or hypertrophy Chamber geometry Neurohormonal activation	Hemodynamic load (preload and afterload) Pericardium (effusions, constriction) Ventricular interdependence (e.g., RV dilatation)

*Other determinants of diastolic function are heart rate, mitral valve area, LA function.
LA, left atrial; LV, left ventricular; RV, right ventricular.

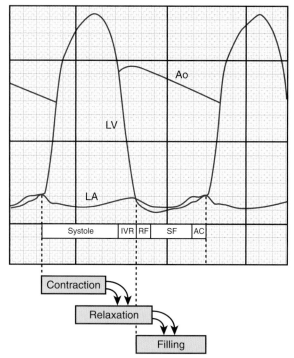

Figure 6-51. In the classic system, the diastole is divided in four phases: isovolumic relaxation (IVR), rapid filling (RF), diastasis or slow filling (SF), and atrial contraction (AC). A more simplified approach divides cardiac cycle in three phases: contraction, relaxation, and filling. The schematic also represents the pressure tracings in the aorta (Ao), LV, and LA.

- Diastasis or slow filling occurs during the midportion of diastole when the pressures between the LA and the LV equilibrate and the flow across the MV ceases.
- Atrial contraction results in a second pressure gradient between the LA and the

LV, leading to late LV filling. In young healthy individuals, atrial contraction may usually contribute up to 20% of the LV filling.
- A simplified approach divides the cardiac cycle into three phases: contraction, relaxation, and diastolic filling. Of note is that LV relaxation begins before the closure of the AV and continues into the early filling phase of diastole.

Physiologic Determinants of Diastolic Function
Left Ventricle Relaxation
- The process during which the myocardium returns to its initial resting length and tension.
- This begins during midsystole and continues throughout the first third of diastole.
- It is dependent on the reuptake of the cytosolic calcium into the sarcoplasmic reticulum (SR), which is an active process, requiring energy accomplished by the SR calcium pump.

Left Ventricle Compliance
- Described as the passive properties of the LV during diastolic filling.
- It is defined as the change in pressure over the change in volume ($\Delta P/\Delta V$) (Table 6-3)

Pathophysiology
The pathophysiology of diastolic dysfunction is primarily described in terms of LV filling patterns (Table 6-4).

TABLE 6-4　GRADING OF LEFT VENTRICULAR DIASTOLIC FUNCTION

Grade of Diastolic Dysfunction	Underlying Mechanism	Pathophysiology
Grade I (impaired relaxation)	Impaired LV relaxation	Decreased early transmitral pressure gradient Decreased LV filling during early filling phase Compensatory increased LV filling during atrial contraction
Grade II (pseudonormal)	Impaired LV relaxation Elevated LA pressure	"Pseudonormal" early transmitral pressure gradient Improved LV filling during early filling phase "Pseudonormalization" of diastolic filling pattern Elevated LA pressure
Grade III (restrictive)	Impaired LV relaxation Decreased LV compliance Highly elevated LV filling pressures	Elevated early transmitral pressure gradient Limited LV filling at high blood velocities Elevated LV filling pressures

LA, left atrial; LV, left ventricular.

TABLE 6-5　EVALUATION OF LEFT VENTRICULAR DIASTOLIC FUNCTION

Echocardiographic Method	Measurements	Comments
Transmitral flow (TMF) (Figure 6-52)	IVRT	Depends on LV relaxation, LA pressure
	Early filling peak velocity (E wave)	Reflects LV-LA pressure gradient in early diastole Depends on LV relaxation, LV compliance
	E wave DT	Depends on LV compliance
	Late filling deceleration time (A-wave)	Depends on LV compliance, LA function
	A-wave duration	Useful in assessment of filling pressures
Pulmonary vein flow (PVF) (Figure 6-53)	Peak systolic flow velocity (S-wave)	May have two components S1 and S2 Depends on LA relaxation, pulmonary vein flow
	Peak diastolic flow velocity (D-wave)	Depends on LV relaxation, LV compliance
	Peak atrial reversal flow velocity (AR wave)	Depends on LA function, LA compliance, LV compliance
	AR wave duration (ARdur)	Useful in assessing filling pressures
Tissue Doppler imaging (TDI) (Figure 6-54)	Early diastolic velocity (E' wave)	Corresponds to the E-wave of TMF Measures myocardial velocities at lateral or septal mitral annulus
	Late diastolic velocity (A' wave)	Corresponds to the A-wave of the TMF
	Systolic velocity (S' wave)	Due to mitral annulus descent during LV systole
Propagation velocity (Vp) (Figure 6-55)	Vp	Measures velocities along a scan line from the mitral annulus to LV apex Correlates well with LV relaxation

DT, deceleration time; IVRT, isovolumic relaxation time; LA, left atrial; LV, left ventricular.

Overview of Echocardiographic Approach (Table 6-5)

Anatomic Imaging

- Anatomic imaging is an integral part of diastolic function evaluation by providing information on LA size, LV size and wall thickness, LV systolic function, and valvular and pericardial pathology.
- LVH is a common reason for impaired diastolic function
  - Concentric LVH occurs in situations of pressure overload (hypertension, aortic valve stenosis).

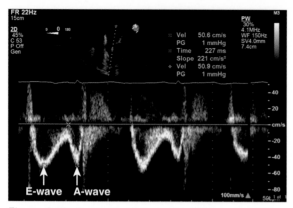

Figure 6-52. Transmitral inflow. The PW Doppler TMF velocity profile shows two distinct waveforms below the baseline-early filling peak velocity (E-wave) and late filling peak velocity (A-wave).

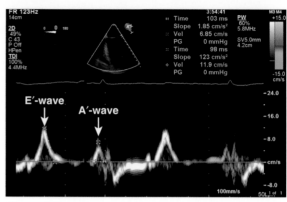

Figure 6-54. Myocardial velocity. The spectral Doppler tissue velocity profile shows an upward motion in early diastole, marking the E' wave, followed by a late diastolic A' wave due to atrial contraction.

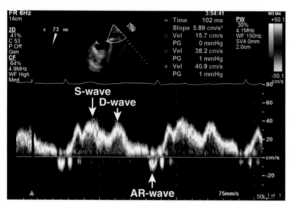

Figure 6-53. Pulmonary vein (PV) flow. The PW Doppler PV velocity profile shows three distinct waveforms. There is a forward flow in systole (S-wave) followed by an early forward diastolic flow (D-wave) into the LA. In late diastole, atrial contraction results in a reversed flow (AR) into the PV.

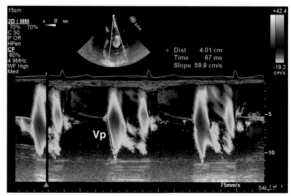

Figure 6-55. Myocardial propagation velocity (Vp), normal profile.

- Eccentric LVH occurs in situations of volume overload (regurgitant valvular lesions, depressed systolic function).
- In the absence of primary atrial pathology or valvular disease, LA enlargement may be a marker of the chronicity and severity of diastolic dysfunction and a sign of chronic elevation of atrial pressure.

Physiologic Data
Acquisition
- Transmitral inflow (TMF) is obtained by employing PW Doppler in the ME 4C view (Figure 6-56).
- Isovolumic relaxation time (IVRT) is obtained by employing CW Doppler in the TG deep LAX view (Figure 6-57).
- Pulmonary venous flow is obtained by employing PW Doppler in the left or

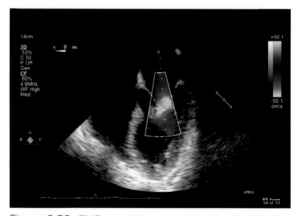

Figure 6-56. TMF velocities are obtained in the ME 4C view by employing PW Doppler and placing the sample volume at the level of the tips of the MV leaflets. Color flow Doppler of the blood flow through the MV may be helpful in better aligning the ultrasound beam with the blood flow.

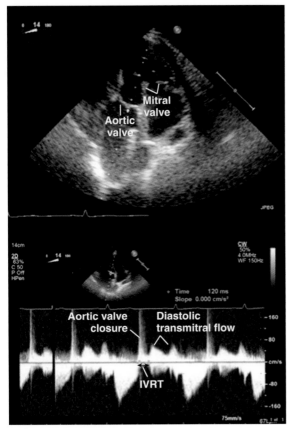

Figure 6-57. IVRT is the time interval between aortic valve closure and MV opening. It is usually recorded in the deep TG LAX view by employing CW Doppler **(top panel)**. The ultrasound beam aligned with the blood flow across the aortic valve will also intercept the blood flow across the MV resulting in the spectral Doppler velocity display shown in the **bottom panel.**

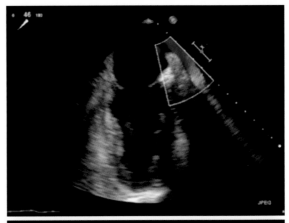

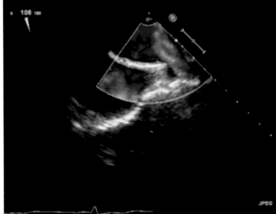

Figure 6-58. The PV Doppler flow velocity profile can be obtained by PW Doppler interrogation of the blood flow in the PVs with the sample volume placed 1 to 2 cm from the opening of the PV in the LA. Both the left upper **(top)** and the right upper **(bottom)** PVs can be interrogated, because they lie almost parallel with the ultrasound beam.

right upper pulmonary veins (PVs; Figure 6-58).

- Myocardial velocity TDI is obtained by employing PW Doppler in the ME 4C view with the TDI function of the TEE machine activated (Figure 6-59).
- Propagation velocity (Vp) is obtained by employing M-mode and CF Doppler in the ME 4C view (Figure 6-60).

Analysis (Tables 6-6 and 6-7)

- Estimation of LV filling pressure
  - AR velocity greater than 35 cm/s, and AR duration greater than A duration by more than 30 ms are indicative of a left ventricular end-diastolic pressure (LVEDP) greater than 15 mm Hg, regardless of the systolic function.
  - An E/E′ ratio greater than 15 is highly specific for LA pressures higher than

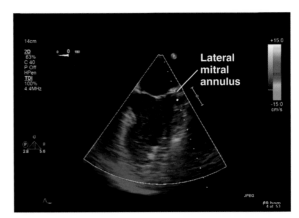

Figure 6-59. The myocardial velocities of the mitral annulus can be recorded with TDI by placing the PW Doppler sample gate at the level of the lateral or septal mitral annulus in the ME 4C view. Minimal angulation should be present between the ultrasound beam and the plane of cardiac motion.

TABLE 6-6   GRADING OF DIASTOLIC FUNCTION*

Grade Diastolic Dysfunction	TMF	PVF	TDI	Vp
Grade I (impaired relaxation) Composite image	↓ E velocity ↑ A velocity ↑ E wave DT ↓ E/A	S < D Normal AR velocity Normal AR duration	↓ E' velocity Normal E/E'	↓ Vp
Grade II* (pseudonormal) Composite image	Normal E velocity Normal DT Normal E/A	S > D ↑ AR velocity AR duration > A duration	↓ E' velocity ↑ E/E' ratio	↓ Vp
Grade III (restrictive) Composite image	↑↑ E velocity ↓ A velocity ↓↓ DT ↑↑ E/A	S >> D ↑ AR velocity AR duration > A duration	↓ E' velocity ↑ E/E' ratio	↓ Vp

*The "pseudonormal" pattern can be differentiated from the normal pattern by reducing the preload and LA pressure, which will unmask the underlying, altered relaxation by changing the pseudonormal pattern to an impaired relaxation pattern.

AR, aortic regurgitation; DT, deceleration time; LA, left atrial; PVF, pulmonary venous flow; TDI, tissue Doppler imaging; TMF, transmitral inflow; Vp, propagation velocity.

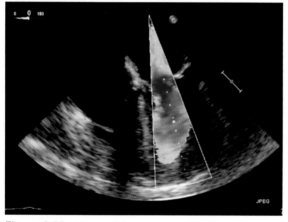

Figure 6-60. Myocardial propagation velocity is obtained in the ME 4C view. A narrow color sector map extending from the mitral annulus to the LV apex is selected and the M-mode cursor is aligned with the mitral inflow. The color scale baseline is reduced to about 20 cm/s in order to enable visualization of the first aliasing velocity. Vp is measured by drawing a line from the mitral annulus at the first aliasing velocity during early filling to 4 cm distally toward the LV apex.

15 mm Hg and a ratio of less than 8 is highly specific for normal LA pressures.
- E/Vp ratio greater than 2.5 predicts a pulmonary capillary wedge pressure greater than 15 mm Hg.

Pitfalls
- TMF velocities are highly dependent on age, HR, and loading conditions.
- With aging, there is a gradual decline in the rate of myocardial relaxation resulting in reduced early LV filling and increased contribution of the atrial contraction to LV filling (E < A).
- Tachycardia results in an increase in the A-wave velocity and fusion of the E- and A-waves, because atrial contraction occurs before early filling is complete.
- Associated valvular lesions can affect measurements of diastolic function.
  - Severe MR may result in a restrictive TMF pattern in the absence of diastolic dysfunction and in the blunting or reversal of the PV S-wave.
  - Severe acute aortic insufficiency may lead to a restrictive TMF pattern due to a rapid increase in LV pressure.
  - Mitral stenosis increases TMF velocities and causes a fusion of the E- and A-waves, with an increase in deceleration time (DT).
  - E' velocity is reduced in patients with mitral annular calcifications, mitral stenosis, mitral annuloplasty, or prosthetic MVs.
- E' may not reflect accurately LV relaxation when there are WMAs in the basal segments of the septal and lateral LV walls.

Alternative Approaches
- Emerging technologies for evaluation of diastolic function include speckle tracking rotation, "untwist" parameters, and more sensitive techniques for discerning subtle diastolic abnormalities.

TABLE 6-7   QUANTITATIVE GRADING OF LEFT VENTRICULAR DIASTOLIC FUNCTION

Echocardiographic Method	Normal	Grade I Impaired relaxation	Grade II Pseudonormal	Grade III Restrictive filling
TMF				
E/A	1–2	<0.8	0.8-1.5	≥2
DT (ms)	150–220	>200	150–220	<160
IVRT (ms)	60–100	>100	>100	<60
PVF				
PV-S/PV-D	>1	>1	<1	<1
PV-AR (cm/s)	<35	<35	>35	>35
ARdur – Adur	<30	<30	>30	>30
Vp	>55	<45	<45	<45
E'	>8 (septal) >10 (lateral)	>8 (septal) >10 (lateral)	<8 (septal) <10 (lateral)	<8 (septal) <10 (lateral)
E/E'	<8 (septal) <8 (lateral)	<8 (septal) <8 (lateral)	9-12 (average)	>15 (septal) >12 (lateral)

DT, deceleration time; IVRT, isovolumic relaxation time; PV-AR, pulmonary vein, aortic regurgitation; PV-D, pulmonary vein, diastolic; PVF, pulmonary venous flow; PV-S, pulmonary vein, systolic; TMF, transmitral inflow; Vp, propagation velocity.

KEY POINTS

- Diastolic dysfunction is a common condition with a high risk of acute decompensation during the perioperative period due to tachyarrhythmias, ischemia, and fluctuating loading conditions.
- Echocardiographic methods that can be used to evaluate diastolic function perioperatively include
  - PW Doppler of TMF and PVs.
  - TDI of the mitral annulus.
  - Color M-mode of Vp.
- Assessment of diastolic dysfunction should be integrated into a comprehensive 2D examination.

- RV diastolic filling time is slightly shorter than LV diastolic filling time and the larger tricuspid annulus results in lower maximal velocities.
- RV diastolic function patterns have been investigated in various diseases including heart failure, chronic obstructive pulmonary disease with pulmonary hypertension, and restrictive cardiomyopathy.
- RV and LV diastolic dysfunction are associated with difficult separation from cardiopulmonary bypass.

RIGHT VENTRICULAR DIASTOLIC FUNCTION

Background

- There is still little information regarding RV diastolic function and numerous gaps remain in our understanding.

Overview of Echocardiographic Approach (Table 6-8)

Anatomic Imaging

- 2D imaging is useful in the evaluation of pathology associated with diastolic dysfunction: RV volume and mass, RVH, and cardiomyopathy.
- During normal breathing, the inferior vena cava (IVC) diameter and diameter variation (collapsibility index) can be used to estimate

TABLE 6-8   EVALUATION OF RIGHT VENTRICULAR DIASTOLIC FUNCTION

Echocardiographic Method	Measurements	Comments
TTF (Figure 6-61)	Early filling peak velocity (E-wave)	Flow velocities may vary during spontaneous respiration by 20%. They increase during inspiration and decrease during expiration. Positive-pressure ventilation may have the opposite effect in comparison with spontaneous ventilation

Continued

TABLE 6-8 EVALUATION OF RIGHT VENTRICULAR DIASTOLIC FUNCTION—cont'd

Echocardiographic Method	Measurements	Comments
	E-wave DT Late filling peak velocity (A-wave) A-wave duration	
HVF (Figure 6-62)	Antegrade systolic flow (S-wave)	Influenced by TV annular motion, RA relaxation, and TR
	Retrograde end-systolic flow (V-wave)	Influenced by RV and RA compliance
	Antegrade diastolic flow (D-wave)	Occurs after TV opening
	Retrograde end-diastolic flow (A-wave)	Occurs during atrial contraction Influenced by RV and RA compliance
Myocardial velocities TDI (Figure 6-63)	Early diastolic velocity (E' wave)	E/E' correlates with RV filling pressures
	E/E' ratio	

DT, deceleration time; HVF, hepatic venous flow; RA, right atrial; RV, right ventricular; TDI, tissue Doppler imaging; TR, tricuspid regurgitation; TTF, transtricuspid flow; TV, tricuspid valve.

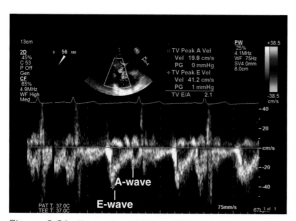

Figure 6-61. Transtricuspid flow (TTF), normal velocity profile.

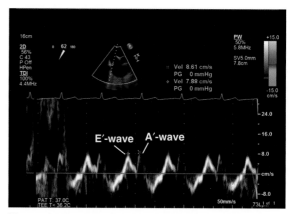

Figure 6-63. Myocardial velocities of the tricuspid annulus by TDI, normal velocity profile.

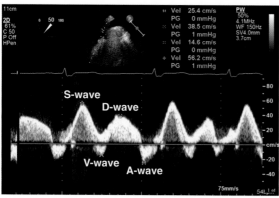

Figure 6-62. Hepatic venous flow, normal velocity profile.

CVP. A reduction in IVC diameter of more than 50% is consistent with a CVP less than 10 mm Hg. A dilated IVC without collapse with inspiration suggests a CVP greater than 15 mm Hg.

- In mechanically ventilated patients, the IVC diameter has also been shown to correlate well with CVP. The IVC diameter is measured at the cavoatrial junction in the ME bicaval view at the end of the T-wave on the electrocardiogram.

Physiologic Data
Acquisition
- Transtricuspid flow is usually obtained with PW Doppler in the ME 4C, ME RV inflow-outflow, or modified bicaval views (Figure 6-64).
- Hepatic vein flow is obtained by employing PW Doppler in the hepatic veins as they empty into the IVC (Figure 6-65).
- Myocardial velocities by TDI are obtained by employing PW Doppler in the ME 4C or ME RV inflow-outflow, or modified bicaval views (Figure 6-66).

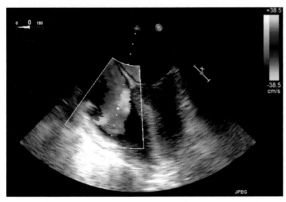

Figure 6-64. TTF velocities are measured in the ME 4C view, ME RV inflow-outflow view, or the ME bicaval view by employing PW Doppler and placing the sample volume at the level of the tips of the TV leaflets. Color flow Doppler may aid alignment of the ultrasound beam with the blood flow through the TV.

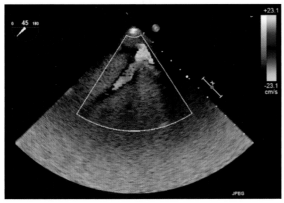

Figure 6-65. Hepatic vein flow velocities are measured by PW Doppler interrogation of the flow in the hepatic veins as they join the intrahepatic IVC tangentially. The hepatic veins can be imaged by advancing and turning the TEE probe to the right from a ME bicaval view.

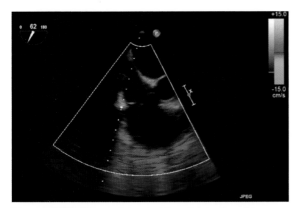

Figure 6-66. Myocardial velocities of the tricuspid annulus can be measured with TDI by placing the PW Doppler sample gate at the septal or lateral tricuspid annulus in the ME 4C view or the ME RV inflow-outflow view.

Analysis

- Transtricuspid flow (TTF)
  - TTF velocities
    - Tend to be lower owing to the larger TV annular size.
    - Although there is no consensus on different patterns or stages of RV diastolic dysfunction, they should resemble corresponding TMF patterns.
- Hepatic vein flow
  - The ratio of total hepatic reverse flow integral to total forward flow
    - Integral $VTI_A + VTI_V / VTI_S + VTI_D$.
    - Can be calculated by measuring the VTI for S-, V-, D-, and A-waves.
  - Prominent V- and A-waves and an increase in the ratio of total hepatic reverse flow integral to total forward flow integral are consistent with a marked decrease in RV compliance and increased filling pressures.
- Myocardial velocities by TDI
  - Tricuspid annular velocities are higher than the mitral annular velocities.
  - E/E′ ratio can be used to estimate RV filling pressures and diastolic function.
  - An RV E/E′ ratio greater than 6 suggests an RA pressure greater than 10 mm Hg.
- Grading of diastolic function
  - Tricuspid E/A ratio less than 0.8 suggests impaired relaxation.
  - Tricuspid E/A ratio of 0.8 to 2.1 with a tricuspid E/E′ ratio more than 6 or diastolic predominance in the hepatic veins suggests pseudonormal filling.
  - Tricuspid ratio more than 2.1 with a deceleration time less than 120 ms suggests restrictive filling.

Pitfalls

- Parallel alignment of the Doppler beam may be difficult with right-sided structures. Transgastric imaging may be helpful.
- RV diastolic function parameters are markedly dependent on loading conditions.
- TTF parameters are dependent on age, similar to the TMF parameters.
- TR has a significant effect on the TTF variable by increasing the E-wave velocity and the E/A ratio.
- TR also results in decreased hepatic vein flow S-wave, S/D ratio, and systolic filling fraction.
- Increased HR decreases diastolic time and results in increased A-wave velocity and atrial filling fraction and decreased E-wave DT and E/A ratio.

Suggested Readings

1. Lang RM, Bierig M, Devereux RB, et al; Chamber Quantification Writing Group; American Society of Echocardiography's Guidelines and Standards Committee; European Association of Echocardiography. Recommendations for chamber quantification: A report from the American Society of Echocardiography's Guidelines and Standards Committee and the Chamber Quantification Writing Group, developed in conjunction with the European Association of Echocardiography, a branch of the European Society of Cardiology. *J Am Soc Echocardiogr.* 2005;18:1440-1463.
2. Nagueh SF, Appleton CP, Gillebert TC, et al. Recommendations for the evaluation of left ventricular diastolic function by echocardiography [review]. *J Am Soc Echocardiogr.* 2009;22:107-133.
3. Rudski LG, Wyman WL, Afilalo J, et al. Guidelines for echocardiographic assessment of the right heart in adults: a report from the American Society of Echocardiography. *J Am Soc Echocardiogr.* 2010;23:685-713.
4. Shanewise JS, Cheung AT, Aronson S, et al. ASE/SCA guidelines for performing a comprehensive intraoperative multiplane transesophageal echocardiography examination: Recommendations of the American Society of Echocardiography Council for Intraoperative Echocardiography and the Society of Cardiovascular Anesthesiologists Task Force for Certification in Perioperative Transesophageal Echocardiography. *Anesth Analg.* 1999;89:870-884.

Diseases of the Aorta

Albert T. Cheung and Stuart J. Weiss

7

ANATOMY OF THE AORTA

The Aortic Wall

- The aortic wall is made up of the adventitia, media, and intima. Under normal conditions, it is not possible to distinguish each of the layers by echocardiography.

Adventitia
- The thin outermost layer, composed mainly of collagen, contains the vasa vasorum and nerves.
- The adventitia has the greatest tensile strength of the three layers of the aorta.
- In aortic dissection, it becomes separated from the intimal layer. In aneurysms, the adventitial layer expands in diameter.

Media
- The thick middle layer between the adventitia and the intima.
- Accounts for up to 80% of the arterial wall thickness and consists of intertwining sheets of elastic tissue and muscle fibers.

Intima
- The thin inner layer of the aorta that consists of a basement membrane lined with endothelial cells in direct contact with the blood.
- The layer that is most susceptible to injury and the site for atherosclerosis and calcification; it may become thickened, calcified, or ulcerated.

Segmental Anatomy of the Aorta

- The aorta begins at the aortic valve and ends at the bifurcation in the abdomen.
- The aorta can be divided into the aortic root, ascending aorta, aortic arch, descending thoracic aorta, and abdominal aorta.

The aortic root consists of the aortic valve annulus, the three aortic valve cusps, the sinuses of Valsalva, and the sinotubular junction where the aortic root joins with the ascending aorta (Figures 7-1 and 7-2).
- The aortic valve cusps and the sinuses of Valsalva are distinguished by their position adjacent to the right coronary ostium, left coronary ostium, or the noncoronary ostium.
- The sinotubular junction (STJ) is distinguished by a narrowing in the vessel as the sinuses of Valsalva join the tubular portion of the ascending aorta.
- The ascending aorta is a tubular portion of the aorta between the STJ and the origin of the innominate artery (Figures 7-2, 7-3, and 7-4).

The aortic arch is the segment containing the origin of the aortic arch branch vessels, the innominate artery, the left carotid artery, and the left subclavian artery (Figures 7-5 and 7-6).
- The descending thoracic aorta is the segment between the origin of the left subclavian artery and the diaphragmatic hiatus (Figures 7-7 and 7-8).
  - The paired intercostal arteries are branch vessels of the descending thoracic aorta.
  - The aortic isthmus is the segment of the proximal descending thoracic aorta just beyond the origin of the left subclavian artery at the site of the ligamentum arteriosum, the vestige of the ductus arteriosus in the fetus.
- The abdominal aorta is the segment of the aorta between the diaphragmatic hiatus and the aortic bifurcation where it becomes the internal iliac arteries.
  - Major branch vessels of the abdominal aorta include the celiac trunk, superior mesenteric artery, renal arteries, inferior mesenteric artery, and the lumbar segmental arteries.

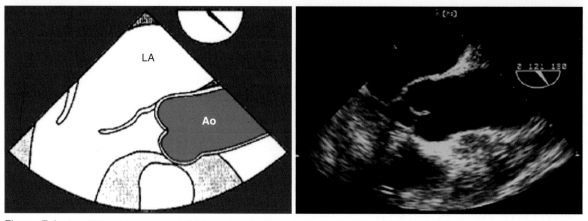

Figure 7-1. The TEE midesophageal (ME) aortic valve long axis image at a multiplane angle between 120 and 160 degrees provides a cross-sectional image of the aortic root for measuring the diameter of the aortic valve annulus, sinuses of Valsalva, and STJ. Ao, aorta; LA, left atrium. *Adapted from Pantin EJ, Cheung AT. Transesophageal echocardiographic evaluation of the aorta and pulmonary artery. In: Konstadt S, Shernan S, Oka Y, eds.* Clinical Transesophageal Echocardiography: A Problem-Oriented Approach. *2nd ed. Philadelphia: Lippincott Williams & Wilkins; 2003:215-244.*

Figure 7-2. TEE ME aortic valve long-axis image at 140 degrees in a patient with a Stanford type A aortic dissection. An intimal flap within the aorta that begins in the aortic root extends into the ascending aorta. Calipers were used to measure the diameter of the aortic valve annulus (A), sinuses of Valsalva (SoV; B), STJ (C), and ascending (ASC) aorta (D).

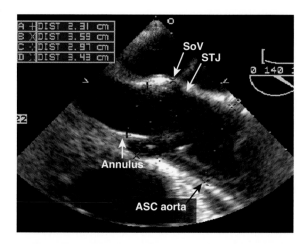

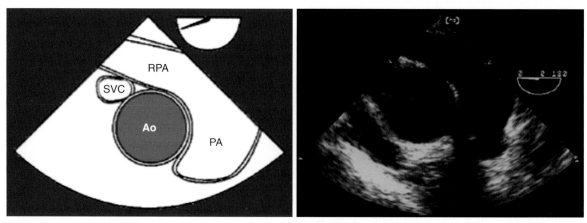

Figure 7-3. The TEE ME ascending aortic short axis image at a multiplane angle between 0 and 60 degrees provides a cross section for measuring the ascending aortic diameter at the level of the RPA. PA, main pulmonary artery; SVC, superior vena cava. *Adapted from Pantin EJ, Cheung AT. Transesophageal echocardiographic evaluation of the aorta and pulmonary artery. In: Konstadt S, Shernan S, Oka Y, eds.* Clinical Transesophageal Echocardiography: A Problem-Oriented Approach. *2nd ed. Philadelphia: Lippincott Williams & Wilkins; 2003:215-244.*

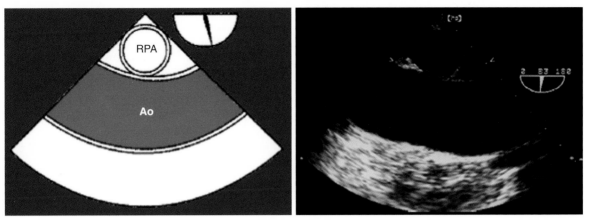

Figure 7-4. The TEE ME ascending aortic long axis image at a multiplane angle between 90 and 150 degrees provides a cross section for measuring the ascending aortic diameter at the level of the RPA. *Adapted from Pantin EJ, Cheung AT. Transesophageal echocardiographic evaluation of the aorta and pulmonary artery. In: Konstadt S, Shernan S, Oka Y, eds.* Clinical Transesophageal Echocardiography: A Problem-Oriented Approach. *2nd ed. Philadelphia: Lippincott Williams & Wilkins; 2003:215-244.*

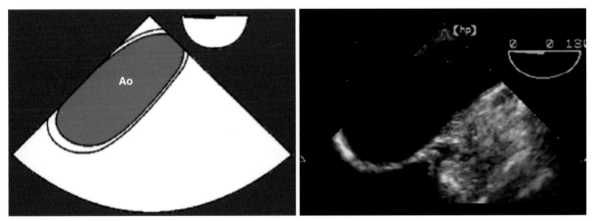

Figure 7-5. The TEE upper esophageal (UE) aortic arch long axis image at a multiplane angle of 0 degrees provides a cross section through the distal aortic arch. *Adapted from Pantin EJ, Cheung AT. Transesophageal echocardiographic evaluation of the aorta and pulmonary artery. In: Konstadt S, Shernan S, Oka Y, eds.* Clinical Transesophageal Echocardiography: A Problem-Oriented Approach. *2nd ed. Philadelphia: Lippincott Williams & Wilkins; 2003:215-244.*

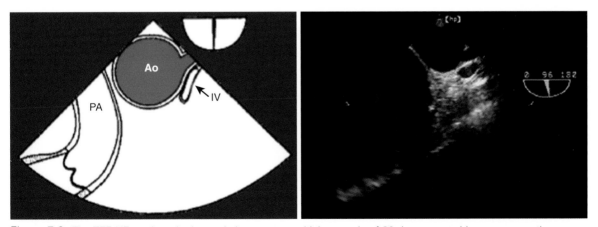

Figure 7-6. The TEE UE aortic arch short axis image at a multiplane angle of 90 degrees provides a cross section through the distal aortic arch that often provides images of the origin of the subclavian artery, the origin of the left carotid artery, the main pulmonary artery, and the innominate vein. IV, innominate vein. *Adapted from Pantin EJ, Cheung AT. Transesophageal echocardiographic evaluation of the aorta and pulmonary artery. In: Konstadt S, Shernan S, Oka Y, eds.* Clinical Transesophageal Echocardiography: A Problem-Oriented Approach. *2nd ed. Philadelphia: Lippincott Williams & Wilkins; 2003:215-244.*

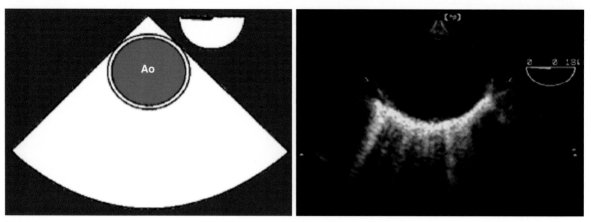

Figure 7-7. The TEE ME descending aortic short axis image at a multiplane angle of 0 degrees provides a cross section for measuring the descending aortic diameter. The entire descending thoracic aorta can be examined by advancing or withdrawing the TEE probe along the length of the descending aorta. *Adapted from Pantin EJ, Cheung AT. Transesophageal echocardiographic evaluation of the aorta and pulmonary artery. In: Konstadt S, Shernan S, Oka Y, eds.* Clinical Transesophageal Echocardiography: A Problem-Oriented Approach. *2nd ed. Philadelphia: Lippincott Williams & Wilkins; 2003:215-244.*

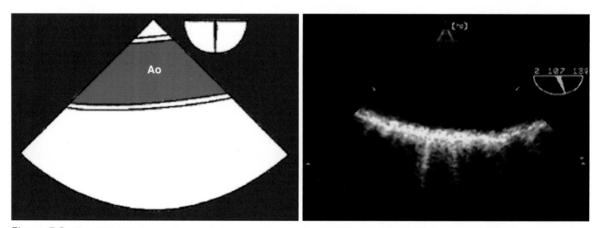

Figure 7-8. The TEE ME descending aorta long axis image at a multiplane angle of 90 degrees provides a cross section for the intimal surface of the descending aorta. *Adapted from Pantin EJ, Cheung AT. Transesophageal echocardiographic evaluation of the aorta and pulmonary artery. In: Konstadt S, Shernan S, Oka Y, eds.* Clinical Transesophageal Echocardiography: A Problem-Oriented Approach. *2nd ed. Philadelphia: Lippincott Williams & Wilkins; 2003:215-244.*

Segmental Anatomy of the Aorta for Thoracic Endovascular Aortic Repair (Figure 7-9)

- The thoracic aorta can be segmented into five anatomic zones for purposes of endovascular repair.
- Zones 2 to 4 are accessible landing zones for descending thoracic aortic endovascular repair procedures, although landing into zone 2 requires coverage of the origin to the left subclavian artery.
- Endovascular stent graft landing in zones 0 and 1 requires debranching of the brachiocephalic vessels to provide cerebral perfusion.
  - Zone 0: ascending aorta and proximal aortic arch to the innominate artery.
  - Zone 1: segment between the innominate artery and left carotid artery.
  - Zone 2: segment between the left common carotid artery and the left subclavian artery.
  - Zone 3: curved segment of the distal aortic arch and proximal descending thoracic aorta beyond the left subclavian artery.
  - Zone 4: the straight portion of the descending thoracic aorta beginning at approximately the level of the fourth thoracic vertebrae.

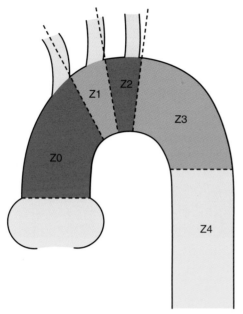

Figure 7-9. The thoracic aorta can be segmented into five anatomic zones for purposes of endovascular repair: Zone 0, the ascending aorta and proximal arch to the innominate artery; zone 1, the segment between the innominate artery and the left common carotid artery; zone 2, the segment between the left common carotid and left subclavian arteries; zone 3, the segment beyond the left subclavian along the curved portion of the distal arch; and zone 4, the straight portion of the descending thoracic aorta starting at the level of the fourth thoracic vertebrae. *From Desai ND, Szeto WY. Complex aortic arch aneurysm and dissections: Hybrid techniques for surgical and endovascular therapy. Curr Opin Cardiol. 2009;24:521-527.*

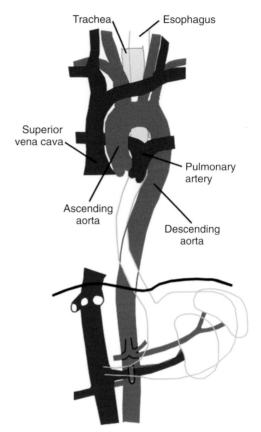

Figure 7-10. The anatomic relationships among the thoracic aorta *(red)*, the main PA *(blue)*, the left pulmonary artery, the RPA, the SVC *(blue)*, the inferior vena cava, the esophagus *(yellow)*, the trachea *(gray)*, and the left mainstem bronchus. The descending thoracic aorta is anterior to the esophagus near the aortic arch, lateral to the esophagus in the mid-thorax, then posterior to the esophagus at the diaphragmatic hiatus. The distal trachea and left mainstem bronchus lies between the esophagus and the aortic arch. *From Pantin EJ, Cheung AT. Transesophageal echocardiographic evaluation of the aorta and pulmonary artery. In: Konstadt S, Shernan S, Oka Y, eds. Clinical Transesophageal Echocardiography: A Problem-Oriented Approach. 2nd ed. Philadelphia: Lippincott Williams & Wilkins; 2003:215-244.*

Position of the Aorta in Relation to the Esophagus and Other Structures

- The aortic root and proximal ascending aorta lie within the pericardial sac. The aortic root is anterior to the esophagus and left atrium (see Figure 7-1).
- The ascending aorta is anterior to the esophagus. The right pulmonary artery (RPA) lies between the esophagus and the proximal ascending aorta (Figure 7-10; see also Figures 7-1 and 7-3).
- The distal trachea and left mainstem bronchus lies between the esophagus and the distal ascending aorta and proximal aortic arch (see Figure 7-10).
- The proximal descending thoracic aorta is initially anterior to the esophagus, then lateral to the esophagus in the midthorax, then posterior to the esophagus at the diaphragmatic hiatus (see Figure 7-10).

- The left atrium provides an acoustic window for TEE imaging of the aortic valve, aortic root, and proximal ascending aorta (see Figure 7-1).
- The RPA provides an acoustic window and anatomic reference for transesophageal echocardiography (TEE) imaging of the proximal and mid ascending aorta (see Figures 7-3 and 7-4).
- The distal trachea and left mainstem bronchus obstruct TEE imaging of the distal ascending aorta and proximal aortic arch (see Figure 7-10).

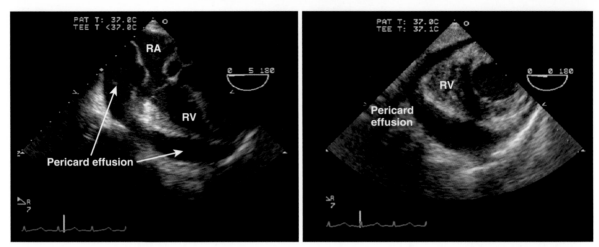

Figure 7-11. TEE ME four-chamber view **(left)** and transgastric left ventricular short axis view **(right)** in a patient with hypotension associated with a Stanford type A aortic dissection. The circumferential pericardial effusion seen on the short axis image of the left ventricle was diagnostic for rupture of the ascending aorta causing hemopericardium **(right)**. Collapse of the right atrium (RA) at the beginning of systole seen in the four-chamber view was diagnostic for cardiac tamponade **(left)**. RV, right ventricle.

TABLE 7-1   NORMAL ADULT THORACIC AORTIC DIAMETERS

Aortic Segment	Men Mean ± SD (cm)	Women Mean ± SD (cm)	Assessment Method
Aortic valve annulus	2.6 ± 0.3	2.3 ± 0.2	Echo
Sinuses of Valsalva	3.4 ± 0.3	3.0 ± 0.3	Echo
Sinotubular junction	2.9 ± 0.3	2.6 ± 0.3	Echo
Proximal ascending aorta	3.0 ± 0.4	2.7 ± 0.4	Echo
Mid descending aorta	2.7 ± 0.3	2.5 ± 0.3	CT

CT, computed tomography; Echo, echocardiography; SD, standard deviation.
Data from Roman MJ, Devereux RB, Kramer-Fox R, et al. Two-dimensional echocardiographic aortic root dimensions in normal children and adults. *Am J Cardiol.* 1989;64:507-512.

- Rupture of the aortic root or proximal ascending aorta will cause cardiac tamponade because it lies within the pericardial sac (Figure 7-11).

The Normal Size of the Aorta

- The diameter of the aorta is greatest at the sinus of Valsalva in the aortic root and then tapers gradually along its length beyond the STJ (Table 7-1).
  - The normal range for aortic diameters for each segment of the aorta varies according to age, gender, and body size (see Table 7-1).
  - Measurement of aortic diameter should be made perpendicular to the direction of blood flow (Figure 7-12).
  - Echocardiographic measurements of aortic diameter are typically slightly less than computed tomography (CT) measurements

of aortic diameter by 1 to 3 mm (see Figure 7-12).
  - According to convention, echocardiographic measurements typically measure the internal diameter of the aorta (intima to intima) whereas CT typically measures the external diameter of the aorta (adventitia to adventitia).

STEP-BY-STEP APPROACH TO TRANSESOPHAGEAL ECHOCARDIOGRAPHIC IMAGING OF THE THORACIC AORTA (Box 7-1)

Step 1: Image the Aortic Valve in Short Axis

- Identify the aortic valve cusps and the presence and pattern of calcification and estimate the aortic valve opening or the aortic valve area.

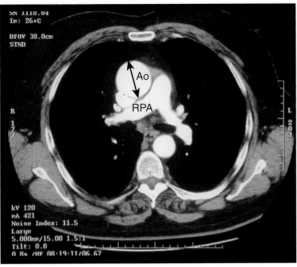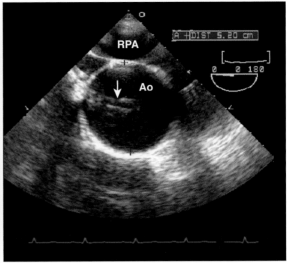

Figure 7-12. CT angiogram **(left)** of an axial slice through the ascending aorta (Ao) at the level of the RPA compared with a TEE ME ascending aorta short axis image **(right)** at the level of the RPA in the same patient with a dilated ascending aorta. Ascending aortic diameter measured from the adventitia to the adventitia was 5.4 cm by CT angiogram. Ascending aortic diameter measured from intima to intima was 5.2 cm by TEE. Linear imaging artifacts *(arrow)* as a consequence of reverberation and side lobe artifacts appear in the lumen of the ascending aorta on the TEE image. Linear imaging artifacts within the ascending aorta on TEE examination may appear in up to 40% of patients with a dilated ascending aorta and can be mistaken for an intimal flap as seen in aortic dissection.

BOX 7-1 Comprehensive Reporting of the Transesophageal Echocardiographic Examination of the Thoracic Aorta

- Pathologic findings including a description of anatomic location and extent according to thoracic aortic segments (see "Segmental Anatomy of the Aorta").
- Maximum diameter and anatomic location of dilated segments of thoracic aorta measured perpendicular to the axis of blood flow.*
- Diameters of the aortic valve annulus, sinus of Valsalva, sinotubular junction, ascending aorta at the level of the right pulmonary artery, distal aortic arch, and descending thoracic aorta.*
- Aortic regurgitation, if present, and its severity (described in Chapter 3).
- Atherosclerosis, if present, and its severity (see Table 7-3).
- Mural thrombus, if present, and its anatomic location.
- Calcification of the vessel wall, if present, and its anatomic location.
- Presence of pleural effusion, pericardial effusion, or perivascular hematoma that may indicate aortic rupture.

*Specify whether aortic diameter was measured from intima to intima or adventitia to adventitia.

- Assess the motion of the aortic valve cusps.
- Apply color flow Doppler imaging to detect aortic regurgitation (AR) and the site of AR in relation to the coaptation of the valve cusps.
- Image the origins of the right and left coronary ostia.

Step 2: Image the Aortic Valve in Long Axis (see Figure 7-1)

- Measure the diameter of the aortic valve annulus, the sinus of Valsalva, and the STJ (see Figure 7-2).
  - Assess whether the STJ is well defined or effaced.
  - Assess for the presence of calcification involving the aortic valve, annulus, or aortic root. Assess the motion of the aortic valve cusps and their separation in systole.
  - Apply color flow Doppler imaging to detect AR.

Step 3: Image the Proximal Ascending Aorta in Short Axis at the Level of the Right Pulmonary Artery

- Anteflex and withdraw the TEE probe from the level of the aortic valve (see Figure 7-3).

- Measure the diameter of the ascending aorta and the RPA at the level of the RPA.
- Assess for the presence of atheroma.
- The distal ascending aorta and proximal aortic arch cannot usually be imaged by TEE because the air-filled trachea or left mainstem bronchus lies between the esophagus and these segments of the thoracic aorta.

Step 4: Image the Proximal Ascending Aorta at the Level of the Right Pulmonary Artery in Long Axis

- Rotate the transducer forward to 90 degrees (see Figure 7-4).
  - Measure the diameter of the ascending aorta at the level of the RPA.
  - Assess for the presence and severity of atherosclerosis.

Step 5: Image the Descending Thoracic Aorta in Short Axis

- Measure the diameter of the mid descending aorta.
  - Assess for the presence of atherosclerosis or pleural effusion (see Figure 7-7).

Step 6: Image the Descending Thoracic Aorta in Long Axis

- Rotate the transducer forward to 90 degrees to provide a long axis cross section of the descending thoracic aorta

- Examine the intimal surface of the aorta longitudinally (see Figure 7-8).
- Advance the TEE probe while turning the probe counterclockwise to examine the distal descending thoracic aorta to the level of the diaphragm.
- Withdraw the TEE probe while turning the probe clockwise to examine the proximal descending thoracic aorta.
- The distal aortic arch is typically at a depth of 20 to 25 cm from the incisors, the mid descending thoracic aorta at 30 to 35 cm from the incisors, and the diaphragmatic hiatus at 40 to 50 cm from the incisors.

Step 7: Image the Distal Aortic Arch

- The distal aortic arch will appear as the TEE probe is withdrawn from the level of the mid descending thoracic aorta.
  - The distal aortic arch long axis image will appear at a multiplane angle of 0 degrees (see Figure 7-5).
- Rotate the transducer forward to 90 degrees to display the distal aortic arch in short axis (see Figure 7-6).
- Rotate the TEE probe from left to right in a clockwise direction to display the origins of the left subclavian and possibly the left carotid and innominate arteries.
- The upper esophageal aortic arch short axis imaging plane will also display the main pulmonary artery and pulmonic valve in long axis and the innominate vein in short axis (Figure 7-13).

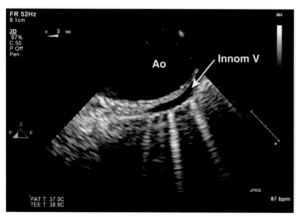
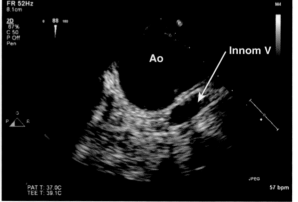

Figure 7-13. TEE UE aortic arch long axis view (**left**) and aortic arch short axis view (**right**) demonstrate the relationship between the aorta (Ao) and the innominate vein (Innom V). The anterior wall of the aorta against the adjacent innominate vein can mimic the appearance of an intimal flap and be mistaken for aortic dissection.

- Measure the diameter of the distal aortic arch and assess for the presence of atherosclerosis.

ECHOCARDIOGRAPHIC IMAGING ARTIFACTS

- Ultrasound imaging artifacts can produce linear artifacts within the lumen of the ascending aorta in up to 40% of patients, especially if the aorta is dilated.
- Ultrasound imaging artifacts, often in combination with motion artifacts on the CT images can sometimes be mistaken for aortic dissection.

Linear Artifacts

- Linear artifacts are generated by reverberations between vessel or chamber walls.
- Ultrasound reverberation between the posterior and the anterior walls of the left atrium or RPA may create a linear artifact that appears within the lumen of the ascending aorta in both the short axis and the long axis imaging planes that can mimic the appearance of an intimal flap within the aorta (see Figure 7-12).
- Linear artifacts within the aortic lumen can also be created by ultrasound reverberation between a vessel or chamber wall and a vascular catheter such as a pulmonary artery catheter in the RPA.

Side Lobe Artifacts

- Side lobe artifacts are generated by calcified plaques on the aortic wall or by vascular catheters such as a pulmonary artery catheter within the RPA (see Videos 7-3G and H on the Expert Consult website).
- They can produce linear artifacts within the aortic lumen.
- Linear artifacts from side lobes appear as curvilinear shadows at a constant depth and may extend across and beyond the wall of the aorta.

Mirroring Artifacts

- Mirroring artifacts are created by ultrasound reflection off acoustic interfaces such as the walls of the aorta that produces a mirror image

of the vessel on the other side of the interface.
- A mirror image artifact of the descending thoracic aorta adjacent to the actual descending aorta can mimic aortic dissection (see Video 7-3A on the Expert Consult website).

KEY POINTS: ECHOCARDIOGRAPHIC IMAGING PITFALLS

- Fluid-filled structures adjacent to the aortic wall can mimic the appearance of an aortic dissection.
- The innominate or brachiocephalic vein is adjacent to the aortic arch in the upper esophageal short and long axis images of the aortic arch (see Figure 7-13). It can be distinguished from aortic dissection by injecting echocontrast into a peripheral vein in the left arm and observing the appearance of the contrast agent in the lumen of the innominate vein.
- A left pleural effusion adjacent to the descending thoracic aorta can be distinguished from aortic dissection by imaging the descending aorta in short axis and noting the characteristic crescent-shaped effusion in the left pleural cavity (Figure 7-15). A right pleural effusion can be detected by turning the TEE probe to the right and noting the presence of a crescent-shaped fluid density oriented in the opposite direction.

AORTIC DISEASES

Aortic Dissection

- Aortic dissection is defined as a separation of the layers of the aorta.
  - In most cases, disruption or a tear in the intimal layer causes blood to enter the medial layer causing the intima to separate from the adventitia.
  - The characteristic appearance of aortic dissection on echocardiographic examination is an intimal flap within the lumen of the aorta separating the true lumen of the vessel from the false lumen (see Figures 7-2 and 7-14).
  - Color flow Doppler imaging may detect one or several intimal tears by demonstrating blood flow across the intimal flap at the site of the tear (Figure 7-15).
- Intramural hematoma is a variant of aortic dissection.

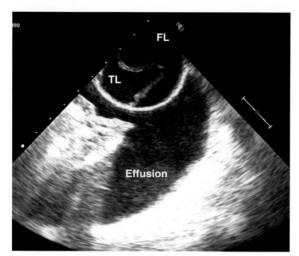

Figure 7-14. TEE ME descending aorta short axis view demonstrates aortic dissection with an intimal flap separating the true lumen (TL) from the false lumen (FL) of the aorta. A pleural effusion in the left pleural cavity (effusion) can indicate rupture of the descending aorta or heart failure.

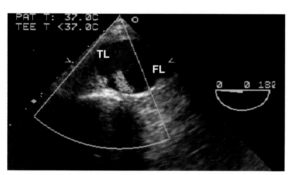

Figure 7-15. TEE ME descending aorta short axis view demonstrates aortic dissection with an intimal flap separating the TL from the FL of the aorta. Color flow Doppler imaging demonstrated two fenestrations in the intimal flap in this cross section indicating intimal tears with blood flow directed from the TL into the FL.

- It is characterized by separation of the intima from the adventitia and the presence of hematoma within the medial layer (Figure 7-16).
- An intimal tear cannot usually be identified by echocardiography in intramural hematoma.
- The echocardiographic characteristic of intramural hematoma is a crescent-shaped thickening of the wall of the aorta.
- Sometimes, the intramural hematoma will contain regions that are echolucent, indicating the presence of noncoagulated blood within the hematoma.

KEY POINTS

- The diagnostic accuracy of TEE in suspected aortic dissection is similar to helical CT and magnetic resonance imaging (MRI) with a sensitivity of 95% to 99% and a specificity of 92% to 97%.
- Because TEE is portable and can be performed at the bedside or in the operating room, it is useful for the evaluation of hemodynamically unstable patients admitted with suspected acute aortic dissection (Figure 7-17).
- In surgical patients in whom the diagnosis of aortic dissection has been confirmed by other imaging studies, intraoperative TEE has clinical utility for detecting complications of aortic dissection and guiding surgical management (Figure 7-18; and see Videos 7-1A through 7-3F on the Expert Consult website).

- Aortic dissection may be classified in several ways:
  - According to type, extent of involvement of the aorta, and the location of intimal tears.
  - Classification of aortic dissection is important for prognosis and determining whether emergent surgical repair should be performed (Figures 7-18 and 7-19).
- DeBakey classification (see Figure 7-19)
  - Type I: Intimal tear within the ascending aorta with dissection involving the ascending aorta, the aortic arch, and at least part of the descending aorta (surgical repair is recommended).
  - Type II: Intimal tear within the ascending aorta with dissection confined to the ascending aorta (surgical repair is recommended).
  - Type III: Intimal tear within the descending thoracic aorta with dissection confined to the descending aorta and no involvement of the ascending aorta or aortic arch (medical management is recommended).
  - Type IIIa: Dissection confined to the descending thoracic aorta.
  - Type IIIb: Dissection of the descending aorta extending below the diaphragm.
- Stanford classification (see Figure 7-19)
  - Type A: Any dissection involving the ascending aorta regardless of the site of intimal tear (surgical repair is recommended).
  - Type B: Dissection that does not involve the ascending aorta (medical management is recommended).

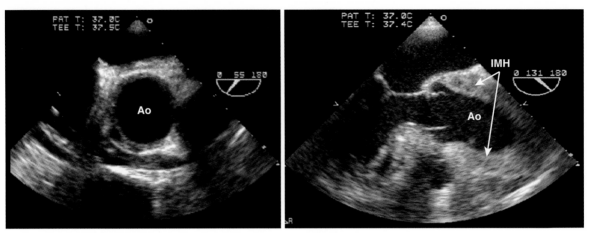

Figure 7-16. **Left,** Intramural hematoma is a variant of aortic dissection and appears as a circumferential or crescent-shaped thickening of the aortic wall on the TEE ME ascending aorta short axis image. In acute intramural hematoma, blood may appear within the intramural hematoma on the short axis image of the aorta (Ao) as lucent cavities within the wall of the vessel. **Right,** TEE ME aortic valve long axis image at 131 degrees demonstrates longitudinal thickening of the wall of the aortic root and ascending aorta caused by intramural hematoma.

ROLE OF TEE FOR THE EVALUATION AND DIAGNOSIS OF
AORTIC DISSECTION

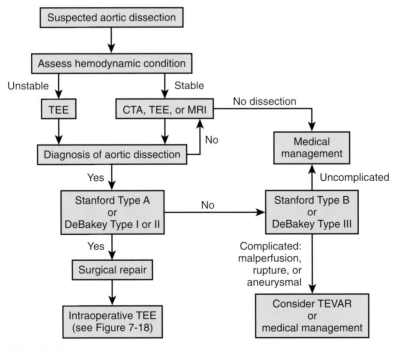

Abbreviations:
CTA = Computed tomographic angiogram
MRI = Magnetic resonance imaging
TEVAR = thoracic endovascular aortic repair

Figure 7-17. Role of TEE for the evaluation and diagnosis of aortic dissection.

INTRAOPERATIVE TEE EXAMINATION FOR AORTIC DISSECTION

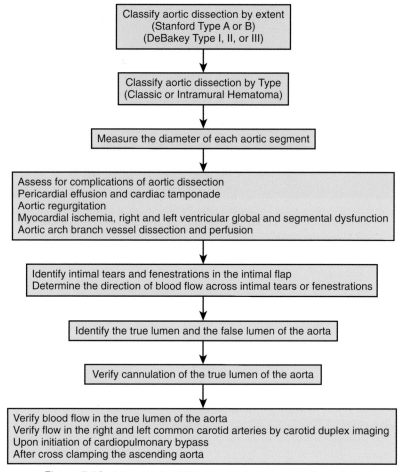

Classify aortic dissection by extent
(Stanford Type A or B)
(DeBakey Type I, II, or III)

↓

Classify aortic dissection by Type
(Classic or Intramural Hematoma)

↓

Measure the diameter of each aortic segment

↓

Assess for complications of aortic dissection
Pericardial effusion and cardiac tamponade
Aortic regurgitation
Myocardial ischemia, right and left ventricular global and segmental dysfunction
Aortic arch branch vessel dissection and perfusion

↓

Identify intimal tears and fenestrations in the intimal flap
Determine the direction of blood flow across intimal tears or fenestrations

↓

Identify the true lumen and the false lumen of the aorta

↓

Verify cannulation of the true lumen of the aorta

↓

Verify blood flow in the true lumen of the aorta
Verify flow in the right and left common carotid arteries by carotid duplex imaging
Upon initiation of cardiopulmonary bypass
After cross clamping the ascending aorta

Figure 7-18. Intraoperative TEE examination for aortic dissection.

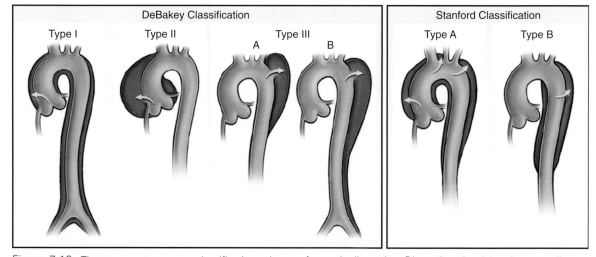

Figure 7-19. The two most common classification schemes for aortic dissection. Dissections involving the ascending aorta are usually considered surgical emergencies. *From Kouchoukos NT, Dougenis D. Surgery of the thoracic aorta.* N Engl J Med. *1997;336:1878-1888.*

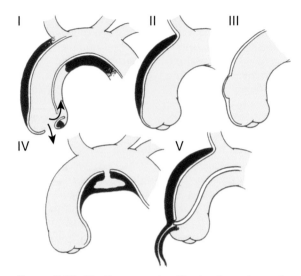

Figure 7-20. The European classification for variants of aortic dissection. Class I, classic aortic dissection; class II, intramural hematoma; class III, subtle discrete aortic dissection; class IV, plaque rupture or ulceration; class V, traumatic or iatrogenic aortic dissection. *Adapted from Erbel R, Alfonso F, Boileau C, et al. Diagnosis and management of aortic dissection: Recommendations of the Task Force on Aortic Dissection, European Society of Cardiology. Eur Heart J 2001;22:1642-1681.*

- European classification (Figure 7-20)
  - Class I: Classic aortic dissection with intimal tear and formation of an intimal flap separating the true and false lumina of the aorta.
  - Class II: Intramural hematoma with hematoma formation within the medial layer. An intimal tear is not usually detected by echocardiography.
  - Class III: Limited dissection confined to a short segment of the aorta. A rupture or partial tear of the inner wall of the vessel is called a *subtle dissection*. Scar formation at the site of the partial tear is called an *abortive discrete dissection.*
  - Class IV: Penetrating atherosclerotic ulcer with localized hematoma or pseudoaneurysm.
  - Class V: Traumatic or iatrogenic aortic dissection caused by catheter or surgical instrumentation of the aorta.

Intramural Hematoma
- Intramural hematoma is a variant of aortic dissection that occurs in approximately 10% to 30% of patients presenting with acute aortic dissection (see Figure 7-16).

- Intramural hematoma tends to affect patients who are elderly or have a long history of peripheral vascular disease.
- Risk factors for hospital mortality that may also serve as indications for surgical repair are involvement of the ascending aorta (Stanford type A), ascending aortic diameter of 4.8 cm or greater, or hematoma thickness of 11 mm or greater.

Echocardiographic Diagnosis of Complications of Aortic Dissection
Cardiac Tamponade
- Cardiac tamponade is caused by rupture of the ascending aorta or aortic root within the pericardium.
- Cardiac tamponade is a frequent cause of early death in acute Stanford type A, DeBakey type I, or DeBakey type II aortic dissection.
- Hemopericardium associated with aortic dissection appears as a circumferential pericardial effusion by echocardiography (see Figure 7-11).
- Sometimes free-floating hematoma or thrombus can be observed within the pericardial space.
- Cardiac tamponade is manifested by external atrial compression and a small left ventricular cavity size in diastole.

Aortic Regurgitation
- AR can be caused by Stanford type A, DeBakey type I, or DeBakey type II aortic dissection. If severe AR is acute, it is often associated with heart failure or cardiogenic shock.
- Causes of AR include dilatation of the aortic root, dissection within the aortic root involving the suspension of the aortic valve cusps, or prolapse of the intimal flap through the aortic valve (Figure 7-21).

Coronary Artery Malperfusion
- Coronary artery malperfusion can occur in Stanford type A, DeBakey type I, or DeBakey type II aortic dissection if the dissection extends into the aortic root and coronary ostia.
- Echocardiographic signs of right coronary artery malperfusion include right ventricular dysfunction and left ventricular inferior segmental wall motion abnormality.

Carotid Artery Malperfusion
- Carotid artery malperfusion is caused by extension of the dissection into the aortic arch branch vessels or obstruction of the origins of

the aortic arch branch vessels by the intimal flap within the aortic arch. Aortic arch branch vessel malperfusion is often associated with upper extremity pulse deficits or acute ischemic stroke.

- Carotid duplex examination can be used to detect a dissection flap or compromised blood flow within the common carotid artery (Figure 7-22).

KEY POINTS

- Hemopericardium, acute severe AR, coronary malperfusion, and aortic arch branch vessel malperfusion associated with aortic dissection are surgical emergencies.

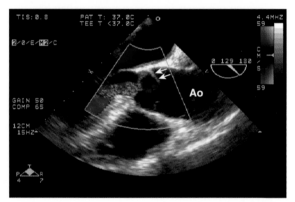

Figure 7-21. TEE ME aortic valve long axis image at 129 degrees with color flow Doppler imaging in a patient with a Stanford type A aortic dissection and AR. An intimal flap *(arrows)* is present in the aorta (Ao) that extends to the base of the aortic valve cusps within the aortic root.

Cardiopulmonary Bypass

- Intraoperative TEE can be used to guide aortic cannulation for cardiopulmonary bypass during operation to decrease the risk of malperfusion (see Figure 7-18; see Videos 7-1A thru 7-3F on the Expert Consult website). Intraoperative TEE is used to identify the true lumen and the false lumen of the aorta and then verify guidewire insertion into the true lumen before aortic cannulation.
- In general, the true lumen of the aorta is typically smaller than the false lumen, expands during systole, and has a rounded border.
- The false lumen is typically crescent-shaped. Blood flows from the true lumen into the false lumen across an intimal tear.
- Variations in the echocardiographic appearance of the aorta can make it difficult to distinguish the true lumen from the false lumen in patients with aortic dissection.
- Intraoperative carotid Duplex imaging can be used to verify blood flow or perfusion in the common carotid arteries after aortic cannulation, start of cardiopulmonary bypass, and after application of the aortic cross-clamp (see Figure 7-22).

Aortic Aneurysm

- Aortic aneurysm is defined as an abnormal dilatation of the aorta with a vessel diameter that is 50% greater than the normal diameter of the aorta.

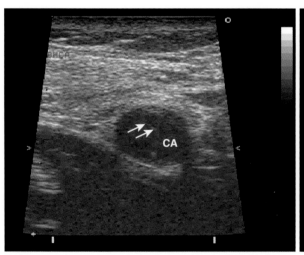
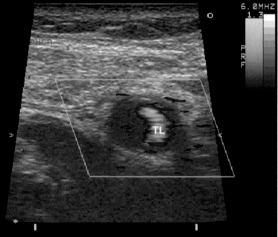

Figure 7-22. Surface ultrasound imaging of the right neck in a patient with a Stanford type A aortic dissection and extension of the dissection into the innominate artery and right common carotid artery. **Left,** An intimal flap *(arrows)* was imaged in the right carotid artery (CA). **Right,** Power Doppler demonstrated flow in the TL of the carotid artery during cardiopulmonary bypass.

TABLE 7-2 INDICATIONS FOR SURGICAL REPAIR FOR THORACIC AORTIC ANEURYSM ACCORDING TO DISEASE CHARACTERISTICS AND AORTIC DIAMETER

Conditions	Indication for Surgical Repair
Degenerative aneurysm	Asc Ao ≥ 5.5 cm Asc Ao < 5.5 cm and growth rate > 0.5 cm/yr Desc Ao > 6.0 cm Desc Ao > 5.5 cm and candidate for TEVAR Saccular aneurysm Pseudoaneurysm
Marfan's	Asc Ao 4.0-5.0 cm
Ehlers-Danlos	Asc Ao 4.0-5.0 cm and family history of aortic dissection
Turner's	Asc Ao 4.0-5.0 cm and rapidly expanding aneurysm
Bicuspid aortic valve	Asc Ao 4.0-5.0 cm and planned pregnancy
Familial TAA	Asc Ao 4.0-5.0 cm and significant aortic regurgitation
Familial dissection	Desc Ao > 5.5 cm
Loeys-Dietz syndrome	Asc Ao ≥ 4.2 cm by TEE Asc Ao ≥ 4.4 cm by CT or MRI
Aortic valve repair or replacement	Asc Ao > 4.5 cm

Asc Ao, ascending aortic diameter; CT, computed tomography; Desc Ao, descending aortic diameter; MRI, magnetic resonance imaging; TAA, thoracic aortic aneurysm; TEVAR, thoracic endovascular aortic repair.
Adapted from Hiratzka LF, Bakris GL, Beckman JA, et al. 2010 ACC/AHA/AATS/ACR/ASA/SCA/SCAI/SIR/STS/SVM Guidelines for the diagnosis and management of patients with thoracic aortic disease. *Circulation.* 2010;121:e266-e369.

- Etiologies for thoracic aortic aneurysms (TAAs) include atherosclerotic disease, collagen vascular diseases, congenital and genetic syndromes, inflammatory diseases, infection, and trauma (Table 7-2).
- Aortic aneurysm can be classified according to its shape as fusiform or saccular.
- True aneurysms involve all three layers of the aorta. Pseudoaneurysms do not involve all three layers of the aorta and arise from defects in the aortic wall as a consequence of surgical instrumentation, vascular anastomosis, trauma, penetrating atherosclerotic ulcer, or infection (Figure 7-23).
- TEE can be used to characterize TAAs according to size, shape, location, and extent.
  - TEE characterization of aneurysm size, location, and extent is important for surgical decision making.
  - TEE can also detect mural thrombus within the aneurysm or associated aortic dissection. The presence of spontaneous echo contrast within the aneurysm by TEE suggests low flow within the aneurysm.
- Aneurysm diameter is important for prognosis and a risk factor for rupture.
  - TEE measurement of aortic diameter typically underestimates aortic diameter by several millimeters compared with CT measurements because TEE

measurements of aortic diameter are typically performed from intima to intima whereas CT measurements are performed from adventitia to adventitia (see Figure 7-12 and Table 7-2).
- For an aortic aneurysm of any given diameter, association with bicuspid aortic valve, collagen vascular disease, or a familial history of aortic aneurysm increases the risk for rupture (see Table 7-2).
- Aneurysm type is also an important risk factor for rupture. Compared with fusiform aneurysms, saccular aneurysms and pseudoaneurysms are at greater risk for rupturing.

Giant Ascending Aortic or Aortic Arch Aneurysms

- Giant ascending aortic or aortic arch aneurysms may cause a mediastinal mass effect with external compression of the RPA, left mainstem bronchus, trachea, esophagus, right ventricular outflow tract, or the superior vena cava (Figure 7-24).
- They may be associated with bicuspid aortic valve.
- Aneurysm of the aortic root or ascending aorta can contribute to AR.
- TEE should be performed cautiously in patients with evidence of a mediastinal mass effect because the volume of the TEE probe

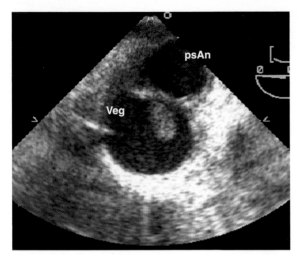

Figure 7-23. TEE ME descending thoracic aortic short axis image in a patient with endocarditis and a mycotic aneurysm. A mobile vegetation (veg) was imaged in the lumen of the descending thoracic aorta adjacent to a pseudoaneurysm (psAn).

in the esophagus has the potential to cause airway obstruction or circulatory collapse.
- Simultaneous compression of the RPA and left mainstem bronchus may cause hypoxemia.
- The TEE probe should not be advanced into the esophagus if resistance is encountered (see Figure 7-10, see Video 7-3I on the companion website).

Descending Thoracic Aortic Aneurysms
- The descending thoracic aorta is adjacent to the esophagus and the esophagus may be distorted or involved in patients with large descending TAAs.
- TEE should be performed with caution in patients with large descending TAAs because instrumentation of the esophagus could injure the esophagus or rupture the aneurysm (see Figure 7-10).

Endovascular Aortic Repair
- TEE can be used to evaluate the proximal and distal landing zones for thoracic endovascular aortic repairs and to detect the presence of endovascular leak after stent graft deployment.
- The detection of blood flow within the excluded aneurysm cavity by color flow Doppler imaging or the presence of swirling spontaneous echo contrast by TEE after endovascular stent deployment indicates the presence of an endovascular leak (Figure 7-25).

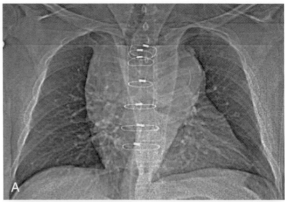

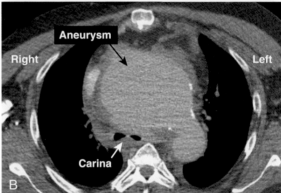

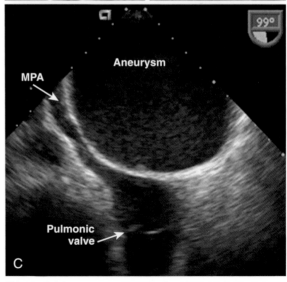

Figure 7-24. Chest roentgenogram (CXR; **A**), CTA with radiocontrast (**B**), and TEE (**C**) in a patient with a giant ascending aorta and aortic arch aneurysm. **A,** The CXR was notable for a widened mediastinum and rightward deviation of the trachea. **B,** The CTA showed the aneurysm and rightward deviation of the carina. **C,** The TEE UE short axis view of the aortic arch at a multiplane angle of 99 degrees demonstrated extrinsic compression of the main pulmonary artery (MPA) by the aortic arch aneurysm.

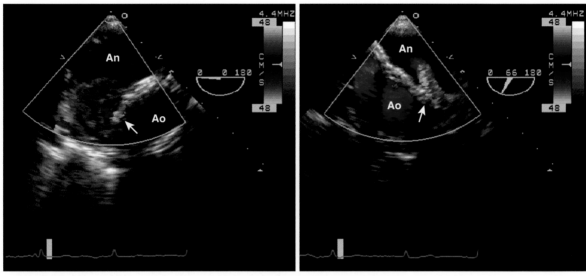

Figure 7-25. TEE ME short axis **(left)** and long axis **(right)** images of the descending thoracic aorta demonstrate the aortic lumen (Ao) and the excluded aneurysm (An) after endovascular stent deployment. Thrombus and swirling spontaneous echo contrast was imaged within the excluded aneurysm cavity. Color flow Doppler imaging demonstrated an endovascular leak with flow from the aortic lumen into the excluded aneurysm cavity *(arrow)*.

- TEE or intravascular ultrasound can be applied for thoracic endovascular aortic repair to decrease the need or the amount of radiographic contrast agents to accomplish the procedure.
- TEE can be used to detect vulnerable atheromas in the aortic arch and descending thoracic aorta in patients undergoing thoracic endovascular aortic repairs at risk for thromboembolic complications.
- TEE can be used to identify location of atheromas that are vulnerable to atheroembolism for guiding intravascular wire manipulation and endovascular stent deployment to decrease the risk of thromboembolism (Figure 7-26).

Traumatic Aortic Injury
- The advantages of TEE for the diagnosis of traumatic aortic injury are:
- That it is portable, can be performed at the bedside or in the operating room, and can provide an immediate diagnosis.
- That it can also detect cardiac tamponade, hypovolemia, or ventricular dysfunction from myocardial contusion.
- The most common survivable aortic injuries result from blunt chest trauma or rapid deceleration.

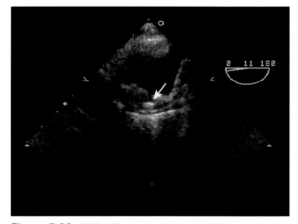

Figure 7-26. TEE ME short axis image of the proximal descending thoracic aorta in a patient undergoing thoracic endovascular aortic repair. TEE demonstrated severe atherosclerosis (grade V) with mobile atheroma at the proximal landing zone for the stent graft. TEE was used to reposition a guidewire *(arrow)* to prevent dislodgment of the atheroma prior to stent graft deployment.

- The most common site of injury is at the aortic isthmus between the aortic arch and the descending thoracic aorta (Figure 7-27).
- The echocardiographic features of traumatic aortic injury are evidence of intimal disruption and perivascular hematoma confined to a short segment of the aorta.

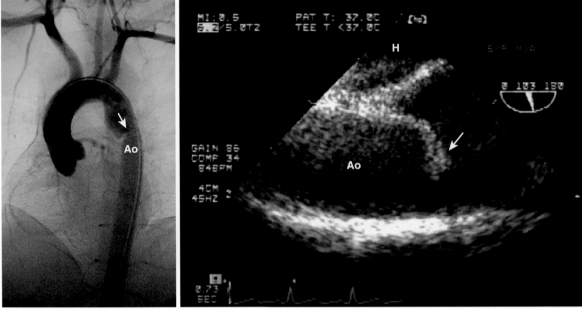

Figure 7-27. Aortic angiogram **(left)** and TEE proximal descending aorta long axis image **(right)** at a multiplane angle of 103 degrees in a patient with traumatic aortic injury involving the region of the aortic isthmus as a consequence of a motor vehicle accident. Both the angiogram and the TEE image demonstrated the presence of a thick mural flap *(arrow)* within the lumen of the descending aorta (Ao) that indicated a disruption of the aortic wall. The TEE image also demonstrated the presence of hematoma (H) in the space between the descending thoracic aorta and the esophagus that indicated a contained rupture.

KEY POINTS

- In suspected aortic injury, the proximal descending aorta should be examined carefully with TEE because the most common site for aortic injuries in patients arriving alive to a hospital are isolated in the region of the aortic isthmus (see Figure 7-27). However, aortic injury can occur at other sites in the thoracic aorta, including segments of the distal ascending aorta and aortic arch that cannot be reliably imaged by TEE.
- Intimal disruption from traumatic injury typically produces a thick mural flap within the aortic lumen confined to a 1 or 2 cm length of the aorta (see Figure 7-27). The mural flap is usually less mobile than the intimal flap associated with classic aortic dissection. Intimal disruption can also appear as a small defect or discontinuity along the intimal surface of the aortic lumen.
- The reported diagnostic accuracy of TEE for diagnosis of traumatic aortic injury ranges from a sensitivity of 57% to 100% and a specificity of 88% to 100%.
- Intramural hematoma indicates a contained rupture at the site of aortic injury and appears as a regional thickening of the aortic wall.

KEY POINTS—cont'd

Perivascular hematoma from a contained rupture appears as a tissue density surrounding the aorta at the site of injury. Perivascular hematoma may cause a separation between the TEE probe tip in the esophagus and the posterolateral wall of the aortic isthmus or a distortion of the vessel wall (see Figure 7-26). Free rupture or leaking into the pleural space will produce a hemothorax that can be detected by TEE as an effusion with thrombus within the left pleural cavity (see Figure 7-14).

Aortic Atherosclerosis

- TEE is useful for detecting and grading the severity of aortic atherosclerosis to estimate the risk of thromboembolic complications and stroke.
- TEE or epiaortic ultrasound scanning to define the location and size of aortic atheroma is also important to decrease the risk of

TABLE 7-3   GRADING OF AORTIC ATHEROSCLEROSIS BY TRANSESOPHAGEAL ECHOCARDIOGRAPHY

Grade	Severity	Description
I	Normal	Normal to mild intimal thickening
II	Mild	Intimal thickening ≤ 3 mm without irregularities
III	Moderate	Sessile atheroma protruding < 5 mm into the lumen
IV	Severe	Sessile atheroma protruding ≥ 5 mm into the lumen
V	Severe	Any size atheroma with mobile components

Adapted from Katz ES, Tunick PA, Rusinek H, et al. Protruding aortic atheromas predict stroke risk in elderly patients undergoing cardiopulmonary bypass: experience with intraoperative transesophageal echocardiography. *J Am Coll Cardiol.* 1992;20:70-77.

thromboembolism during operations that involve instrumentation of the thoracic aorta (see Figure 7-26).

- Atheromas appear on echocardiographic examination as irregular thickening along the intimal surface of the aorta (see Figure 7-26).
- The increased density of atherosclerotic plaques causes it to appear brighter on ultrasound imaging compared with normal regions of the vessel wall.
- Calcified plaques will produce ultrasound shadowing.
- The severity of atherosclerotic disease is graded according to the thickness of the plaque, the length that the atheroma protrudes into the vessel lumen, and the presence of mobile atheroma (Table 7-3).

KEY POINTS

- Significant atherosclerotic disease of the thoracic aorta is an independent risk factor for stroke and mortality in patients undergoing coronary artery bypass grafting and other cardiac operations.
- The burden of atherosclerotic disease within the aorta is typically progressively greater in vessel segments more distal from the heart.
- Epiaortic ultrasound is more sensitive than manual palpation or TEE for detecting atherosclerosis of the ascending aorta (see discussion in Chapter 9).

KEY POINTS—cont'd

- Severe atherosclerosis of the aortic arch or mobile atheroma detected by TEE in the aortic arch have been shown to be an important risk factor for perioperative stroke in patients undergoing thoracic endovascular aortic repairs involving the distal aortic arch or proximal descending thoracic aorta (see Figure 7-25). This finding indicates that severe atherosclerosis or mobile atheroma detected by TEE represent atheroma vulnerable to thromboembolism as a consequence of surgical or intravascular instrumentation.
- TEE can also be performed to assess the burden of atherosclerosis in the descending thoracic aorta for intra-aortic balloon insertion. TEE can also be used to position the tip of the intra-aortic balloon catheter just distal to the origin of the left subclavian artery.

Aortic Coarctation

- Coarctation of the aorta can range from a localized deformity or narrowing of the aorta to complete interruption of the aorta.
- In adults, the location of the coarctation is typically postductal, just beyond the origin of the subclavian artery or distal to the insertion of the ligamentum arteriosum.
- TEE diagnosis and characterization of aortic coarctation is difficult, because it is not possible to image the narrowed region adjacent to normal segments of the aorta.
- On TEE examination in patients with aortic coarctation, the proximal descending aorta appears to be interrupted as the TEE probe is withdrawn while tracking the descending aorta into the aortic arch.
- TEE color flow Doppler imaging may demonstrate high velocity turbulent flow at the site of coarctation, but it is difficult to estimate the pressure gradient across the stenosis because the ultrasound beam cannot be aligned along the direction of maximum flow.

Patent Ductus Arteriosus

- A patent ductus arteriosus (PDA) is the persistence of the ductus arteriosus connecting the pulmonary artery to

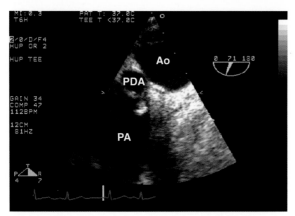

Figure 7-28. TEE UE aortic arch short axis image at a multiplane angle of 71 degrees demonstrates a PDA between the aortic arch (Ao) in short axis and the main PA in long axis.

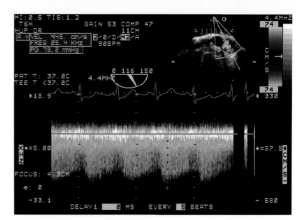

Figure 7-30. TEE UE aortic arch short axis image at a multiplane angle of 116 degrees in a patient with a PDA. Continuous wave Doppler demonstrated that blood flow through the PDA from the aorta to the PA was continuous throughout the cardiac cycle with a phasic component.

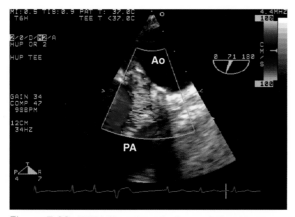

Figure 7-29. TEE UE aortic arch short axis image at a multiplane angle of 71 degrees with color flow Doppler imaging demonstrates blood flow in diastole from the aortic arch (Ao) in short axis into the main PA in long axis through a PDA.

the descending aorta in the fetus (Figure 7-28).
• TEE can detect the presence of a PDA in adolescents and adults by demonstrating flow from the aorta to the pulmonary artery using color flow Doppler imaging in the upper esophageal aortic arch long or short axis views (Figure 7-29).
• With a restrictive PDA, pressure in the aorta is greater than the pressure in the pulmonary artery throughout the cardiac cycle resulting in high velocity continuous flow through the

PDA with a velocity in the range of 2 to 5 m/s (Figure 7-30).
• Longstanding left-to-right shunting through a PDA may cause pulmonary hypertension with associated right ventricular dilatation or hypertrophy that can be detected by echocardiography.

Aortic Tumors and Masses

Thrombus
• Thrombus can occur within the aorta.
• Mural thrombus within an aortic aneurysm appears as an eccentric, crescent-shaped density within the aortic lumen against the aneurysm wall.
• Free-floating thrombus can sometimes be detected within a pseudoaneurysm or within the false lumen of an aortic dissection.
• Complete thrombosis within the aorta causing cardiovascular collapse has also been diagnosed by TEE.

Bacterial Endocarditis
• Vegetations isolated to the descending aorta have been diagnosed using TEE (see Figure 7-23); however, TEE cannot reliably distinguish vegetations caused by infection from mobile atheromas in patients with severe atherosclerotic disease of the aorta.

Tumors

- Tumors can present as a mass within the aortic lumen.
- Tumors can invade the aortic lumen from adjacent organs such as in the case of lung cancer.
- Primary aortic tumors such as leiomyosarcoma, fibroelastoma, or malignant endotheliomas are very rare.

Suggested Readings

1. Shanewise JS, Cheung AT, Aronson S, et al. ASE/SCA guidelines for performing a comprehensive intraoperative multiplane transesophageal echocardiography examination: Recommendations of the American Society of Echocardiography Council for Intraoperative Echocardiography and the Society of Cardiovascular Anesthesiologists Task Force for Certification in Perioperative Transesophageal Echocardiography. *Anesth Analg.* 1999;89:870-884.

2. Pantin EJ, Cheung AT. Transesophageal echocardiographic evaluation of the aorta and pulmonary artery. In: Konstadt S, Shernan S, Oka Y, eds. *Clinical Transesophageal Echocardiography: A Problem-Oriented Approach.* 2nd ed. Philadelphia: Lippincott Williams & Wilkins; 2003:215-244.
A textbook chapter that outlines the TEE examination of the great vessels. Excellent illustrations and images that detail the views to use and the measurements of clinical importance.

3. Hiratzka LF, Bakris GL, Beckman JA, et al. 2010 ACCF/AHA/AATS/ACR/ASA/SCA/SCAI/SIR/STS/SVM guidelines for the diagnosis and management of patients with thoracic aortic disease: A report of the American College of Cardiology Foundation/American Heart Association Task Force on Practice Guidelines, American Association for Thoracic Surgery, American College of Radiology, American Stroke Association, Society of Cardiovascular Anesthesiologists, Society for Cardiovascular Angiography and Interventions, Society of Interventional Radiology, Society of Thoracic Surgeons, and Society for Vascular Medicine. *Circulation.* 2010;121:e266-e369.

4. Coady MA, Ikonomidis JS, Cheung AT, et al, on behalf of the American Heart Association. Surgical management of descending thoracic aortic disease: Open and endovascular approaches. A scientific statement from the American Heart Council on Cardiovascular Surgery and Anesthesia and Council on Peripheral Vascular Disease. *Circulation.* 2010;121:2780-2804.

5. Erbel R, Alfonso F, Boileau C, et al. Diagnosis and management of aortic dissection: Recommendations of the Task Force on Aortic Dissection, European Society of Cardiology. *Eur Heart J.* 2001;22:1642-1681.
Three references which detail the positions of major cardiothoracic societies on the management of patients with thoracic aortic disease.

6. Glas KE, Swaminathan M, Reeves ST, et al. Council for Intraoperative Echocardiography of the American Society of Echocardiography. Society of Cardiovascular Anesthesiologists. Guidelines for the performance of a comprehensive intraoperative epiaortic ultrasonographic examination: Recommendations of the American Society of Echocardiography and the Society of Cardiovascular Anesthesiologists; endorsed by the Society of Thoracic Surgeons. *J Am Soc Echocardiogr.* 2007;20:1227-1235.

7. Nienaber CA, Eagle KA. Aortic dissection: New frontiers in diagnosis and management: Part I: From etiology to diagnostic strategies. *Circulation.* 2003;108:628-635.

8. Moore AG, Eagle KA, Bruckman D, et al. Choice of computed tomography, transesophageal echocardiography, magnetic resonance imaging, and aortography in acute aortic dissection: International Registry of Acute Aortic Dissection (IRAD). *Am J Cardiol.* 2002;89:1235-1238.

9. Movsowitz HD, Levine RA, Hilgenberg AD, et al. Transesophageal echocardiographic description of the mechanisms of aortic regurgitation in acute type A aortic dissection: Implications for aortic valve repair. *J Am Coll Cardiol.* 2000;36:884-890.
Excellent review detailing the pathophysiology of aortic regurgitation in aortic dissection and how knowledge of the mechanisms allows the use of TEE in predicting repairability.

10. Nienaber CA, Kodolitsch Y, Petresen B, et al. Intramural hemorrhage of the thoracic aorta: Diagnostic and therapeutic implications. *Circulation.* 1995;92:1465-1472.

11. Mohr-Kahaly S, Erbel R, Kearney P, et al. Aortic intramural hemorrhage visualized by transesophageal echocardiography: Findings and prognostic implications. *J Am Coll Cardiol.* 1994;23:658-664.

12. von Kodolitsch Y, Csösz SK, Koschyk DH, et al. Intramural hematoma of the aorta: Predictors of progression to dissection and rupture. *Circulation.* 2003;107:1158-1163.
An observational study that details the pathophysiology of intramural hematoma. In cases without dissection, it outlines the early and late progression and prognosis.

13. Shiga T, Wajima Z, Apfel CC, et al. Diagnostic accuracy of transesophageal echocardiography, helical computed tomography, and magnetic resonance imaging for suspected thoracic aortic dissection: systematic review and meta-analysis. *Arch Intern Med.* 2006;166:1350-1356.

14. Vignon P, Boncoeur MP, Francois B, et al. Comparison of multiplane transesophageal echocardiography and contrast-enhanced helical CT in the diagnosis of blunt traumatic cardiovascular injuries. *Anesthesiology.* 2001;94:615-622.
Two papers comparing various diagnostic modalities and their accuracy in dissection and traumatic aortic injuries.

15. Vignon P, Gueret P, Vedrinne JM, et al. Role of transesophageal echocardiography in the diagnosis and management of traumatic aortic disruption. *Circulation.* 1995;92:2959-2968.

16. Appelbe AF, Walker PG, Yeoh JK, et al. Clinical significance and origin of artifacts in transesophageal echocardiography of the thoracic aorta. *J Am Coll Cardiol.* 1993;21:754-760.
An important paper in the understanding of how the aorta is a rich source of artifacts and the underlying mechanisms.

17. Vignon P, Spencer KT, Rambaud G, et al. Differential transesophageal echocardiographic diagnosis between linear artifacts and intraluminal flap of aortic dissection and disruption. *Chest.* 2001;119:1778-1790.

18. Katz ES, Tunick PA, Rusinek H, et al. Protruding aortic atheromas predict stroke in elderly patients undergoing cardiopulmonary bypass: Experience with intraoperative transesophageal echocardiography. *J Am Coll Cardiol.* 1992;20:70-77.

19. Hartman GS, Yao FF, Bruefach M III, et al. Severity of aortic atheromatous disease diagnosed by

transesophageal echocardiography predicts stroke and other outcomes associated with coronary artery surgery: A prospective study. *Anesth Analg.* 1996;83:701-708.
Helps one appreciate the morbidity and mortality when aortic atheromas are seen in the setting of cardiac surgery and how TEE helps in the planning of cannulation and clamping strategies.

20. Desai ND, Szeto WY. Complex aortic arch aneurysm and dissections: Hybrid techniques for surgical and endovascular therapy. *Curr Opin Cardiol.* 2009;24:521-527.

21. Gutsche JT, Cheung AT, McGarvey ML, et al. Risk factors for perioperative stroke after thoracic endovascular aortic repair. *Ann Thorac Surg.* 2007;84:1195-1200.

22. Swaminathan M, Mackensen GB, Podgoreanu MV, et al. Spontaneous echocardiographic contrast indicating successful endoleak management. *Anesth Analg.* 2007;104:1037-1039.
Three nice papers describing the diagnostic approach and imaging in endovascular aortic repair.

Congenital Heart Disease

8

Denise Joffe

- There are now more adults than children with congenital heart disease (CHD).
- Many present for reoperative procedures; they were treated in an era when there was a long interval between palliative procedures and complete repair. Their hearts were exposed to prolonged pressure and volume loads, cyanosis, abnormal rhythms, and other physiologic stresses.
- A smaller number of adult patients require surgery for unrepaired simple or complex CHD.
- Patients with CHD also require noncardiac surgery.
- In order to interpret an intraoperative transesophageal echocardiography (TEE) examination, it is critical to have a detailed appreciation of the patient's history, including all cardiac surgical/interventional procedures. The echocardiographer must understand the long-term risks and complications of the defect and treatments.
- For optimal management, most of these procedures including noncardiac surgery should be performed in centers with the expertise and resources to care for these complex patients.
- Many of these patients have had exhaustive studies to delineate their anatomy and residual defects before elective surgery. Intraoperative TEE can confirm the preoperative diagnosis, assess the surgical repair, and help guide the hemodynamic management of the patient.

ATRIAL SEPTAL DEFECTS

KEY POINTS

All Atrial Septal Defects (ASD)
(Tables 8-1 and 8-2)
- Adult presentation is not uncommon.
- Presentation may be shortness of breath (SOB), congestive heart failure (CHF), arrhythmias, and/or right heart enlargement.

KEY POINTS—cont'd

- Symptoms worsen with age because the decrease in left ventricular (LV) compliance increases left to right (L→R) shunt.

Primum Atrial Septal Defects (Figure 8-1A)
- Cleft mitral valve (MV) is almost always present (see Figure 8-1B).
- Secondary changes to the MV from prolonged mitral regurgitation (MR) can result in annular dilatation, thickened leaflets, and restricted motion and complicate the repair.
- Left ventricular outflow tract obstruction (LVOTO) can develop because of:
  - A deficient LV inlet compared with the LV outlet causing long tunnel-like LVOTO ("gooseneck deformity").
  - A discrete membrane causing stenosis (Figure 8-2A).
  - Aberrant chords inserting into the interventricular septum (IVS) obstructing outflow (see Figure 8-2B).
- **Reoperations** for new/recurrent MR/LVOTO.

Secundum Atrial Septal Defects
(see Figure 8-1C)
- Associated defects include MV prolapse, left superior vena cava (LSVC), pulmonic stenosis (PS), and partial anomalous pulmonary venous drainage (PAPVD).
- If left untreated, approximately 5% develop Eisenmenger's syndrome (irreversible pulmonary vascular disease).

Sinus Venosus Atrial Septal Defects
(Figure 8-3)
- Most are superior sinus venosus (SV) ASDs and are associated with anomalous right pulmonary vein drainage into the right atrium (RA) or superior vena cava (SVC).
- Inferior defects are very rare.
- Scimitar syndrome is anomalous pulmonary vein (PV) drainage of part or all of the right lung to the inferior vena cava (IVC). Associated defects include secundum ASD,

Continued

right lung hypoplasia, and aortopulmonary collaterals supplying the right lung.
- **Reoperations** for obstruction of the SVC/PVs/ASD baffle.

Coronary Sinus Atrial Septal Defects (Figure 8-4)
- The coronary sinus (CS) opens into the floor of the left atrium (LA) causing a L→R shunt. The defect may involve part or the whole CS.
- There is a high association with an LSVC and it alters the surgical repair (Figure 8-5).
- Associated defects: PAPVD, LSVC.

Principles of Surgical/Interventional Management

- Concomitant tricuspid valve (TV) repair may be necessary if right ventricular (RV) dilatation/hypertension has caused moderate to severe tricuspid regurgitation (TR).

Secundum Atrial Septal Defects
- Defect closed with a device in catheterization laboratory or with surgical closure using a pericardial patch or simple stitch closure.

Primum Atrial Septal Defects
- Surgical patch closure of the primum ASD.
- The MV cleft is usually stitch closed even if there is no MR.
- If the MR is more complex or in cases of re-operation, repair may involve annular reduction, commissurotomy, or patch augmentation of deficient leaflet tissue. If the valve cannot be repaired a MVR (mitral valve replacement) is performed in the older patient.

Sinus Venosus Atrial Septal Defects
- Patch closure of defect with anomalous PV baffled to the LA (see Figure 8-3C).
- SVC-RA junction may require augmentation with a pericardial patch to avoid SVC obstruction: "two-patch technique," one to baffle the PV and one to augment the SVC.
- A Warden procedure may be necessary when the PVs drain into the high SVC or if there is difficulty making an unobstructed baffle. The SVC is disconnected and reattached to the right atrial appendage (RAA). The PV "stump" (cardiac end of the SVC containing the anomalous PV) is baffle closed to the LA.

Scimitar Syndrome
- Several surgical techniques can be used.
  1. The scimitar vein is baffled from its origin in the IVC to the LA through an existing patent foramen ovale (PFO)/ASD or a

---

TABLE 8-1   BASIC ECHOCARDIOGRAPHIC PRINCIPLES WHEN IMAGING PATIENTS WITH AN ATRIAL SEPTAL DEFECT

Defect	What to Look for on 2D	CF and Spectral Doppler
All ASDs	• Measure ASD size. • Examine MV structure and function. Look for prolapse/cleft. • Examine TV for prolapse. Measure annulus. • Examine PV drainage especially right-sided PVs. • Assess for RAE, RVE. • Assess biventricular function. • Examine morphology/function of PulmV. Look for number of leaflets, doming leaflets, commissural fusion, restricted motion (ME AV SAX, ME asc aortic SAX, ME RV inflow-outflow, UE aortic arch, SAX). • Elevated PAP, RVH, R→L shunt, flat or leftward orientation of IAS in systole may indicate Eisenmenger's. • Look for an LSVC, located between the LUPV and the LAA (see Figure 8-5) (ME 2C, ME 4C).	• CF/PW Doppler for direction of flow (L→R in uncomplicated ASDs) (Figure 8-6). • CF/CW Doppler to grade MR, TR. • PW of PVs may show higher baseline velocities second to high PBF but pulsatility is preserved and peak and mean velocities are not significantly elevated. • Estimate PAP if TR is present RVP = PAP = $4V_{TR}^2$ + RAP (ME inflow-outflow, ME 4C). • CF/CW Doppler to assess for PS. Velocities up to 2.5 m/s may result from ASD flow alone.

asc, ascending; ASD, atrial septal defect; AV aortic valve; 4C, four-chamber; CF, color flow; IAS, interatrial septum; L, left; LAA, left atrial appendage; LSVC, left superior vena cava; LUPV, left upper pulmonary vein; ME, midesophageal; MR, mitral regurgitation; MV, mitral valve; PAP, pulmonary artery pressure; PBF, pulmonary blood flow; PS, pulmonic stenosis; PulmV, pulmonary valve; PV, pulmonary vein; PW, pulsed wave; R, right; RAE, right atrial enlargement; RV, right ventricular; RVE, right ventricular enlargement; RVH, right ventricular hypertrophy; RVP, right ventricular pressure; SAX, short axis; TR, tricuspid regurgitation; TV, tricuspid valve; 2C, two-chamber; 2D, two-dimensional; UE, upper esophageal.

TABLE 8-2 BASIC ECHOCARDIOGRAPHIC PRINCIPLES WHEN IMAGING SPECIFIC ATRIAL SEPTAL DEFECTS

Defect	Best TEE Views	What to Look for on 2D	CF and Spectral Doppler
Secundum ASD		• Defect in the area of the FO (ME 4C, ME bicaval, ME AV SAX and ME RV inflow-outflow, deep TG LAX with 90-degree rotation (deep TG bicaval equivalent).	

Continued

TABLE 8-2   BASIC ECHOCARDIOGRAPHIC PRINCIPLES WHEN IMAGING SPECIFIC ATRIAL SEPTAL DEFECTS—cont'd

Defect	Best TEE Views	What to Look for on 2D	CF and Spectral Doppler
Primum ASD	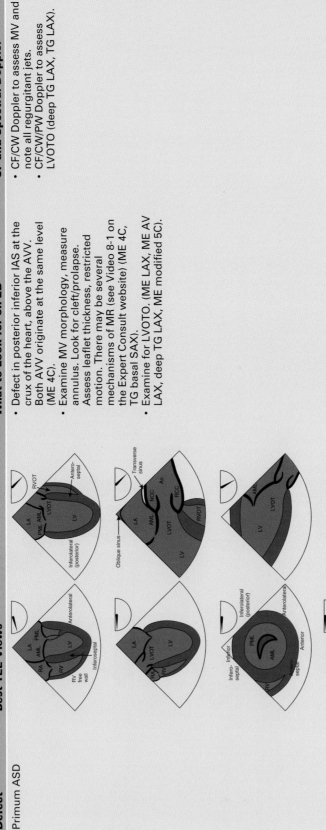	• Defect in posterior inferior IAS at the crux of the heart, above the AVV. Both AVV originate at the same level (ME 4C). • Examine MV morphology, measure annulus. Look for cleft/prolapse. Assess leaflet thickness, restricted motion. There may be several mechanisms of MR (see Video 8-1 on the Expert Consult website) (ME 4C, TG basal SAX). • Examine for LVOTO. (ME LAX, ME AV LAX, deep TG LAX, ME modified 5C).	• CF/CW Doppler to assess MV and note all regurgitant jets. • CF/CW/PW Doppler to assess LVOTO (deep TG LAX, TG LAX).

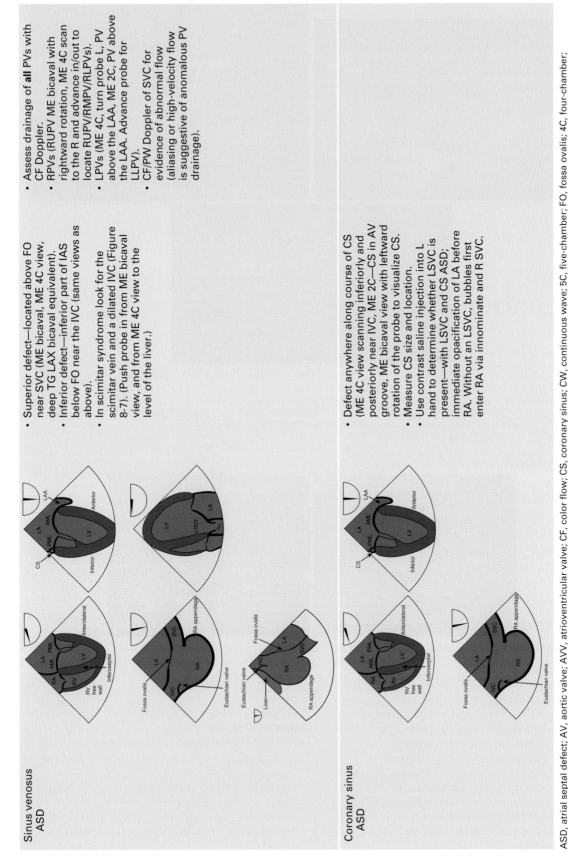

Sinus venosus ASD

- Superior defect—located above FO near SVC (ME bicaval, ME 4C view, deep TG LAX bicaval equivalent).
- Inferior defect—inferior part of IAS below FO near the IVC (same views as above).
- In scimitar syndrome look for the scimitar vein and a dilated IVC (Figure 8-7). (Push probe in from ME bicaval view, and from ME 4C view to the level of the liver.)

- Assess drainage of **all** PVs with CF Doppler.
- RPVs (RUPV ME bicaval with rightward rotation, ME 4C scan to the R and advance in/out to locate RUPV/RMPV/RLPVs).
- LPVs (ME 4C, turn probe L, PV above the LAA, ME 2C, PV above the LAA. Advance probe for LLPV).
- CF/PW Doppler of SVC for evidence of abnormal flow (aliasing or high-velocity flow is suggestive of anomalous PV drainage).

Coronary sinus ASD

- Defect anywhere along course of CS (ME 4C view scanning inferiorly and posteriorly near IVC, ME 2C—CS in AV groove, ME bicaval view with leftward rotation of the probe to visualize CS.
- Measure CS size and location.
- Use contrast saline injection into L hand to determine whether LSVC is present—with LSVC and CS ASD; immediate opacification of LA before RA. Without an LSVC, bubbles first enter RA via innominate and R SVC.

ASD, atrial septal defect; AV, aortic valve; AVV, atrioventricular valve; CF, color flow; CS, coronary sinus; CW, continuous wave; 5C, five-chamber; FO, fossa ovalis; 4C, four-chamber; IAS, interatrial septum; IVC, inferior vena cava; L, left; LA, left atrium; LAX, long axis; LLPV, lower left pulmonary vein; LPV, left pulmonary vein; LSVC, left superior vena cava; LVOTO, left ventricular outflow tract obstruction; ME, midesophageal; MR, mitral regurgitation; MV, mitral valve; PW, pulsed wave; R, right; RA, right atrium; RLPV, right lower pulmonary vein; RMPV, right middle pulmonary vein; RPV, right pulmonary vein; RUPV, right upper pulmonary vein; RV, right ventricular; SAX, short axis; SVC, superior vena cava; 2D, two-dimensional.

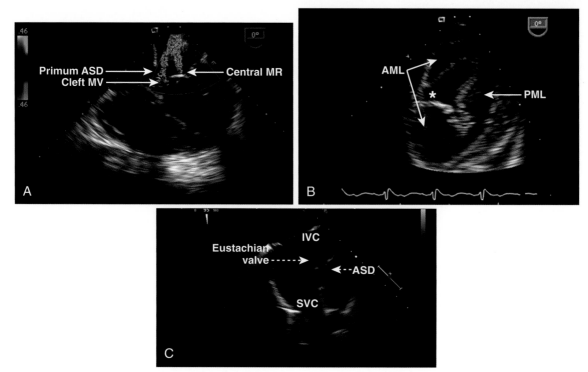

Figure 8-1. **A,** Primum ASD. ME 4C view with CF Doppler demonstrates a defect in the inferior part of the IAS and two jets of MR. More imaging suggested that the medial jet originated from the medial aspect of the cleft and the second, more central jet of MR was likely a coaptation defect from annular dilatation. Note also that both AVVs originate at the same level from the center (crux) of the heart. **B,** TG basal SAX view showing a large cleft *(asterisk)* in the anterior mitral leaflet (AML). **C,** Secundum ASD. Deep TG view at 90 degrees with rightward rotation (deep TG bicaval equivalent) shows a defect in the area of the fossa ovalis (FO).

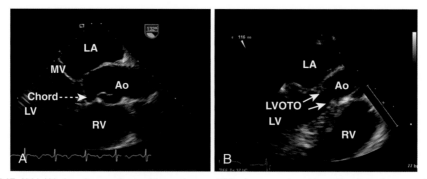

Figure 8-2. **A,** ME AV LAX view in a patient with a primum ASD shows a chord inserting into the ventricular septum. **B,** ME AV LAX in a patient 2 years post primum ASD repair shows a long segment tunnel-like LVOTO that required surgical repair.

surgically created ASD. The baffle is usually long and makes a sharp turn at its origin with a risk of obstruction.

2. The preceding procedure is employed except that the vein is reattached to the RA before the intracardiac baffle. The baffle is shorter and the baffle angle is less.

3. A direct anastomosis to the LA. It is not always possible to mobilize the vein for this approach.

Coronary Sinus Atrial Septal Defects

- Simple patch closure of the CS orifice. The CS drains into the LA, resulting in minimal cyanosis (R→L shunt).
- With an LSVC, the roof of the CS is covered and allowed to drain into the RA. If an LSVC is not recognized, simple patch closure of the CS ostium will result in unacceptable cyanosis.

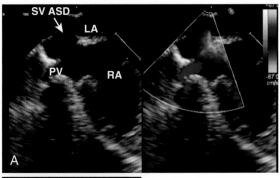

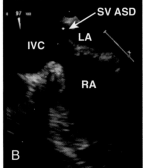

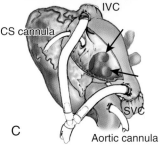

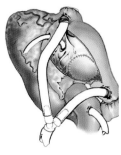

Figure 8-3. **A,** Superior SV ASD. 2D and CF Doppler ME 4C view with the probe withdrawn slightly demonstrates a defect in the superior aspect of the IAS. The RUPV is seen to drain into the RA and flow is left to right through the ASD. **B,** Inferior SV ASD. 2D ME bicaval view shows a defect in the inferior part of the IAS. Note the enlarged IVC. **C,** Schematic drawing with the SV ASD straddling the right upper and lower pulmonary veins (*arrows*). In the right hand frame, the defect was closed using a double-patch repair technique, while assuring that the right pulmonary veins drained into the left atrium. *Courtesy of Starr Kaplan.*

Postoperative TEE Assessment after Atrial Septal Defect Repair

Step 1: Verify ASD closure
- Bubble contrast study is often a helpful adjunct to visualize residual shunts.

Step 2: Assess MV function
- After a primum repair, MR can be eccentric and composed of multiple jets. Grading can be difficult. Less than mild MR is necessary for a durable repair but more significant MR

is often tolerated in children to avoid early mitral valve repair (MVR).

Step 3: Assess TV function
- If a repair/annuloplasty ring was performed, mild residual TR is ideal.

Step 4: Specific ASDs
- SV ASD. Confirm appropriate drainage of PVs into the LA without narrowing of PV/SVC/SVC baffle/SVC-RAA anastomosis (Figure 8-8). PV flow should be pulsatile and of low velocity.
- CS ASD. In patients without an LSVC, confirm closure of the CS. In those with an LSVC, the CS drains into the RA and the CS appears normal (covered) in the midesophageal (ME) two-chamber (2C) view.
- Scimitar syndrome. Confirm unobstructed drainage of the scimitar vein to the LA after repair. If a baffle was used, assess for obstruction at the baffle origin and along its course to the LA.

VENTRICULAR SEPTAL DEFECTS

KEY POINTS

All Ventricular Septal Defects
(Tables 8-3 to 8-5)
- Adult presentation is rare unless the ventricular septal defect (VSD) is small or there are coexisting defects that restrict pulmonary blood flow (PBF). A high incidence of Eisenmenger's occurs in unrepaired moderate to large VSDs.
- Cardiac catheterization must be performed when there is PHTN to evaluate pulmonary vascular resistance (PVR) and suitability for VSD closure.
- Associated lesions: ASDs, double-chamber right ventricle (DCRV), coarctation, subaortic obstruction, other complex CHDs (see Video 8-2 on the Expert Consult website).
- PHTN may occasionally progress even in those with early repair.

Perimembranous Defects
(Figure 8-9A)
- Also known as infracristal, subaortic, paramembraneous, conoventricular.
- Owing to the Venturi effect from VSD flow, the right coronary cusp (RCC) and noncoronary cusp (NCC) are at risk of prolapse with the development of aortic insufficiency (AI).
- Defect may be partially/completely closed with TV tissue that appears aneurysmal

Continued

Text continued on p. 198

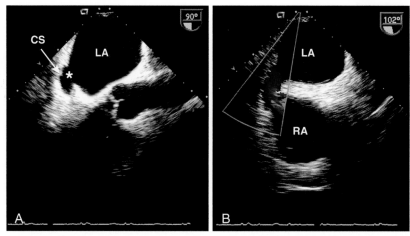

Figure 8-4. **A,** CS ASD. ME AV LAX shows the CS opening into the LA *(asterisk)*. The extent of the defect cannot be determined in this view. **B,** Flow is going left to right through the defect.

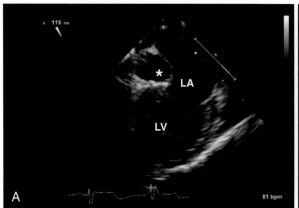
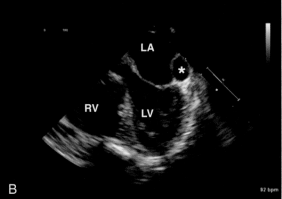

Figure 8-5. **A,** ME modified 2C view shows an enlarged CS in the atrioventricular groove (enlarged CS marked with an *asterisk*). **B,** ME modified 5C view shows the LSVC. Always rule out an LSVC in the presence of a dilated CS (>1 cm).

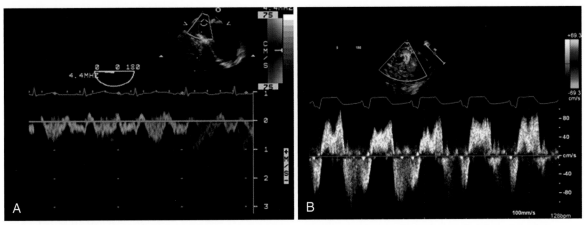

Figure 8-6. PW Doppler of ASD flow in a ME 4C view with rightward rotation. **A,** There is mostly left to right flow. **B,** PW Doppler shows bidirectional flow through an ASD. There is right to left flow during systole and left to right flow during diastole. Although it is not possible to calculate PVR by echocardiography, a careful examination of the heart for signs of pulmonary hypertension (PHTN) should be performed (see note on Eisenmenger's).

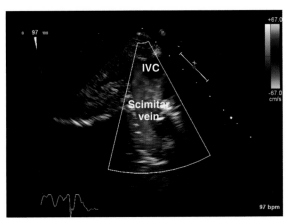

Figure 8-7. CF Doppler view at 97 degrees with insertion of the probe to the level of the liver shows the scimitar vein joining the IVC slightly inferior to the RA.

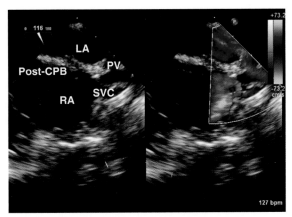

Figure 8-8. 2D and CF Doppler ME bicaval view shows the PV baffle directing RUPV flow to the LA. It is important to verify unobstructed PV and SVC flow.

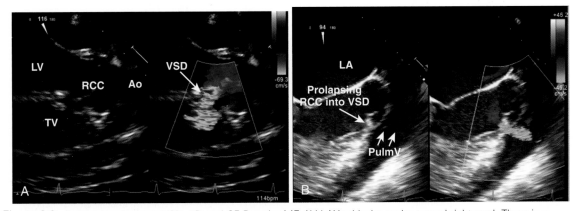

Figure 8-9. **A,** Perimembranous VSD. 2D and CF Doppler ME AV LAX with the probe turned rightward. There is a high-velocity restrictive VSD adjacent to the RCC in the LV and the TV in the RV. Note that the RCC is prolapsing into the defect. Ao, aorta. **B,** Outlet VSD. 2D and CF Doppler modified ME AV SAX demonstrates a VSD immediately underneath the PulmV. The RCC is prolapsing into the defect, although there is no AI seen (clip taken in diastole).

TABLE 8-3   SURGICAL APPROACH TO VENTRICULAR SEPTAL DEFECT CLOSURE

Most Common Surgical Approach	Defect	Additional Facts
RA	• Inlet, perimembranous, anterior malaligned VSD.	• Preferable because it is the most innocuous approach. • Retraction of TV necessary. Occasionally partial removal and then resuspension of TV is employed.
RV	• Anterior malaligned (TOF) • Perimembranous/inlet if cannot be closed via RA approach.	• Division/resection of muscle bundles easily performed from RV. • Risk of RV dysfunction or dysrhythmias.
Transpulmonary	• Outlet	
Transaortic	• VSD associated with DORV or when concomitant aortic valve repair (valvuloplasty) or subaortic resection is needed.	• Higher incidence of heart block when VSD closed via this approach.
LV	• Rarely muscular	• Risk of LV dysfunction or dysrhythmias.

DORV, double-outlet right ventricle; LV, left ventricle; LV, left ventricular; RA, right atrium; RA, right atrial; RV, right ventricle; RV, right ventricular; TOF, tetralogy of Fallot; TV, tricuspid valve; VSD, ventricular septal defect.

TABLE 8-4   BASIC ECHOCARDIOGRAPHIC PRINCIPLES WHEN IMAGING PATIENTS WITH A VENTRICULAR SEPTAL DEFECT

Defect	What to Look for on 2D	CF and Spectral Doppler
All VSDs	• Measure VSD size. • Scan complete septum for multiple VSDs. • Look for ASD/PFO. • Assess for LAE and LVE. • Assess biventricular function. • PHTN, RVH and R→L ventricular shunt may indicate Eisenmenger's syndrome. • Look for subpulmonary obstruction or subaortic membrane. • Examine AV. Look for the mechanism of AI.	• CF/CW Doppler to evaluate VSD size, direction of shunt/RVP. 　• **Size:** 2D/CF Doppler. Defects < 25% size of aortic annulus small, 25-75% mod, >75% large. 　• **Direction:** In an *uncomplicated* VSD, flow is predominantly L→R during systole. Often there is a small reversal of flow (R→L) during the early part of diastole. Bidirectional or R→L flow suggests PHTN/RVOTO. 　• **Velocity:** High-velocity flow with aliasing consistent with a restrictive defect. Low-velocity VSD flow consistent with a large unrestrictive defect or RVOTO and a small VSD. RVP = RVOT gradient + PAP. 　• **RVP:** CW Doppler used measure $RVP = SBP - 4V_{vsd}^2$ (Figure 8-13), $RVP = 4V_{TR}^2 + RAP$. *Ensure VSD jet is not confused with TR jet or PAPs may be factitiously elevated.* (Measure V_{vsd} in ME 4C, ME AV SAX, ME AV LAX, ME RV inflow-outflow, TG mid SAX.) • CF Doppler to assess intracavitary RV obstruction, DCRV, or RVOTO, although Doppler may be hard to align for accurate gradient (ME RV inflow-outflow, deep TG LAX turn the probe leftward with slight anteflexion). • CF/CW Doppler to assess for LVOTO/AI. The AI jet is usually directed away from the prolapsed leaflet (deep TG LAX, TG LAX).

AI, aortic insufficiency; ASD, atrial septal defect; AV, aortic valve; CF, color flow; CW, continuous wave; 4C, four-chamber; DCRV, double-chamber right ventricle; L, left; LAE, left atrial enlargement; LAX, long axis; LVE, left ventricular enlargement; ME, midesophageal; PAP, pulmonary artery pressure; PFO, patent foramen ovale; PHTN, pulmonary hypertension; R, right; RAP, right atrial pressure; RV, right ventricular; RVH, right ventricular hypertrophy; RVOT, right ventricular outflow tract; RVOTO, right ventricular outflow tract obstruction; RVP, right ventricular pressure; SAX, short axis; SBP, systolic blood pressure; TG, transgastric; TR, tricuspid regurgitation; 2D, two-dimensional; VSD, ventricular septal defect.

TABLE 8-5 BASIC ECHOCARDIOGRAPHIC PRINCIPLES WHEN IMAGING SPECIFIC VENTRICULAR SEPTAL DEFECTS

Defect	Best TEE Views	What to Look for on 2D	CD and Spectral Doppler
Perimembranous VSD		• From RV: defect adjacent to the septal leaflet of the TV. • From LV: defect adjacent to the RCC and NCC (ME 4C, ME AV SAX, ME RV inflow-outflow, modified 5C view—obtained by withdrawing and flexing the probe slightly from the ME 4C view). • Examine the septal leaflet of the TV for aneurysm formation, although it rarely causes TV dysfunction. • Examine AV cusp for thickness or prolapse (RCC/NCC).	• CF/CW Doppler to assess AI.

Continued

TABLE 8-5 BASIC ECHOCARDIOGRAPHIC PRINCIPLES WHEN IMAGING SPECIFIC VENTRICULAR SEPTAL DEFECTS—cont'd

Defect	Best TEE Views	What to Look for on 2D	CD and Spectral Doppler
Inlet VSD		• Located inferiorly and posteriorly in the inlet septum adjacent to AVV (ME 4C, or leftward rotation from ME RV inflow-outflow view or rightward rotation from ME LAX—see absent, scooped-out appearance of septum). • Often part of CAVC defect. • A SV repair is performed if an AVV overrides (>50% of the valve originates from the opposite ventricle) or for straddling chords that cross the IVS and insert in the opposite ventricle (ME 4C). • Examine for LVOTO.	• CF/CW Doppler to assess for AVVR/stenosis. • CF/CW Doppler to assess LVOTO (deep TG LAX, TG LAX).

Continued

Outlet VSD

- From RV: defect anterior & adjacent to PulmV in RV outlet (ME AV SAX, deep TG LAX, ME RV inflow-outflow).
- From LV: defect between LCC and RCC (ME AV LAX with rightward rotation).
- Examine AV cusp (RCC) for prolapse (ME RV inflow-outflow, ME AV LAX with rightward rotation).
- CF/CW Doppler to assess AI

TABLE 8-5   BASIC ECHOCARDIOGRAPHIC PRINCIPLES WHEN IMAGING SPECIFIC VENTRICULAR SEPTAL DEFECTS—cont'd

Defect	Best TEE Views	What to Look for on 2D	CD and Spectral Doppler
Muscular		• Defect in muscular inlet, outlet or midventricular or apical septum.	• CF/CW Doppler to examine IVS for multiple VSDs.
Malalignment type		• Anterior deviation typical of VSD in TOF (see section on TOF). • Posterior deviation typical of patient with interrupted aortic arch and results in subaortic stenosis.	

AI, aortic insufficiency; AV, aortic valve; AVV, atrioventricular valve; AVVR, atrioventricular valve repair; CAVC, complete atrioventricular canal; CF, color flow; CW, continuous wave; 5C, five-chamber; 4C, four-chamber; IVS, interventricular septum; LAX, long axis; LV, left ventricle; LVOTO, left ventricular outflow tract obstruction; ME, midesophageal; NCC, noncoronary cusp; PulmV, pulmonary valve; PV, pulmonary vein; RCC, right coronary cusp; RV, right ventricle; SAX, short axis; SV, single ventricle; TEE, transesophageal echocardiography; TG, transgastric; TOF, tetralogy of Fallot; TV, tricuspid valve; 2D, two-dimensional; VSD, ventricular septal defect.

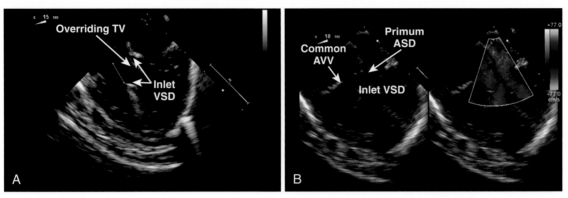

Figure 8-10. **A,** Inlet VSD. ME 4C view shows a defect immediately underneath the AVV. There is an overriding TV with more than 50% of the TV opening into the LV (the *stippled yellow line* marks where the crest of the septum would line up with the AVV). There are also straddling chords that are not well seen in this image (see text). **B,** Inlet VSD as part of an AVC defect. 2D and CF Doppler ME 4C views show an inlet VSD and the associated primum ASD and common AVV. The direction of flow through the VSD is away from the LV (L→R).

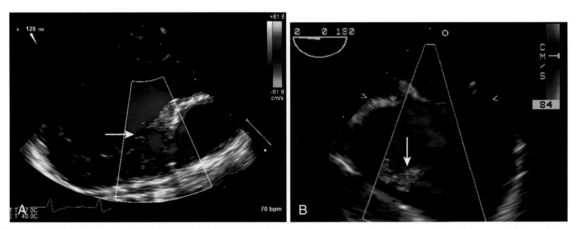

Figure 8-11. **A,** Muscular VSD. CF Doppler ME AV LAX view shows a muscular VSD in a heavily trabeculated part of the mid septum. There is a left to right shunt and it is likely large given the low-velocity flow. Note also there is LV enlargement. **B,** CF Doppler ME 4C view shows a high-velocity restrictive VSD in the mid septum.

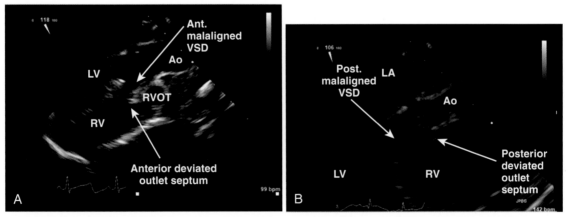

Figure 8-12. **A,** Anterior malaligned VSD. ME AV LAX shows the outlet septum deviated anteriorly resulting in a VSD and RVOTO. This patient had TOF. **B,** Posterior malaligned VSD. ME AV LAX view shows the outlet septum deviated posteriorly into the LVOT resulting in a VSD and LVOTO. This patient had an interrupted aortic arch.

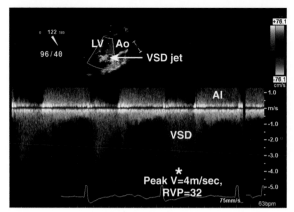

Figure 8-13. CW Doppler of ME AV LAX view in a patient with a perimembranous VSD. CW is aligned as parallel as possible to the direction of the jet and the peak velocity is used to calculate RVP = LVP − $4V_{vsd}^2$. SBP is used as LVP, assuming there is no LVOTO. As RVP nears LVP, the defect becomes unrestrictive and the velocity decreases.

Principles of Surgical Management

- TV repair/annuloplasty ring may be necessary if RV dilation/hypertension has caused moderate to severe TR.
- Aortic prolapse can usually be repaired but occasionally requires valve replacement.
- Surgical closure of VSD is with a synthetic patch via a right atrial (RA), RV, infundibular (transpulmonary), transaortic, and rarely, LV approach (see Table 8-3).
- Devices are not yet approved for routine closure of VSDs, although devices for closure of muscular and perimembranous defects are available. Hybrid approach with catheter access through a right ventriculotomy with TEE guidance is useful in some cases of apical muscular VSD.

Postoperative TEE Assessment after Primary or Revision Ventricular Septal Defect Repair

Step 1: Look for evidence of a residual VSD
- Residual VSD flow should be high velocity with right ventricular pressure (RVP)/left ventricular pressure (LVP) less than 0.5 to 0.6 and a size less than 25% of the diameter of the aortic annulus are ideal. Reexamine the entire IVS because the decrease in RVP can "unmask" another VSD or DCRV.
Step 2: Examine the TV apparatus, PulmV and aortic valve (AV) for evidence of injury or inadequate repair

- Look for prolapse, perforation of a cusp, or poor resuspension of TV around annulus. Less than mild AI, TR is ideal after repair.
Step 3: Examine biventricular function especially after ventriculotomies
- New or worsening ventricular dysfunction can be secondary to the ventriculotomy or injury to a coronary artery.
Step 4: Measure pulmonary artery pressure (PAP)

ATRIOVENTRICULAR CANAL DEFECTS (TABLE 8-6)

KEY POINTS

Primum ASD
- Also called a partial AVC (see "Atrial Septal Defects" section)

Transitional Canal
- Adult presentation possible.
- Includes primum ASD, cleft MV, restrictive VSD (Figure 8-14).
- Reoperations for atrioventricular valve repair (AVVR), LVOTO

Common Atrioventricular Canal
- Includes a primum ASD, a large inlet VSD, and a common atrioventricular valve (AVV).
- Common in trisomy 21. Surgery between 4 and 6 months of age. Early development of Eisenmenger's in nonoperated patients. Adult presentation only if patient has concomitant RVOTO.
- Single AVV has multiple leaflets: an anterior (superior) and posterior (inferior) leaflet that bridge the IVS and several lateral leaflets (see Figure 8-14; see Video 8-4 on the Expert Consult website).
- AVV is often described as right- or left-sided AVV.
- SV repair is necessary in patients with straddling chords or in patients with an unbalanced AVC (the VSD separates the heart unevenly so that one ventricle, usually the LV, is too small).
- Associated lesions: tetralogy of Fallot (TOF), heterotaxy syndrome.
- **Reoperations** for residual VSD, AVVR, LVOTO.

Principles of Surgical Management

- A one- or two-patch technique or the so-called Australian technique (stitch closure of VSD with patch closure of ASD) is used to close

TABLE 8-6 BASIC ECHOCARDIOGRAPHIC PRINCIPLES WHEN IMAGING PATIENTS WITH REPAIRED OR UNREPAIRED ATRIOVENTRICULAR CANAL DEFECTS

Best TEE Views	What to Look for on 2D	CF and Spectral Doppler
	• Examine the IAS for primum defect. • Look for PFO or secundum ASD. • Examine the configuration of the AVV. Look for a cleft MV, prolapse, restricted motion. Measure the annulus. • Examine the IVS for a VSD. • Evaluate biventricular size/function (ME 4C, TG mid SAX). • Examine LVOT for chords, membranes, tunnel-like obstruction. • Look for an LSVC.	• CF/CW Doppler to evaluate ASD size/direction of flow (L→R in uncomplicated AVC). • CF/CW Doppler to evaluate VSD size/direction of flow (L→R in uncomplicated AVC. In an adult presentation, a small restrictive VSD, RVOTO or Eisenmenger's would be present). • Measure RVP = PAP if TR or VSD jet present. • An LV to RA jet may be difficult to distinguish from a TR jet and would make the RVP (PAP) appear systemic. • Grade AVVR/stenosis. • CF/CW Doppler to identify/measure LVOTO (deep TG LAX, TG LAX, ME LAX).

ASD, atrial septal defect; AVC, atrioventricular canal; AVV, atrioventricular valve; AVVR, atrioventricular valve regurgitation; CF, color flow; CW, continuous wave; 4C, four-chamber; IAS, interatrial septum; IVS, interventricular septum; L, left; LAX, long axis; LSVC, left superior vena cava; LV, left ventricle; LVOT, left ventricular outflow tract; LVOTO, left ventricular outflow tract obstruction; MV, mitral valve; PAP, pulmonary artery pressure; PFO, patent foramen ovale; R, right; RA, right atrium; RVOTO, right ventricular outflow tract obstruction; RVP, right ventricular pressure; SAX, short axis; TG, transgastric; TR, tricuspid regurgitation; 2D, two-dimensional; VSD, ventricular septal defect.

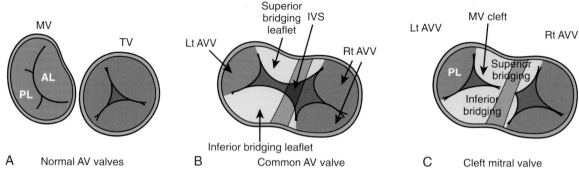

Figure 8-14. Schematic of the AVVs. **A,** A normal heart. **B,** CAVC defects. In the most common configuration, there is a common AVV with five leaflets including two right-sided lateral leaflets, one left-sided lateral leaflet, and superior and inferior leaflets that bridge the IVS. During surgical repair, the atrial and ventricular defects are closed and are fashioned to separate the valves. In addition, the cleft is closed. **C,** Primum and transitional AVC defects. There is a cleft in the left-sided AVV, which is usually closed during repair. IVS, interventricular septum; Lt AVV, left atrioventricular valve; Rt AVV, right atrioventricular valve; PL, posterior leaflet (of the MV). *A and B, Modified and reprinted with permission from Seale A, Shinebourne EA. Cardiac problems in Down's syndrome. Curr Paediatr. 2004;14:33-38.*

the septal defects and bridge the anterior and posterior leaflets.

- The atrial patch is usually placed so that the CS drains into the LA. An LSVC draining to the CS would preclude that.
- MV clefts are usually closed unless it would result in significant mitral stenosis (MS).
- When repaired in infancy, may have to accept even moderate residual regurgitation in order to avoid AVV stenosis or early valve replacement because morbidity/mortality is significantly increased when MVR is performed at less than 2 years. Approximately 15% of patients require reoperations for AVVR. Complex techniques often required for revision MVR (see section on "Primum Atrial Septal

Defect"). MVR may be necessary in older patients.
- Significant LVOTO may require a simple resection or more aggressive intervention (see section on "Left Ventricular Outflow Tract Obstruction").

Postoperative TEE Assessment after Atrioventricular Canal Repair

Step 1: Visualize the ASD/VSD patch
- Verify the absence of atrial/ventricular level shunts.
- AVV without stenosis or regurgitation. At most, trace regurgitation is ideal.

Step 2: Measure PAP if TR is present

Step 3: Assess biventricular function
- LVOTO without significant stenosis.

TETRALOGY OF FALLOT

KEY POINTS

All Tetralogy of Fallot (Tables 8-7 and 8-8)
- Consists of RVOTO, an anterior malaligned VSD, right ventricular hypertrophy (RVH), and overriding aorta (<50% overrides the VSD). The VSD is almost always large and unrestrictive. There may be additional muscular VSDs (Figure 8-15).
- RVOTO may be multifactorial including a subpulmonary component, infundibular narrowing, PulmV annular hypoplasia, PS, and PA or branch PA hypoplasia. Rarely, there is also DCRV.
- Associated defects: PFO, ASD, additional muscular VSDs, aortopulmonary collateral arteries (APCs).

- There is a 25% incidence of right aortic arch (the arch goes over the right bronchus, but this is not seen by TEE).
- Coronary artery anomalies are common. In approximately 3%, the left anterior descending (LAD) comes from the right coronary artery (RCA) and crosses the RVOTO.
- Patients with conotruncal abnormalities (TOF, transposition of the great arteries [TGA], truncus arteriosus) can develop dilatation of the ascending aorta, which may progress and become a risk for rupture or dissection. It may also cause AI.

Continued

TABLE 8-7 PRINCIPLES OF SURGICAL/INTERVENTIONAL MANAGEMENT

Defect	Most Common Surgical Approach
All TOF (except TOF-PA)	• Complete repair consists of VSD closure, division (occasionally resection) of obstructing RV muscle bundles, pulmonary valvotomy and commissurotomy, a transannular patch or PA plasty if indicated. RA or RV approach for VSD. May require a separate infundibular incision for obstructing outlet components. • An RV-PA conduit may be necessary if aberrant coronary anatomy interferes with the ability to relieve RVOTO. • After repair, variable degree of PI results from valvotomy/transannular patch (mild to 4+) • A small atrial fenestration/PFO often left as "pop off" because of decreased RV diastolic function. • **Reoperations/reinterventions** for residual VSDs, persistent/recurrent RVOTO, PA stenosis, PV/AV and RV-PA conduit replacements, ASD/PFO closure, dilated ascending aorta. • Long-term RV function can be compromised by residual volume/pressure loads/ventriculotomy as a result of the disease and/or repair. Many patients returning for reoperation have decreased RV function. • The natural history of isolated root dilatation (without AI) is not known in this disease; some recommend surgery when the ascending aorta is greater than 50 to 55 cm. The optimal procedure can include aortic reduction, a valve-sparing root replacement, or a Bentall.
TOF-PS	• The norm is complete repair as an infant. This may be preceded by an aortopulmonary shunt in some patients. • Adult patients having primary repair would benefit from PulmV placement (or valved RV-PA conduit) at the time of the repair in order to reduce the volume load on the RV.
TOF-PA	• Surgical strategy is complex and often requires staged procedures. • Cardiac catheterization is necessary for adequate assessment of distal PAs and MAPCAs. • **Reoperations/reinterventions.** Patients require life-long interventions including repeat PA dilatations/stent placements/late VSD/ASD closure because of persistent RVOTO secondary to hypoplastic PAs. They may also have PHTN in some lung segments.
TOF-AVC	• Both lesions are usually repaired simultaneously as an infant. • **Reoperations/reinterventions** for R- or L-sided AVVR/stenosis/PulmV replacement, residual VSD/RVOTO obstruction.
TOF-APV	• In addition to standard TOF repair, may require translocation and/or plication of PAs or placement of a valved RV-PA conduit. • **Reoperation/reintervention:** see TOF.
DORV	• The spectrum of repairs for DORV varies from a TOF-like repair to an arterial switch procedure and occasionally other options. • In the TOF spectrum, the VSD closure involves placing the patch in such a way that left ventricular outflow is baffled out the aorta. • **Reoperation/reintervention:** see TOF. The intracardiac baffle may also result in subaortic obstruction.

AI, aortic insufficiency; APV, absent pulmonary valve; ASD, atrial septal defect; AV, aortic valve; AVC, atrioventricular canal; AVVR, atrioventricular valve regurgitation; DORV, double-outlet right ventricle; L, left; MAPCAs, multiple aortopulmonary collateral arteries; PA, pulmonary artery; PFO, patent foramen ovale; PI, pulmonic insufficiency; PS, pulmonic stenosis; PulmV, pulmonary valve; R, right; RA, right atrial; RV, right ventricle; RV, right ventricular; RVOTO, right ventricular outflow tract obstruction; TOF, tetralogy of Fallot; VSD, ventricular septal defect.

TABLE 8-8 BASIC ECHOCARDIOGRAPHIC PRINCIPLES WHEN IMAGING REPAIRED/UNREPAIRED TETRALOGY OF FALLOT

Best TEE Views	What to Look for on 2D	CF and Spectral Doppler
	• Assess atrial size. • Examine IAS for ASD/PFO. • Assess VSD location(s) and size (ME AV LAX, ME LAX, ME 5C, ME RV inflow-outflow, ME AV SAX, deep TG LAX). • Assess RV size/function/RVH (ME 4C, TG mid SAX, ME RV inflow-outflow). • Look for etiology of RVOTO. Examine RV, RVOT, measure pulmonary annulus, and PAs as far distally as possible, assess morphology and function of PulmV/conduit (ME 4C, ME RV inflow-outflow, deep TG LAX, deep TG RVOTO; turn probe to the left and anteflex slightly, ME asc aortic SAX, UE aortic arch SAX). • Examine AVV: (1) Look for TV dysfunction secondary to RV systolic/diastolic dysfunction, (2) look at both AVVs after TOF AVC repair. • Examine LV size/function. • Examine origin and course of coronary arteries. • Measure aortic root dimensions. • Look for abnormalities in the course of the descending aorta (Figure 8-16).	• CF/PW Doppler to identify presence and size of atrial level shunts. • CF/CW Doppler to identify size/location of VSDs. In unrepaired TOF, direction of flow may be dynamic depending on degree of RVOTO. • CF/CW Doppler to quantitate RVOTO and identify PI (Figure 8-17). • Peak gradient greater than 50 mm Hg or RVP/LVP greater than 0.6 severe (ME RV inflow-outflow, deep TG LAX turn leftward and anteflex slightly, ME asc aortic SAX, UE aortic arch SAX). • CF/CW Doppler to grade AVVR/stenosis. • CF/CW Doppler to evaluate/quantitate AI/LVOTO. • Continuous flow signals suggestive of the presence of aortopulmonary collaterals (catheterization diagnosis).

AI, aortic insufficiency; asc, ascending; ASD, atrial septal defect; AV, aortic valve; AVC, atrioventricular canal; AVV, atrioventricular valve; AVVR, atrioventricular valve repair; CF, color flow; CW, continuous wave; 5C, five-chamber; 4C, four-chamber; IAS, interatrial septum; LAX, long axis; LV, left ventricle; LVOTO, left ventricular outflow tract obstruction; LVP, left ventricular pressure; ME, midesophageal; PA, pulmonary artery; PFO, patent foramen ovale; PI, pulmonic insufficiency; PulmV, pulmonary valve; PW, pulsed wave; RV, right ventricle; RV, right ventricular; RVH, right ventricular hypertrophy; RVOTO, right ventricular outflow tract obstruction; RVP, right ventricular pressure; SAX, short axis; TEE, transesophageal echocardiography; TG, transgastric; TOF, tetralogy of Fallot; 2D, two-dimensional; UE, upper esophageal; VSD, ventricular septal defect.

KEY POINTS—cont'd

Tetralogy of Fallot with Pulmonic Stenosis
- The most common location of PA hypoplasia is the left pulmonary artery (LPA), which is not well seen by TEE.
- APCs very rare.
- Patients rarely present with unrepaired disease as an adult.

Tetralogy of Fallot with Pulmonary Atresia
- Atresia may be limited to the valve or may involve the subpulmonary infundibulum.
- Usually variable degrees of hypoplasia of the main or branch PAs often with multiple aortopulmonary collateral arteries (MAPCAs) supplying lung segments.
- Adult presentation of unrepaired TOF-pulmonary atresia possible if MAPCAs supply enough PBF.

Tetralogy of Fallot with Atrioventricular Canal
- Patients have components of both diseases.

Tetralogy of Fallot with Absent Pulmonary Valve
- The pulmonary annulus is usually hypoplastic and there are no real PV leaflets, resulting in severe pulmonic insufficiency (PI). PAs are large and frequently aneurysmal. Often severe RV dilatation.
- The degree of airway compromise in these patients is the overriding determinant of prognosis.

Double-Outlet Right Ventricle–Tetralogy of Fallot Spectrum
- When the aorta overrides the ventricular septum by more than 50%, the patient is said to have double-outlet right ventricle (DORV).
- When associated with a subaortic VSD and subpulmonary obstruction, the patient has physiology that resembles TOF. The intracardiac anatomy resembles TOF except that the aorta is more rightward and there is no aorta-MV continuity.

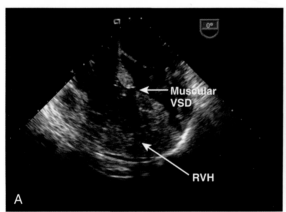
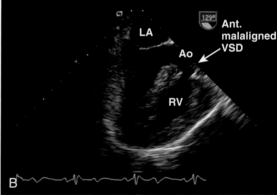

Figure 8-15. Primary TOF repair in a 40-year-old patient. **A,** ME 4C view shows RVH and an additional muscular VSD. **B,** ME AV LAX with slight rightward rotation shows the anterior malaligned VSD with an overriding aorta.

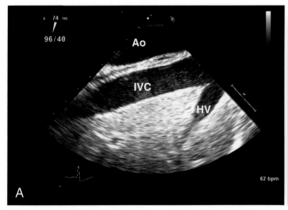
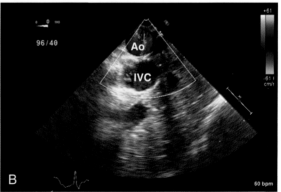

Figure 8-16. ME longitudinal (**A**) and transverse (**B**) views at the level of the liver show the descending aorta and IVC on the right side. Abnormalities in the course of the descending aorta should increase the suspicion of a right aortic arch. A left aortic arch can exist with a right descending aorta, but it is unusual. HV, hepatic vein.

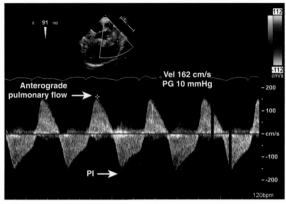

Figure 8-17. CW Doppler of RVOT/PulmV after TOF repair in ME AV SAX view. There is no significant RVOTO (peak gradient < 10 mm Hg) and wide-open PI lasting throughout diastole.

Postoperative TEE Assessment after Primary Repair/Reoperation of Tetralogy of Fallot

Step 1: Look for a residual VSD and reexamine the entire IVS because a drop in RVP may unmask additional VSDs

Step 2: Look for RVOTO and identify etiology
  • RVP/LVP should be less than 0.6 (lower is ideal).

Step 3: Assess PulmV/RV-PA valved conduits
  • Gradients should be within manufacturer's expected estimate and PI should be minimal. Conduits may be hard to visualize but flow is usually visible.

Step 4: Assess biventricular systolic and diastolic dysfunction
  • Circumflex coronary at risk of injury during PulmV replacement.

Step 5: Note the predominant direction of flow through the atrial defect
  • Flow that is R→L provides a crude indication of the degree of restrictive RV dysfunction and also provides an explanation for systemic desaturation.

Step 6: Assess AV/ascending aorta after AVR/ ascending aorta repair or replacement/Bentall

TRANSPOSITION OF THE GREAT ARTERIES

Surgical Management

• Contemporary management for D-transposition of the great arteries (D-TGA) is the ASO in which the PA and branches are brought anterior and connected to the RV (Lecompte's maneuver) and the aorta is moved posteriorly to the LV. The coronary arteries are translocated to the aorta. Any intracardiac shunt is closed and the arch is repaired if necessary.
• Coronary abnormalities are very common in TGA (Figure 8-18). Typically, the coronaries

TABLE 8-9 BASIC ECHOCARDIOGRAPHIC PRINCIPLES WHEN IMAGING REPAIRED D-TRANSPOSITION OF THE GREAT ARTERIES

Best TEE Views	What to Look for on 2D	CF and Spectral Doppler
	• Look for a residual VSD. • Assess biventricular size/function. Include a detailed assessment of RWMA. • Examine MV morphology/function. Look for evidence of papillary muscle dysfunction, tethered chords, annular dilatation secondary to ischemia. • Examine both outflow tracts/semilunar valves for morphology, function, and outflow tract obstruction. • Assess for PA branch stenosis (especially the RPA). Bifurcation of main PA is anterior to aorta. (ME asc aortic SAX). • Note the origin and course of the coronary arteries (see below). • Measure aortic dimensions. D-TGA treated with atrial switch: • Assess RV size/function. • Assess TV size/function. • Examine atrial baffle course and look for obstruction at the SVC/RA > IVC/RA junctions or PV baffle or baffle leaks (ME 2C 4C, ME LAX, LE AV LAX). CTGA treated with double switch: • Similar considerations as ASO and atrial switch. • May have Ebstein-like malformation of systemic TV.	• CF/CW Doppler to assess VSD location/size. • CF/CW Doppler to examine both outflow tracts for aliasing and measure any gradients. • CF/CW Doppler to examine both semilunar valves for stenosis or insufficiency. • CF/PW Doppler to examine coronary flow for evidence of stenosis. • CF/CW Doppler to grade TR/MR. • CF/PW Doppler to assess flow through baffle or leaks.

asc, ascending; AV, aortic valve; CF, color flow; CTGA, congenitally corrected transposition of the great arteries; CW, continuous wave; D-TGA, D-transposition of the great arteries; 4C, four-chamber; IVC, inferior vena cava; LAX, long axis; ME, midesophageal; MR, mitral regurgitation; MV, mitral valve; PA, pulmonary artery; PV, pulmonary vein; PW, pulsed wave; RA, right atrium; RPA, right pulmonary artery; RV, right ventricle; RWMA, regional wall motion abnormalities; SAX, short axis; SVC, superior vena cava; TEE, transesophageal echocardiography; TR, tricuspid regurgitation; TV, tricuspid valve; 2C, two-chamber; VSD, ventricular septal defect.

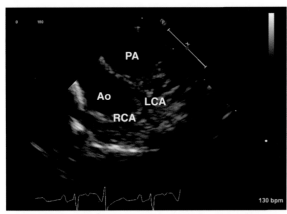

Figure 8-18. ME ascending aortic SAX view before an ASO shows a single coronary giving rise to the RCA and the LCA. Not well seen is the LCA dividing into the LAD and the Cx. Coronary anomalies are common and include intramural and interarterial segments.

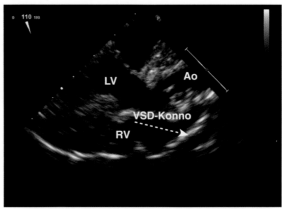

Figure 8-19. ME AV LAX view post Nikaidoh procedure. This patient had TGA with a VSD and PS. The anterior aortic root was translocated posteriorly and is now the LV outflow vessel. The LVOT was enlarged (Konno procedure, see "Left Ventricular Outflow Tract Abnormalities") and the VSD patch is clearly seen. The *stippled arrow* is where a patch is placed had a Rastelli been performed (in which case, the great vessels are not switched). The VSD patch is oriented in a more anatomic position with a Nikaidoh. The RV-PA conduit is not visible in this view (see text).

originate from the aortic sinuses that face the PA. The most common arrangement is the anterior sinus gives rise to the right coronary artery (RCA) and the posterior sinus to the left coronary artery (LCA). Intramural and interarterial segments can also occur (see "Coronary Anomalies"). During the ASO, the coronaries are translocated to the closest area on the PulmV (neoaorta), usually the anterior/posterior right side *above* the respective sinus.

- Coronary insufficiency may be a result of ostial stenosis or may involve more distal stenosis. Ostial stenosis generally requires surgical intervention and balloon dilatations. Stent placement are options for more distal disease.
- Supravalvar PS or aortic stenosis (AS) may be treated with balloon dilatation/surgical repair.
- An atrial switch (Mustard's or Senning's procedure), which involves intra-atrial baffling of systemic and PV flow to the opposite atrium, is no longer a standard treatment for d-TGA because of early RV failure and arrhythmias.
- Baffle obstruction and leaks or PS from septal shift causing RVOTO as a result of elevated RVP may occur after an atrial switch. Baffle issues can usually be treated in the catheterization laboratory.
- A Rastelli, Nikaidoh, or ASO with left ventricular outflow tract (LVOT) enlargement are surgical options for patients with d-TGA, VSD, and PS.

- The Rastelli procedure has been the standard treatment and involves baffling the VSD so that LV outflow is routed to the anterior aorta. The PA is disconnected from the RV and an RV-PA conduit is usually used. Long-term survival is poor as a result of LVOTO/RVOTO from the intracardiac baffle and from repeated reoperations on the conduit/baffle.
- A Nikaidoh procedure involves switching the aorta along with the valve so that the aortic root, coronaries, and aorta are moved to the LV. An RV-PA conduit is also required but it is in a more favorable position than in a Rastelli. The procedure has components of a Ross, Konno, and ASO (Figure 8-19).
- The treatment of CTGA is controversial:
  1. Perform repair of associated defects and "disregard" the CTGA (Figure 8-20A). This is not optimal because the RV/TV remain in the systemic ventricle, and there is a high risk of heart block, systemic ventricular failure, and TR. TR should be managed very aggressively with early valve repair/replacement.
  2. Perform a double switch in early life (see Figure 8-20B). An atrial switch and ASO are performed after a preliminary PA band.
  3. Heart transplant.

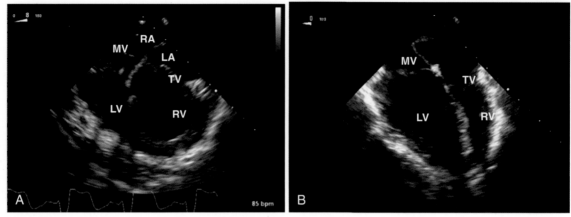

Figure 8-20. **A,** ME 4C view in a patient with CTGA treated with "disregard" for the CTGA. There was a VSD, which was closed, and the VSD patch is clearly visible. Note the IVS bows toward the LV because the RV is the systemic ventricle. Also note that the patient is in heart block and is paced. **B,** ME 4C view shows a patient who has been managed with a double switch. The IVS bows toward the RV because the LV is the systemic ventricle. There is an interatrial baffle. In this patient, there is significant apical displacement of the TV consistent with Ebstein's anomaly of the left-sided TV.

TOTAL ANOMALOUS PULMONARY VENOUS DRAINAGE (TABLE 8-10)

KEY POINTS

- All PVs drain to a location other than the LA.
- PV usually drains to a horizontal confluence behind the LA and then to a vertical vein that drains to a systemic vein, most commonly the innominate vein. However, drainage may be to the SVC, azygos, CS, IVC, or other veins (Figure 8-21).
- Supracardiac total anomalous pulmonary venous drainage (TAPVD). The most common type. Drainage is usually to the innominate vein.
- Cardiac TAPVD. Drainage is usually to the CS. CS can be so large that it obstructs mitral inflow.
- Infracardiac TAPVD. Confluence is more vertically oriented. Drainage is usually to a vertical vein that descends to join the ductus venosus. Usually associated with pulmonary venous obstruction requiring emergent surgery as a newborn.
- Mixed TAPVD. A combination of these.
- A PFO/ASD is necessary for survival.
- TAPVD usually an isolated finding except when associated with heterotaxy syndrome.
- Adult presentation can occur with unobstructed TAPVD. Patients present with symptoms/signs of a large L→R shunt, cyanosis, and often PHTN.
- **Reoperation/reintervention** for PV stenosis, closure of ASD.

Surgical Management

- The surgical management of TAPVD involves ligating the vertical vein and opening the pulmonary vein confluence (PVC) into the LA (incising the floor of the LA, which is the roof of the PVC).
- In newborns at risk of PHTN, a PFO may be left open to serve as a "pop-off."
- In the case of cardiac TAPVD to the CS, the procedure involves "unroofing" the CS into the LA and closing the ostium of the CS with a patch (Figure 8-22). Unroofing is performed by incising the floor of the LA (roof of the CS) so that the CS (and anomalous PVs) drain into the LA.

Reoperations/Reinterventions

- Patients may develop symptoms of recurrent PV obstruction. They usually present in childhood but may occur later.
- Obstruction can occur:
  1. At the anastomosis of the PVC and the LA (Figure 8-23).
  2. Involving the PV itself. It may be extensive and involve multiple veins. The etiology is thought to be an inflammatory reaction related to the surgery/intrinsic vasculopathy.

TABLE 8-10 BASIC ECHOCARDIOGRAPHIC PRINCIPLES WHEN IMAGING PRIMARY/REVISION TOTAL ANOMALOUS PULMONARY VENOUS DRAINAGE

Best TEE Views	What to Look for on 2D	CF and Spectral Doppler
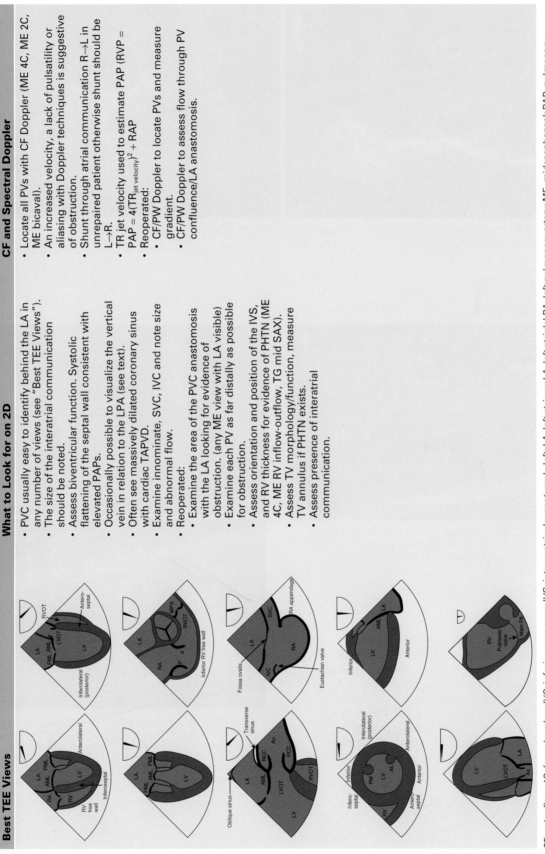	• PVC usually easy to identify behind the LA in any number of views (see "Best TEE Views"). • The size of the interatrial communication should be noted. • Assess biventricular function. Systolic flattening of the septal wall consistent with elevated PAPs. • Occasionally possible to visualize the vertical vein in relation to the LPA (see text). • Often see massively dilated coronary sinus with cardiac TAPVD. • Examine innominate, SVC, IVC and note size and abnormal flow. • Reoperated: • Examine the area of the PVC anastomosis with the LA looking for evidence of obstruction. (any ME view with LA visible) • Examine each PV as far distally as possible for obstruction. • Assess orientation and position of the IVS, and RV thickness for evidence of PHTN (ME 4C, ME RV inflow-outflow, TG mid SAX). • Assess TV morphology/function, measure TV annulus if PHTN exists. • Assess presence of interatrial communication.	• Locate all PVs with CF Doppler (ME 4C, ME 2C, ME bicaval). • An increased velocity, a lack of pulsatility or aliasing with Doppler techniques is suggestive of obstruction. • Shunt through atrial communication R→L in unrepaired patient otherwise shunt should be L→R. • TR jet velocity used to estimate PAP (RVP = PAP = $4(TR_{jet\ velocity})^2$ + RAP • Reoperated: • CF/PW Doppler to locate PVs and measure gradient. • CF/PW Doppler to assess flow through PV confluence/LA anastomosis.

CF, color flow; 4C, four-chamber; IVC, inferior vena cava; IVS, interventricular septum; L, left; LA, left atrial; LA, left atrium; LPA, left pulmonary artery; ME, midesophageal; PAP, pulmonary artery pressure; PHTN, pulmonary hypertension; PV, pulmonary vein; PVC, pulmonary vein confluence; PW, pulsed wave; R, right; RAP, right atrial pressure; RV, right ventricular; RVP, right ventricular pressure; SAX, short axis; SVC, superior vena cava; TAPVD, total anomalous pulmonary venous discharge; TEE, transesophageal echocardiography; TG, transgastric; TR, tricuspid regurgitation; TV, tricuspid valve; 2C, two-chamber; 2D, two-dimensional.

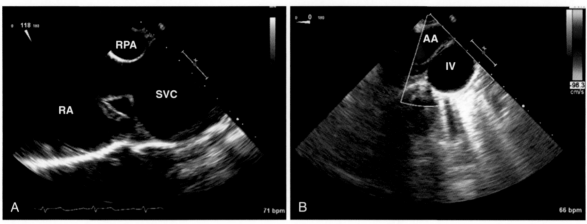

Figure 8-21. **A,** ME bicaval view shows an enlarged SVC from TAPVD. **B,** CF Doppler UE aortic arch (AA) LAX view shows an enlarged innominate vein in a patient with TAPVD.

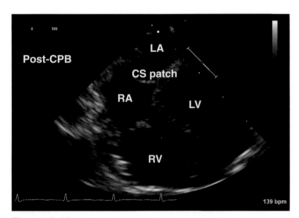

Figure 8-22. ME 4C view with probe advancement in a patient with TAPVD to the CS shows a patch over the CS. The PVs and CS now drain into the LA.

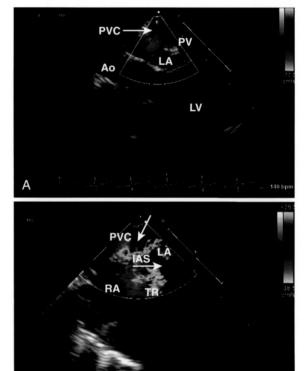

Catheterization is usually necessary to delineate the extent. Revision surgery may involve enlarging the anastomosis, alone or in combination with a "sutureless" technique of PV repair. This involves filleting the PV as distally as necessary and the pericardium is folded over and sutured to the atrium and used to "capture" PV flow. Extensive involvement may not respond well to therapy.

Figure 8-23. **A,** ME modified 5C view shows the LUPV drain to the PVC. A widely patent anastomosis with low-velocity flow is seen. **B,** ME 4C view with the probe turned to the LA. The PVC is seen entering the LA. There is turbulence at the anastomotic site *(arrow)* that required surgical revision. Note there is also mild TR.

TRUNCUS ARTERIOSUS
(TABLE 8-11)

KEY POINTS

- Truncus arteriosus is classified according to the location of the origin of the main PA or (if absent) the separate PAs off the truncus (common great vessel exiting the heart) (see Video 8-6 on the companion website).
- Abnormal truncal valve (neoaortic valve) very common with more than three leaflets. Can be regurgitant, rarely stenotic.
- Associated defects include a subaortic VSD, interrupted aortic arch (10-15%), right aortic arch (25%), and aberrant right subclavian artery (5-10%).
- Abnormal coronary anatomy is common.
- There is very early development of pulmonary vascular disease in unrepaired patients. Adult presentation is very unlikely unless there is PS or Eisenmenger's.
- **Reoperations and reinterventions** for truncal valve disease, residual VSD, RV-PA conduit replacement, and dilated ascending aorta.

Surgical and Interventional Management

Complete early repair consists of removing the PAs from the truncus, VSD closure, and placement of an RV-PA conduit. When possible, a valved conduit is used. A PFO or fenestrated atrial communication is left.

- The management of moderate to severe truncal valve regurgitation is usually attempted with a valve repair with the understanding that residual regurgitation is likely and so is future prosthetic valve replacement. When repair is not possible, a homograft AV replacement is necessary in the neonatal period.
- The placement of PA bands as palliation before complete repair was performed in the past but results were poor. Adequate PA band placement was rare and patients develop early PVD, or PA stenosis.
- Percutaneous balloon dilatation/stent placement/valve replacement (Melody valve) may be possible in some cases of conduit obstruction/regurgitation. Otherwise, reoperations are necessary for RV-PA conduit replacements and truncal (aortic) valve repair/replacement. Dilatation of the ascending aorta may require root replacement, with or without a Bental procedure.

SINGLE VENTRICLE

KEY POINTS

- Includes hypoplastic left heart syndrome (HLHS) (Figure 8-24A), single ventricle (SV; double-inlet left ventricle [DILV] most common variant), tricuspid atresia, unbalanced AVC, pulmonary atresia with intact septum (PAIVS), heterotaxy syndrome (Table 8-12).
- In double-inlet ventricle, both AVVs empty into the ventricle. A VSD (also referred to by its embryologic name, the *bulboventricular foramen*) leads to the outlet chamber (see Figure 8-24B). The ventricles are often transposed, as are the great vessels. There is often obstruction to one or, rarely, both great vessels.
- In tricuspid atresia, there is no effective TV orifice. The RV is frequently very hypoplastic. A VSD may be present and the vessels are often transposed.
- In PAIVS, the TV and RV are often hypoplastic. RVP may be suprasystemic. In severe cases, there are coronary artery sinusoids/fistulae and nonatherosclerotic proximal coronary artery stenosis so that myocardial perfusion becomes dependent on the right ventricle (RV) providing coronary perfusion via the fistulae. RV decompression may result in acute ischemia/death.
- Heterotaxy syndrome occurs when there is ambiguous differentiation of sidedness of the heart/lungs/visceral organs. Associated with bilateral SVC, PS, unbalanced AVC defects, interrupted IVC with azygos continuation, TAPVD, and unroofed CS. This constellation usually results in SV physiology/management (Figure 8-25).

- A three-stage approach leading to a Fontan procedure is usually necessary (Table 8-13). A stage 1 procedure is usually performed within the first couple of weeks of life unless there is a perfectly "balanced" circulation with an adequate degree of restriction to PBF and no restriction to systemic outflow. Stage 2—bidirectional cavopulmonary anastomosis (Glenn or hemi-Fontan procedure) is usually performed between 4 and 6 months. A stage 3—Fontan procedure—is performed between 18 months and 4 years.
- Occasionally, an adult will present having had only a stage 1 or 2 palliation or rarely no previous surgery.
- The principles of long-term management of patients with SV are to preserve systolic and diastolic ventricular function, and AVV competence and to keep PVR as low as possible.

TABLE 8-11   BASIC ECHOCARDIOGRAPHIC PRINCIPLES WHEN IMAGING PATIENTS AFTER TRUNCUS ARTERIOSUS REPAIR

Best TEE Views	What to Look for on 2D	CF and Spectral Doppler
	• Examine IAS for ASD/PFO. • Look for a residual VSD in the area of the outlet septum. • Assess the RV-PA conduit course/calcification. • Assess biventricular size/function. • Characterize the truncal valve with the number of leaflets, thickness, mobility, the presence of stenosis or regurgitation in order to optimize the potential for surgical repair. • Verify prosthetic AV function. • Measure the aortic root and ascending aorta. • Examine the descending aorta and arch for evidence of obstruction. • Examine the coronary arteries for abnormal origin or course.	• CF/PW Doppler to identify PFO. • CFD/CW to identify residual VSD. • CF/CW Doppler to assess truncal valve regurgitation/stenosis (deep TG LAX, TG LAX, ME LAX, ME AV LAX)

ASD, atrial septal defect; AV, aortic valve; CF, color flow; CW, continuous wave; IAS, interatrial septum; LAX, long axis; ME, midesophageal; PA, pulmonary artery; PFO, patent foramen ovale; PW, pulsed wave; RV, right ventricle; TEE, transesophageal echocardiography; TG, transgastric; 2D, two-dimensional; VSD, ventricular septal defect.

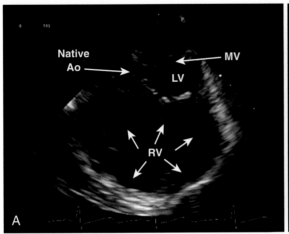 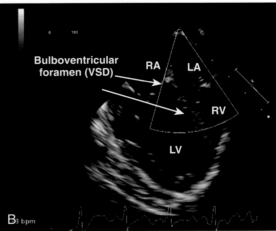

Figure 8-24. **A,** ME 4C view in a patient with HLHS. The mitral annulus and MV are hypoplastic, as are the LV and ascending aorta. In some patients, there is atresia of the MV and aorta so that the ascending aorta and coronary arteries are perfused in a retrograde fashion by the PDA. **B,** ME 4C view in a patient with DILV. The smooth-walled LV is on the right and both inlet valves open into the LV. This patient also has transposed great vessels, which are not seen in this view. The bulboventricular foramen is large and extends from the *lower arrow,* which marks the crest of the IVS, to the *upper arrow,* which marks the crux of the heart.

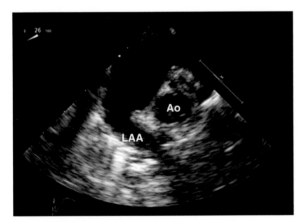

Figure 8-25. A modified ascending aortic view shows a right-sided appendage with a short narrow opening and a "Snoopy ear" appearance characteristic of an LAA.

- Conversion from an atriopulmonary Fontan to an extracardiac Fontan is performed in some older patients with arrhythmias/ recurrent thrombus and massively dilated RAs. They must have preserved systemic ventricular function and low PVR (Figure 8-26).
- Patients with complications related to end-stage heart failure or other SV-specific diseases (e.g., protein-losing enteropathy) may be candidates for cardiac transplantation.

Stage 2
- Glenn/hemi-Fontan: The SVC(s) are connected to the PA so that there is passive flow to the lungs (see Video 8-7 on the Expert Consult website). IVC return is left to enter the heart. The volume work of the ventricle is decreased compared with stage 1.

Stage 3
- The Fontan procedure has undergone significant modifications since the 1970s. Original versions incorporated an atriopulmonary connection that became significantly dilated over time. Contemporary management reroutes IVC flow to the PAs via an extracardiac conduit or a lateral tunnel Fontan.
- Extracardiac Fontan: The cardiac end of the IVC is suture closed and the IVC is anastomosed to the PA via a conduit.
- Lateral tunnel Fontan: An intra-atrial baffle is fashioned from Gore-Tex and directs IVC flow to the PAs *within* the atrium.
- A small 3- to 4-mm fenestration may be placed between the conduit and the atrium in order to serve as a "pop-off" in the event of high SVC/PAP.
- A Kawashima Glenn (K Glenn) is a Glenn performed in a patient with an interrupted IVC and azygos continuation resulting in all lower extremity venous blood returning to the Glenn circuit via the azygos. The stage 3 procedure in those patients reroutes hepatic venous blood to the PAs via a conduit.

TABLE 8-12 BASIC ECHOCARDIOGRAPHIC PRINCIPLES WHEN IMAGING PATIENTS WITH SINGLE VENTRICLES

Best TEE Views	What to Look for on 2D	CF and Spectral Doppler
	• Determine the position and size of the great vessels. Look for obstruction at the ventricular, subvalvar, valvar, or supravalvar level. Ensure a widely patent VSD/BVF if systemic outflow depends on it. • Examine the size/morphology/location/function of the AVV. • Examine the size/function of the systemic ventricle (TG mid SAX, ME 4C). • Attempt to assess the Glenn anastomosis. • Confirm the presence of a large ASD in contemporary Fontan procedures. • Attempt to assess the Fontan circuit. Look for RA size, smoke, thrombus in atriopulmonary Fontan. Verify absence of external atrial compression in extracardiac conduits (see Figure 8-26B). • Assess the PAs for obstruction/stenosis. • Check for a fenestration in the Fontan with CF Doppler or by injecting agitated saline in a lower extremity vein. • Look for anomalous pulmonary venous drainage/obstruction. • Examine the coronaries, look for evidence of coronary sinusoids/fistulae (PAIVS). • Rapid transit of contrast saline injected through an upper extremity vein into the pulmonary venous atrium is suggestive of pulmonary arterial-venous malformations. • Check both pleural spaces for effusions.	• CF/PW Doppler to confirm unrestrictive ASD without a gradient. • CF/CW Doppler to assess/quantitate restriction of the BVF/VSD. • CFD/CW to assess/quantitate outflow tract obstruction. CF/CW Doppler to grade AVVR/stenosis. • CF/PW Doppler to assess for Glenn/PA stenosis. Look for laminar, low-velocity phasic flow in the PAs (see Figure 8-28B). (ME bicaval where the RPA is visible). • CF/PW Doppler to assess IVC/hepatic veins for obstruction (ME asc aortic SAX, ME RV inflow-outflow, UE aortic arch SAX). • CF/PW Doppler to localize/time/characterize flow signals such as coronary arteries/sinusoids/aortopulmonary collaterals.

UE aortic arch SAX

asc, ascending; ASD, atrial septal defect; AVV, atrioventricular valve; AVVR, atrioventricular valve regurgitation; BVF, biventricular function; CF, color flow; CW, continuous wave; 4C, four-chamber; IVC, inferior vena cava; ME, midesophageal; PA, pulmonary artery; PAIVS, pulmonary atresia with intact ventricular septum; PW, pulsed wave; RA, right atrial; RPA, right pulmonary artery; SAX, short axis; TEE, transesophageal echocardiography; TG, transgastric; 2D, two-dimensional; UE, upper esophageal; VSD, ventricular septal defect.

TABLE 8-13   SURGICAL AND INTERVENTIONAL MANAGEMENT FOR STAGE 1

Defect	Surgical Options for Stage 1	Additional Points
HLHS	• Norwood procedure—includes arch augmentation, DKS type of proximal anastomosis, atrial septectomy, and Sano (RV to PA shunt) or BT shunt (Figures 8-27A and 8-28A).	• DKS—the PulmV and proximal main PA, which is the effective systemic outflow vessel, is anastomosed end to side to the aorta.
SV-DILV	1. Norwood/DKS 2. Enlargement of BVF, PA band, arch or coarctation repair if needed (see Figure 8-26B).	• In option 2, the size of the BVF is critical because systemic flow must cross the BVF to reach the aorta. Obstruction at any time adversely affects ventricular function.
Tricuspid atresia	1. BT shunt 2. PA band 3. DKS	• Similar concerns to SV-DILV with the size of the VSD.
Unbalanced AVC	• PA band/nothing	
Pulmonary atresia/ intact septum	• SV, one and one-half-, two-ventricle repair	• Must not decompress the RV in patients with RVDCA circulation. • Natural history of coronary perfusion in patients with RVDCA is not known.
Heterotaxy	• Usually, a SV approach is necessary. Procedure(s) depend on associated defects.	• See below for cases with interrupted IVC and azygos continuation.

AVC, atrioventricular canal; BT, Blalock-Taussig; BVF, biventricular function; DILV, double-inlet left ventricle; DKS, Damus-Kaye-Stansel; HLHS, hypertrophic left heart syndrome; IVC, inferior vena cava; PA, pulmonary artery; PulmV, pulmonary valve; RV, right ventricle; RVDCA, right ventricle-dependent coronary artery; SV, single ventricle.

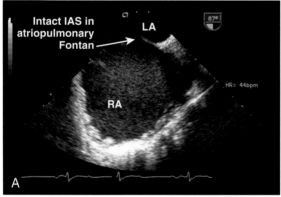
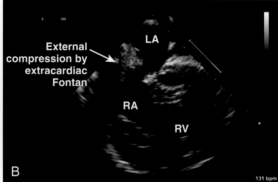

Figure 8-26. **A,** 2D ME bicaval view in a patient with an atriopulmonary Fontan. The RA is massively enlarged. It is important to look for thrombus. Note that the atrial septum must be intact in an atriopulmonary connection. **B,** Modified ME 4C view with the probe turned rightward in a patient with an extracardiac Fontan. External compression of the common atrium is seen and CF/PW Doppler images confirmed flow obstruction. Revision of the extracardiac conduit was required.

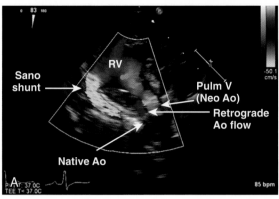
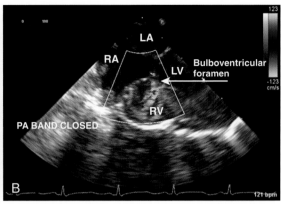

Figure 8-27. **A,** A patient with HLHS after a Norwood procedure. Deep TG LAX shows the RV leading to the PulmV. A DKS anastomosis is used to connect the PA and aorta. Note that there is retrograde flow in the proximal aorta (and coronary arteries). Turbulent flow through the Sano shunt is also seen exiting the RV. A velocity of up to about 3 m/s is often seen in the Sano. **B,** CF Doppler ME 4C view in a patient with DILV and transposed great vessels (not seen). The PA comes off the LV and the aorta off the small RV. Blood MUST pass through the BVF (VSD) in order to get to the aorta. The size of the BVF is borderline and could become restrictive. Surgical options include a DKS type of anastomosis or placement of PA bands and enlargement of the BVF.

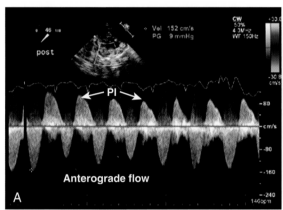
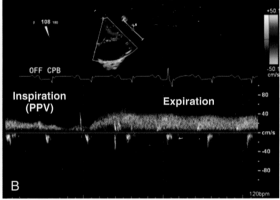

Figure 8-28. **A,** CW Doppler in a ME 4C view with the probe turned toward the RV in a patient with HLHS and a Sano shunt demonstrates a peak velocity of 1.5 m/s. There is also free PI through the valveless conduit. **B,** PW Doppler in a ME bicaval view in a patient with a Glenn. Note the variation in PBF with the respiratory cycle while on a ventilator.

CORONARY ARTERY ABNORMALITIES

KEY POINTS

- The left main coronary artery (LMCA) originates from the left sinus of Valsalva and bifurcates into the anteriorly directed LAD and the posteriorly directed circumflex coronary artery (Cx) just behind the main PA.
- The Cx continues laterally and posteriorly in the AV groove. In patients with a left dominant circulation, the Cx becomes the posterior descending coronary artery.
- The RCA originates anteriorly and slightly superior to the origin of the LCA from the right sinus of Valsalva and courses rightward around the atrioventricular groove to the posterior aspect of the heart. In patients with a right

dominant circulation (75%), the RCA becomes the posterior descending coronary artery.
- Both the LAD and the RCA should be similar in size. A large size discrepancy can occur as a result of aneurysms, coronary fistulae, or compensatory enlargement of one coronary secondary to increased flow when it is providing collateral circulation.
- Coronary abnormalities often exist in patients with CHD (e.g., TOF, TGA, PAIVS).
- Isolated congenital coronary artery abnormalities occur in less than 1.5% of angiograms and 0.3% of autopsies.
- Despite a variety of abnormalities, most are not associated with an increased risk of sudden

Continued

death. High-risk lesions include anomalous origin of the left coronary artery from the pulmonary artery (ALCAPA) or an abnormal origin or course of the coronary artery from the aorta, most commonly from the opposite aortic sinus of Valsalva with an intramural or interarterial course (especially LMCA/LAD and perhaps RCA) (Figures 8-29 and 8-30).

Anomalous Origin of the Coronary Artery from the Aorta

- Commonly have abnormally shaped ostia with stenosis, intramural coronary segments, or an interarterial course (see Figures 8-29 and 8-30B).
- An intramural coronary segment is one in which the coronary courses within the wall of the aorta for some distance before exiting, unlike the normal coronary artery, which exits the aortic wall perpendicularly.
- A coronary with an interarterial segment originates from the opposite aortic sinus and travels in between the great vessels to supply the appropriate territory.
- Presenting symptoms include sudden death, chest pain, and syncope.
- Presentation most commonly in the adolescent/ early adult years.

Anomalous Origin of the Left Coronary Artery from the Pulmonary Artery

- LMCA or, very rarely, both coronary arteries arise from the left or right posterior sinus of the PA, the posterior main PA, or the PA branches (see Figure 8-30A).

- Early in life when the PVR is increased, there is anterograde flow of (deoxygenated) blood from the PA.
- As PVR decreases, reversal of flow in the left coronary system develops and there is retrograde flow into the PA. This results in coronary steal and myocardial ischemia.
- There are often some collateral vessels between the right and left coronary systems with significant enlargement of the RCA, which provides essentially all of the coronary perfusion, including retrograde flow into the PA.
- Patients often present as neonates in cardiogenic shock. Rarely, if enough collateral circulation has developed, they can present later in life with symptoms of a L→R shunt (aorta to coronary artery to PA) or symptoms of myocardial ischemia, including sudden death.

Coronary Artery Fistula

- Originates from either coronary artery but typically empties into the right side of the heart (RA, RV, or less commonly, the PA). Usually solitary fistula.
- Often accompanied by enlargement of the involved coronary because of increased flow and occasionally by aneurysm formation. In addition, it can result in steal of coronary flow from the distal segment of the involved coronary. Also, when large, the fistula results in volume overload of a right-sided structure. There is a small risk of endocarditis, aneurysm formation, and rupture of the fistula.
- Patients present in young adulthood with a murmur or symptoms of myocardial ischemia or right-sided volume overload.

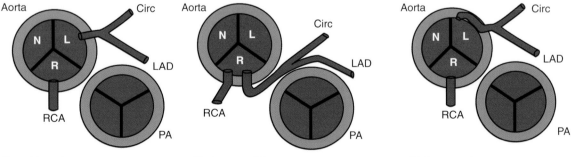

A Normal coronary pattern   B Interarterial coronary pattern   C Intramural coronary pattern

Figure 8-29. Schematics. **A,** A normal coronary pattern. **B,** The LCA originated aberrantly from the RCC with an interarterial course. **C,** The LCA with ostial stenosis and an intramural segment. ***A-C,*** *Modified and reprinted with permission from Eisses M, Verma S, Gurvitz M, Joffe DC. Echo rounds: Intramural left coronary artery. Anesth Analg. 2010;111:354-357.*

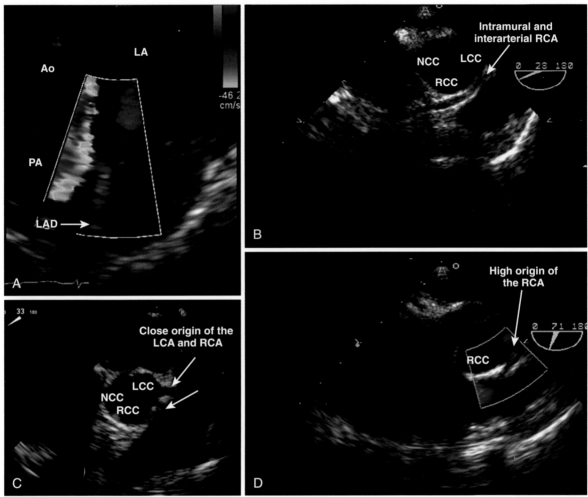

Figure 8-30. **A,** 2D and CF Doppler ME modified AV SAX view in a newborn with ALCAPA shows the LMCA origin from the posterior PA. The vessel is seen to bifurcate into the LAD and the Cx. Retrograde systolic flow is seen in this clip and diastolic anterograde flow was seen in another. **B,** ME AV SAX view shows an aberrant origin of the RCA from the LCC. The RCA has an intramural segment and an interarterial course. The patient was symptomatic and had the coronary unroofed. **C** and **D,** Abnormal coronaries with no known risk: **C,** ME AV SAX view shows an incidental finding of both coronaries originating very closely from the appropriate cusp. **D,** CF Doppler ME AV LAX view shows an incidental finding of a high origin of the RCA above the sinus.

Basic Echocardiographic Principles When Imaging Coronary Arteries (Table 8-14)

- The small size of coronary arteries, cardiac movement, echo drop-out, and other artifacts can make visualization of the coronaries difficult. Despite these limitations, transthoracic echocardiography (TTE) or TEE are often the only diagnostic tools necessary to identify congenital coronary abnormalities. However, cardiac catheterization is often used to confirm the diagnosis and perform a detailed examination of coronary anatomy.

- Decreasing the color scale and using spectral Doppler to time signals can be helpful.

Principles of Surgical/ Interventional Management

- The treatment of coronaries with anomalous origins involves unroofing intramural segments, enlarging abnormal ostia, translocation of the coronary to the appropriate sinus, translocation of the PA, which can compress the aberrantly located coronary or coronary bypass with venous or arterial conduits.

TABLE 8-14　BASIC ECHOCARDIOGRAPHIC PRINCIPLES WHEN IMAGING FOR CONGENITAL CORONARY ARTERY ANOMALIES (see Figure 8-30)

Best TEE Views	What to Look for on 2D	CF and Spectral Doppler
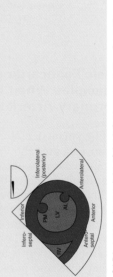	• Origin and course of LCA and RCA. • Left (ME AV SAX, ME RV inflow-outflow, occasionally the ME AV LAX if viewing the left cusp). • Right—withdraw probe slightly from above views, also seen exiting from lowest sinus (right sinus) on ME AV LAX. • The vessel should exit the aorta in a perpendicular fashion. • If ALCAPA is suspected, carefully inspect PulmV or PA for coronary origin. • If a fistula is suspected, right-sided receiving chamber is enlarged.	• CF/PW Doppler used to measure direction and timing of signal. Normal pattern is low-velocity, anterograde flow during diastole. • In ALCAPA may see retrograde flow in the PA. • Continuous coronary flow signal is consistent with a coronary fistula. • Abnormal CF Doppler signal into a right-sided chamber may represent entry point of a coronary fistulae. • CF/CW Doppler to grade MR.
	• Use multiple views to assess biventricular function and size. Attempt to correlate areas of dysfunction with the coronary artery distribution (TG mid SAX, ME 4C, ME LAX, ME 2C). • Assess the MV. Measure annulus size, check for leaflet prolapse, mobility/restriction. Assess the papillary muscles for evidence of retraction/fibrosis (ME 4C, ME LAX, ME 2C).	

ALCAPA, anomalous origin of the left coronary artery from the pulmonary artery; AV, aortic valve; CF, color flow; 4C, four-chamber; LAX, left axis; LCA, left coronary artery; ME, midesophageal; MR, mitral regurgitation; MV, mitral valve; PA, pulmonary artery; PulmV, pulmonary valve; RCA, right coronary artery; RV, right ventricular; SAX, short axis; TEE, transesophageal echocardiography; 2C, two-chamber; 2D, two-dimensional.

- Unroofing a segment that crosses an aortic valve commissure may involve resuspension of the aortic leaflet.
- Contemporary surgical treatment of ALCAPA is to translocate the coronary artery to the aorta. The etiology of the MR is usually a combination of papillary muscle dysfunction from ischemia or annular dilatation from cardiomegaly and, if mild to moderate, may improve as ventricular remodeling occurs. However, moderate to severe MR may require primary repair of the valve, although in neonates, this is rarely necessary (see "Mitral Valve Repair in Ischemic Mitral Regurgitation").
- Most coronary fistulae can be closed using interventional catheter techniques. Rarely, surgical closure is necessary for very large fistulae. The fistula may be closed at its origin or at its entry into the heart.

Postoperative TEE Assessment after Repair of Coronary Anomalies

Step 1: Depending on the repair, verify a suitable origin and course of the repaired coronary
- Verify low-velocity anterograde flow from the ostia without obvious stenosis. Coronary flow may be hard to visualize and indirect assessment of perfusion such as RWMA and MR may be necessary.
Step 2: Confirm there is no prolapse, perforation, or other injury to the PulmV or AV
Step 3: Myocardial function is usually improved but it can be gradual if there is stunned or hibernating myocardium
Step 4: Verify MV function and grade MR (see Chapter 2)

CONGENITAL VALVULAR HEART DISEASE

Tricuspid Valve

KEY POINTS

Ebstein's Anomaly (Table 8-15)
- Ebstein's anomaly is the most common isolated congenital abnormality of the TV.
- Abnormal development of the TV, especially the septal and posterior leaflets, which are dysplastic and apically displaced occupying the ventricle and creating an "atrialized ventricle." There is tethering and shortening of the valve and subvalvar apparatus. The annulus is normally positioned (see Video 8-8 on the companion website).

KEY POINTS—cont'd

- There are variable degrees of TR and effective RV hypoplasia. Massive right heart enlargement can lead to functional pulmonary atresia and LV dysfunction. Structural pulmonary atresia is rare.
- An atrial level shunt is usually present and may be necessary for survival.
- Presentation can vary from severe cardiac compromise in a newborn to mild TR in an adult.

Surgical/Interventional Management (Table 8-16)

- Patients with Ebstein's can have a very variable presentation from severe cardiac disease in the newborn to mild asymptomatic TV disease in older patients.
- Newborn patients who do not improve as their PVR decreases may require TV reconstruction or an RV exclusion procedure leading to an SV strategy. A valved RV-PA conduit or division of the PA may also be required if there is associated PI.
- The older symptomatic patient may require a TV repair with or without a Glenn procedure (functionally a one- and one-half ventricle repair) or a Fontan procedure.

Postoperative TEE Assessment after Primary or Revision Surgery for Ebstein's Anomaly

Step 1: Assess TV after a valve repair
- Trace to minimal TR without inflow obstruction is ideal.
- After TV repair, ensure the valve is well seated and there are no paravalvular leaks.
Step 2: Assess biventricular size and function
- The RCA is at risk of injury especially during complex valve repairs.
Step 3: If a Glenn and TV repair/replacement is being performed, assess the Glenn anastomosis and PA flow and ensure there is only trace to mild TR and adequate RV function for IVC return
- A PFO/atrial communication can be left and closed at a later time as RV function recovers.
Step 4: If the patient had an RV exclusion procedure, there will be a fenestration in the pericardial patch portion of the TV patch and the RV should appear decompressed. Confirm that the ASD is unrestrictive
- Assess LV function.
Step 5: If an RV-PA conduit was replaced, assess RV function/PulmV function

TABLE 8-15 BASIC ECHOCARDIOGRAPHIC FEATURES WHEN IMAGING UNREPAIRED OR PREVIOUSLY REPAIRED EBSTEIN'S ANOMALY

Best TEE Views	What to Look for on 2D	CF and Spectral Doppler
	• Visualize TV morphology and the mechanism of TR. Evaluate the degree of tethering, prolapse, the subvalvar apparatus and the anterior leaflet size; factors important for repair (ME 4C, ME RV inflow-outflow, TG RV inflow). • After an RV exclusion procedure, a fenestrated patch will be seen covering the TV. • Assess RV function and volume (ME 4C, ME RV inflow-outflow, TG SAX). • If there was associated PS or an RV to PA conduit, examine them for obstruction (ME RV inflow-outflow, deep TG LAX, UE aortic arch SAX). • Examine the IAS and verify the presence of a PFO/ASD (see text).	• CF/CW Doppler to assess TR severity by measuring the area of the regurgitant jet, the width of the vena contracta, the spectral Doppler density of the TR jet, and the systolic flow reversal in the hepatic vein. • An enlarged IVC is suggestive of increased RAP. • CF/CW Doppler to assess anterograde flow through RVOT/conduit and PI (ME RV inflow-outflow, deep TG LAX, UE aortic arch SAX). • CF/PW Doppler to assess the direction/size of flow through the PFO/ASD.

ASD, atrial septal defect; CF, color flow; CW, continuous wave; 4C, four-chamber; IAS, interatrial septum; IVC, inferior vena cava; LAX, long axis; ME, midesophageal; PFO, patent foramen ovale; PI, pulmonic insufficiency; PS, pulmonic stenosis; RAP, right atrial pressure; RV, right ventricular; RVOT, right ventricular outflow tract; SAX, short axis; TEE, transesophageal echocardiography; TG, transgastric; TR, tricuspid regurgitation; TV, tricuspid valve; 2D, two-dimensional; UE, upper esophageal.

TABLE 8-16 DETAILS OF THE SURGICAL REPAIR IN PATIENTS WITH EBSTEIN'S ANOMALY

Procedure	Key Facts
Valve repair	• Two main types of TV repair techniques. 　1. Anterior leaflet of the TV is used to form a competent valve 　2. A trileaflet valve that originates at the true annulus is created (the cone technique). • A reduction atrioplasty and a fenestrated atrial communication are performed in both. • The valve repairs may involve a reduction annuloplasty at the anteroposterior commissure, fenestration of the subvalvar apparatus, and/or augmentation of the anterior leaflet with a pericardial patch. • In the older patient, TVR with a bioprosthetic valve is an option.
RV exclusion or Starnes procedure	• The staged approach involves placing a fenestrated patch closure on the TV (a Starnes procedure) (Figure 8-31). • The ASD is enlarged • A reduction atrioplasty is performed. • An aortopulmonary shunt is placed. • If there is PI, the PV is oversewn or the main PA is disconnected. **The goal is to decompress the RV so that it does not interfere with LV function.** • A Glenn and Fontan procedure are performed at the standard time (see "SV" section).
Glenn	• Must be old enough (usually 3 mo minimum). • Usually done in combination with a valve repair. • May need a subsequent Fontan.
One and one-half ventricle repair	• RV function/size cannot provide a full cardiac output (IVC and SVC return). • A Glenn is used for SVC flow; the RV pumps IVC flow to the PA. • ASD is closed.

ASD, atrial septal defect; IVC, inferior vena cava; LV, left ventricular; PA, pulmonary artery; PI, pulmonic insufficiency; PV, pulmonary vein; RV, right ventricle; RV, right ventricular; SV, single ventricle; SVC, superior vena cava; TV, tricuspid valve; TVR, tricuspid valve repair.

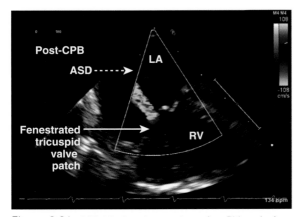

Figure 8-31. ME 4C view in a patient after RV exclusion (Starnes procedure). The TV is closed but a fenestration is left to decompress the RV.

Pulmonary Valve

KEY POINTS

• Isolated PulmV stenosis (PS) is almost always congenital and other than critical PS is often well tolerated.
• PS is due to variable degrees of fusion of the valve leaflets and commissures. The valve may be trileaflet, bicuspid, or unicuspid. There is often post-stenotic dilatation of the main PA that does not regress after treatment and

KEY POINTS—cont'd

poses a negligible risk of rupture, although there is a small risk of compression of surrounding structures.
• PulmV abnormalities are also characteristic of syndromes such as Alagille's, Noonan's, and Williams' syndromes. The valves are often thick and dysplastic and include annular hypoplasia and stenosis of the PAs and other vessels as well.
• PI usually occurs in patients who have had balloon dilatation of congenital PS, in those status post TOF repairs/other procedures requiring RV-PA conduits. RV function may be diminished as a result of years of PI and the effects of multiple surgical procedures.
• Adult presentation of PS/PI is common. Treatment of PS is generally indicated when peak velocity is greater than 3 m/s.

Surgical and Interventional Management

• Balloon valvuloplasty is the treatment of choice for nondysplastic PS. PulmV or conduit replacement is the treatment for PI.
• Balloon dilatation is usually attempted in patients with dysplastic valves but has a lower success rate. Patients may need surgical intervention and transannular

patch placement for relief of annular obstruction.
- Over time, the effects of severe PI may result in RV dysfunction. The decision to replace the valve is mostly dependent on the degree of symptoms and the function and size of the RV. Usually, a bioprosthetic valve is placed in the pulmonary position.
- RV-PA conduits require revision with interventional/surgical procedures several times during the patient's lifetime for conduit stenosis/regurgitation. Percutaneous balloon dilatation with stent placement and valve replacement procedures are possible in some patients.

Basic Echocardiographic Features When Imaging Pulmonary Valve or Conduit Abnormalities
- Given the anterior location of the PulmV and conduit, they may not be well seen by TEE. Color flow (CF) Doppler is helpful in identifying abnormal jets but localization may be difficult. The deep transgastric (TG) long axis (LAX) view is used to measure pressure gradients (Table 8-17).

Postoperative TEE Assessment after Pulmonary Valve or Conduit Replacement
Step 1: Verify that the valve is well positioned and look for paravalvular/transvalvular insufficiency

Step 2: Examine the conduit for obstruction and grade insufficiency

Step 3: Assess biventricular function (the Cx can be injured during the procedure)

Mitral Valve (Table 8-18)

> **KEY POINTS**
>
> - Composed of the mitral annulus, leaflets, chordae, and papillary muscles all attached to the anterolateral and posteromedial LV. Abnormalities in any of these can result in MV disease.
> - Congenital MS consists of a combination of abnormalities of the mitral apparatus including thick, short, webbed chordae with restricted interchordal space (arcade) that produces LV inflow obstruction and often LVOTO. The papillary muscles may connect the leaflets to the ventricle (papillary commissural fusion). There may be a double-orifice MV or a parachute MV (there is only one papillary muscle). The result is often restricted inflow

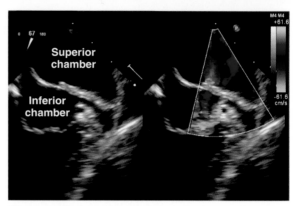

Figure 8-32. 2D and CF Doppler ME 2C view shows the membrane in a patient with cor triatriatum. The atrium is separated into a superior and an inferior chamber. The inferior chamber communicates with the LAA. The ostium of the membrane is not seen in this view.

> **KEY POINTS—cont'd**
>
> and MR (see Videos 8-9 and 8-10 on the Expert Consult website).
> - Supramitral rings and cor triatriatum are anomalous fibromuscular tissue membranes that are located in the LA and can cause obstructive symptoms that mimic MS. A ring is located below the atrial appendage and is thought to be an acquired lesion that results from turbulent flow at the orifice, whereas the membrane of cor triatriatum is above the appendage (Figure 8-32).

Surgical and Interventional Management on the Mitral Valve
- Balloon valvuloplasty is the treatment of choice for rheumatic MS in the young patient, but it has limited success in patients with congenital MS.
- Valve repair is preferable to replacement in any child, even if there is residual mild to moderate disease but especially in the youngest patients (<2 yr) because of a markedly increased morbidity/mortality with MVR. In older patients, less residual disease is acceptable post repair and the lower the threshold for valve replacement.
- Some techniques of valve repair include closure of clefts, chordae lengthening and transfers, triangular resections, commissurotomy, splitting of papillary muscles, fenestrating webbed chords, pericardial patch augmentation of deficient leaflets, and annuloplasty techniques.
- Supraannular placement of a mitral prosthesis may be necessary in young children in order

TABLE 8-17 BASIC ECHOCARDIOGRAPHIC PRINCIPLES WHEN IMAGING PATIENTS WITH PULMONARY VALVE DISEASE

Best TEE Views	What to Look for on 2D	CF and Spectral Doppler
	• Characterize the PulmV morphology and function. A thick, doming valve is common in nondysplastic PS. Calcification is rare (ME RV inflow-outflow and ME AV SAX, deep TG LAX, UE aortic arch SAX). • Examine RVOT/subvalvar area and conduit for obstruction (ME RV inflow-outflow, ME AV SAX, deep TG LAX turn probe to the left and anteflex). • Assess if post stenotic dilatation of the PAs is causing compression of surrounding structures/coronaries. PA aneurysm may cause PI. • Examine the IAS for PFO/ASD. • Assess RV function, volume and thickness.	• CF/CW Doppler—localize area of obstruction and identify PI. • Localize/quantitate any additional RVOTO (deep TG LAX with leftward rotation and mild anteflexion, UE aortic arch SAX view, ME AV SAX). • Assess/quantitate PI by measuring the width of the vena contracta and the deceleration slope of the jet. • An enlarged IVC is suggestive of increased RAP. • Measure PAP.

AV, aortic valve; CF, color flow; CW, continuous wave; IAS, interatrial septum; IVC, inferior vena cava; LAX, long axis; ME, midesophageal; PA, pulmonary artery; PFO, patent foramen ovale; PI, pulmonic insufficiency; PS, pulmonic stenosis; PulmV, pulmonary valve; RAP, right atrial pressure; RV, right ventricular; RVOTO, right ventricular outflow tract obstruction; SAX, short axis; TEE, transesophageal echocardiography; TG, transgastric; 2D, two-dimensional; UE, upper esophageal.

TABLE 8-18　BASIC ECHOCARDIOGRAPHIC FEATURES WHEN IMAGING THE PATIENT WITH A REPAIRED/REPLACED OR UNREPAIRED MITRAL VALVE

Best TEE Views	What to Look for on 2D	CF and Spectral Doppler
	• Characterize the morphology and function of the MV and subvalvar apparatus. Examine the MV apparatus, and mobility of each component. Measure the annulus, examine the leaflets, look for a cleft in the anterior leaflet, and examine the chordal arrangement and the number and location of papillary muscles. Assess the mechanism of MS/MR (ME 4C, ME 2C, ME LAX, ME AV LAX, ME mitral commissural, TG basal SAX, TG 2C). • Status post MVR, the valve may be in the suprannular position. The appendage should be above the prosthesis and appear decompressed. • If the valve is in the annular position, confirm fixation to the annulus without perivalvular/transvalvular regurgitation. • Leaflets should be seen to open and close. • Assess LA/LV size and function. • Examine LAA for evidence of stasis and thrombus. Look for supramitral ring or cor triatriatum.	• CF Doppler—Assess location and degree of MR or mitral inflow obstruction (see Chapter 2). • MR—size of vena contracta, density of MR Doppler signal, increase mitral E wave (>1.2 m/s), and pulmonary venous trace useful in operating room. However, MR is often underestimated under anesthesia. • PW/CW Doppler—Pressure half-time is not a reliable indicator of inflow obstruction in pediatric patients. Mean and peak pressures are flow-related but otherwise reliable indicators of MS severity. Mean gradients greater than 10 to 12 mm Hg are severe. The presence of an atrial level communication with L→R shunting can factitiously decrease the severity of MS as measured by Doppler. • Measure PAP using CW Doppler of TR jet. Systolic PAP greater than 50 mm Hg severe.

AV, aortic valve; CF, color flow; CW, continuous wave; L, left; LA, left atrial; LAA, left atrial appendage; LAX, long axis; LV, left ventricle; ME, midesophageal; MR, mitral regurgitation; MS, mitral stenosis; MV, mitral valve; MVR, mitral valve repair; PAP, pulmonary artery pressure; PW, pulsed wave; PFO, patent foramen ovale; PI, pulmonary insufficiency; PS, pulmonic stenosis; R, right; SAX, short axis; TEE, transesophageal echocardiography; TG, transgastric; 2C, two-chamber; 2D, two-dimensional.

to place an adequate-sized valve. The atrial appendage is left above the prosthesis. The atrium may need augmentation in some cases in order to decrease atrial hypertension.

- Rarely, the Ross II procedure is used. Use the pulmonary autograft in the mitral position and insert a valved conduit in the pulmonary position.
- The "membranes" from supramitral rings and cor triatriatum are resected when obstructive.
- PHTN may resolve over time with vascular remodeling and rarely falls acutely.
- Multiple reinterventions in the form of either repeat balloon valvuloplasties or valve repair/ replacement are the norm for the treatment of MS.
- The reintervention rate for patients who have had an MVR for MR depends on the etiology of the MR and the type of repair but it is not insignificant.
- Reintervention may also be necessary for prosthetic valve endocarditis, thrombosis, dehiscence, leaflet dysfunction, and pannus formation.

Postoperative TEE Assessment after Mitral Valve Repair/Replacement

Step 1: Assess the repair or replacement using techniques described in Chapter 2

Step 2: In addition, in the younger patient:
- Assess for LVOTO and AV dysfunction from an oversized MV.
- Measure PAP, although it seldom falls acutely.

Aortic Valve/Left Ventricular Outflow Tract Abnormalities
(Table 8-19)

KEY POINTS

Aortic Valve
- A bicuspid AV is the most common congenital abnormality with an incidence of 1% to 2%.
- About one third remain asymptomatic, one third develop stenosis, or one third develop insufficiency. Symptoms tend to occur after childhood.
- Critical AS in the newborn is a result of a deformed valve with one to four cusps. Often associated with variable degrees of hypoplastic left-sided structures including the MV, LV, LVOT, and aorta. In addition, there may be associated endocardial fibroelastosis. The latter occurs when fibrous tissue replaces myocardium compromising LV function. Various "grading" schemes have been

---

KEY POINTS—cont'd

developed in an attempt to determine whether a one- or two-ventricle repair is best.

Left Ventricular Outflow Tract
- Subaortic membranes are fibromuscular membranes with attachments to the septum and often to the AV and MV. They may be discrete or long and complex. AI occurs in approximately 50% of patients from injury to the valve as a result of turbulent flow and/or involvement of the AV in the fibromuscular process.

Aorta
- The aorta consists of the aortic root, the ascending aorta, the proximal and distal transverse arch, the isthmus, and the descending aorta.
- The aortic root consists of the aortic annulus, the aortic cusps, the aortic sinuses, and the sinotubular junction (STJ). These structures are part of the AV apparatus and, when diseased, each component should be measured and examined to help determine the etiology and guide the surgical repair.
- The size of the aorta decreases from ascending to descending so that the descending aorta is approximately 40% of the size of the ascending aorta.
- The combination of left heart obstructive lesions including **coarctation, AS, subaortic stenosis,** and a **supramitral ring** or other forms of **congenital MS,** is referred to as **Shone's** complex.
- **Reoperations/reinterventions** for AV/ LVOTO/aortic disease, for recurrent AV and MV dysfunction, prosthetic valve dysfunction, endocarditis, recurrent subaortic obstruction, RV-PA conduit revision, and aortic root dilatation (more common with bicuspid AVs).

Surgical/Interventional Management
- Balloon valvuloplasty is the procedure of choice for treating isolated, noncalcified AS in pediatric patients, adolescents, and young adults (<30 yr). Pediatric patients may return for a repeat balloon valvuloplasty as long as the AI is mild. AI resulting from balloon dilatation can often be treated with a valve repair rather than AV replacement; however, they may require replacement at an older age.
- Options for valve replacements in very small infants include autograft valves (Ross procedure), homografts, and metallic

TABLE 8-19   BASIC ECHOCARDIOGRAPHIC PRINCIPLES WHEN IMAGING THE LEFT VENTRICULAR OUTFLOW TRACT AND AORTIC VALVE

Best TEE Views	What to Look for on 2D	CF and Spectral Doppler
	• Characterize the morphology/function of the AV. A thick, doming valve is common. A calcified valve is uncommon before age 30. Identify areas of perforation/prolapse for potential repair. The most common abnormality in bicuspid valves involves fusion of the left and right cusps followed by the RCC and NCC, rarely the NCC and the LCC. Evaluate the valve in systole. Cusp size is often uneven with an eccentric orifice (ME RV inflow-outflow, ME AV SAX, ME LAX, ME AV LAX, ME asc aortic SAX, TG LAX, deep TG LAX). • Examine LVOT and subvalvular area for evidence of obstruction. • Assess LV function, hypertrophy, and size. • Measure the components of the aortic root and aorta (asc aorta > 4.5 mm with AV disease or > 5 mm without warrants intervention). • Examine origin/course of coronary arteries. • Examine LA for evidence of supramitral ring and cor triatriatum (as a component of Shone's). • Examine MV size, morphology, and function (include subvalvular apparatus). • Examine the IAS for PFO/ASD.	• CF/CW Doppler to quantitate AS. Peak gradient greater than 64, velocity greater than 4 m/s, or mean pressure gradient greater than 40 mm Hg is severe. In older patients, may use the continuity equation to calculate AVA (index to BSA) (deep TG LAX or TG LAX). • CF/CW Doppler to quantitate AI by measuring the width of the vena contracta and the deceleration slope of the jet. Check for flow reversal in the descending aorta. Note direction of jet (eccentric vs. central). • CF/CW Doppler to quantitate LVOTO. The modified Bernoulli equation may not be applicable for multilevel LVOTO. If unable to obtain an LVOT gradient, use CW Doppler to measure MR jet velocity, which can estimate LVP. LVP = $4(MR)^2$ + LAP. LVOT gradient is then LVP – blood pressure. • CF/PW Doppler to check for turbulence/persistent gradient in diastole in desc aortic Doppler trace for evidence of coarctation. • PW/CW Doppler of MV. Measure mean/peak inflow gradients. • Perform "quick" assessment of diastolic function if no obstruction present. • Measure PAP.

AI, aortic insufficiency; AS, aortic stenosis; asc, ascending; ASD, atrial septal defect; AV, aortic valve; AVA, aortic valve area; BSA, body surface area; CF, color flow; CW, continuous wave; desc, descending; IAS, interatrial septum; LA, left atrium; LAP, left atrial pressure; LAX, long axis; LCC, left coronary cusp; LV, left ventricle; LVOT, left ventricular outflow tract; LVP, left ventricular pressure; ME, midesophageal; MR, mitral regurgitation; MV, mitral valve; NCC, noncoronary cusp; PAP, pulmonary artery pressure; PFO, patent foramen ovale; RCC, right coronary cusp; RV, right ventricular; SAX, short axis; TEE, transesophageal echocardiography; TG, transgastric; 2D, two-dimensional.

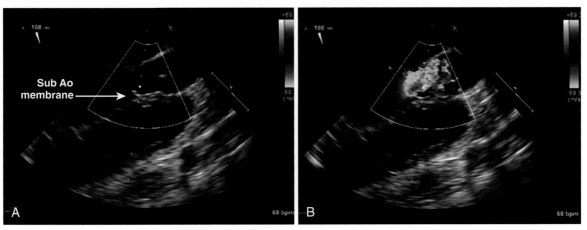

Figure 8-33. **A,** 2D and CF Doppler ME AV LAX view in a patient with a discrete subaortic membrane. **B,** Aliasing begins at the level of the membrane. This patient underwent a simple membrane resection.

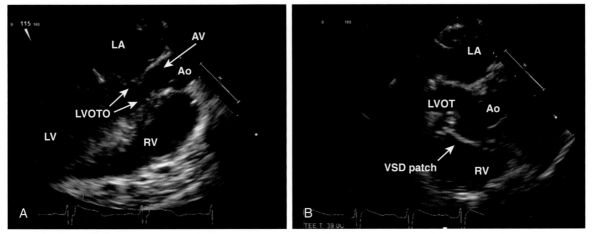

Figure 8-34. **A,** ME AV LAX view demonstrates long segment subaortic stenosis. **B,** Modified ME AV LAX in the same patient post modified Konno procedure that was used to enlarge the LVOT. The pressure gradient decreased to less than 20 mm Hg.

prosthetic valves. The latter has a lower profile (smaller sewing ring) than bioprosthetic valves.

• The Ross procedure can be performed in combination with the modified Konno to enlarge the LVOT as well as the annulus (Ross-Konno). Reinterventions on the neoaortic valve and replacement of the RV-PA conduit are necessary.

• A Konno procedure is performed in patients needing a prosthetic valve replacement and annular enlargement with or without subaortic enlargement. This allows the placement of a larger prosthetic valve (valve can be two or three sizes greater) and reduces LVOTO. The annulus is enlarged "into" the ventricular septum using a surgically created VSD. Much less commonly, the annulus can be enlarged but to a lesser degree posteriorly

toward the MV using the Manougian's or Nick's procedure.

• Simple resection of subaortic membranes has been associated with a high rate of recurrence (10-30%) (Figure 8-33). A peak gradient greater than 50 mm Hg (mean > 30) is an indication to resect the membrane. The risk of AI increases with gradients greater than 50 mm Hg. Very aggressive resection of the membrane on all surfaces in combination with a myomectomy may be associated with a decreased rate of recurrence and a lower incidence of AI. Alternatively, a modified Konno (LVOT enlargement *without* prosthetic valve placement) can be performed if there is more tunnel-like subaortic obstruction or in patients who have had multiple recurrences of the subaortic membrane (Figure 8-34).

Postoperative TEE Assessment after AV or LVOT Surgery

Step 1: Verify integrity and function of the valve repair/replacement

- Acoustic shadowing often makes evaluation of prosthetic valves in the aortic position difficult. Epicardial echocardiography may be helpful. Prosthetic valves have characteristic "signature" regurgitant jets. Identify and grade pathologic paravalvular and transvalvular jets.

Step 2: Confirm that there is an acceptable gradient in order to avoid patient-prosthesis mismatch

- The expected gradient is found in the manufacturer's specifications. This is especially important with small size bioprosthetic valves because the sewing ring is large relative to the valve.

Step 3: Homografts are very fragile; ensure no leaflet perforations occurred during placement

- There should be at most trace AI for an adequate long-term result. Bioprosthetic valves should also have less than mild central AI.

Step 4: If a Nick or Manougian procedure was performed, confirm that there was no injury to the MV resulting in MR

- If a Konno was required, verify that there is no residual VSD.

Step 5: After a subaortic membrane resection, ensure that the membrane is adequately resected and the AV and MV are intact and there is no VSD

Step 6: Examine the coronary arteries especially after procedures that required coronary artery reimplantation such as Ross, Konno, homograft placements, or Bentall procedures

Step 7: Examine ventricular function

- These are complex cases with long bypass/cross-clamp times and the possibility of injury to coronary arteries.

Suggested Readings

1. *Operative Techniques in Thoracic and Cardiovascular Surgery.* Philadelphia: Elsevier Inc.
   An excellent resource with beautiful illustrations. The papers by Richard A. Jonas are detailed descriptions of the common congenital cardiac surgical procedures by a leader in the field. An understanding of the operative techniques facilitates the understanding of the echocardiographic images.
2. Seminars in Thoracic and Cardiovascular Surgery series. Pediatric Cardiac Surgery Annual. Philadelphia: Elsevier Inc.
   Published yearly in this journal. Also replete with illustrations and descriptions of medical and surgical management of congenital cardiac conditions.
3. Warnes CA, Williams RG, Bashore TM, et al. ACC/AHA 2008 guidelines for the management of adults with congenital heart disease: A report of the American College of Cardiology/American Heart Association Task Force on Practice Guidelines (Writing Committee to Develop Guidelines on the Management of Adults With Congenital Heart Disease). Developed in Collaboration With the American Society of Echocardiography, Heart Rhythm Society, International Society for Adult Congenital Heart Disease, Society for Cardiovascular Angiography and Interventions, and Society of Thoracic Surgeons. *J Am Coll Cardiol.* 2008;52:e1-e121. Epub 2008;November 14.
   Important resource. Overall management of the complex adult with congenital cardiac disease.
4. Russell I, Rouine-Rapp K, Stratmann G, Miller-Hance WC. Congenital heart disease in the adult: A review with internet-accessible transesophageal echocardiographic images. *Anesth Analg.* 2006;102:694-723.
5. Lai W, Mertens L, Cohen M, Geva T, eds. *Echocardiography for Pediatric and Congenital Heart Disease.* Boston: Wiley-Blackwell; 2009.
   An outstanding journal article and book, which give the reader a solid basis for understanding echocardiography in pediatric and congenial heart disease.

Epiaortic Ultrasonography and Epicardial Echocardiography

Kathryn E. Glas and Stanton K. Shernan

9

SURFACE IMAGING

Probe Orientation

Probe orientation marker is important for surface imaging techniques.

- Conventional imaging planes are based on transthoracic echocardiography (TTE), because orientation is most similar to TTE windows. As with transesophageal echocardiography (TEE), images on the left side of the monitor screen are on the patient's right and images on the right side are on the patient's left.
- The probe marker is a raised line, indentation, or mark on the probe (Figure 9-1). It is easily hidden by the standoff in the sheath. Thus, alternative methods to identify orientation are frequently needed.
- Images will appear left to right inverted if probe orientation is incorrect (Figure 9-2). Imaging the left ventricle (LV) in reverse could lead to misdiagnosis of regional wall motion abnormalities. An incorrect diagnosis of dextrocardia could be made if images are inverted.
- Within a given image sector, structures progressively appear from anterior (near-field) to posterior (far-field), as opposed to TEE views that start posterior and progress anterior. For example, on epicardial imaging, the right coronary cusp of the aortic valve will be closest to the transducer instead of farthest away (Figure 9-3).

Probe Options

Because the probe is close to the structure being imaged, a high-resolution (i.e., high-frequency) transthoracic or surface probe can be used to optimize images.

- Use a probe that provides a transducer frequency of at least 7.5 MHz. Standard TTE probes are no more than 5 MHz, so a dedicated probe is needed. Pediatric TTE probes have higher resolution than equivalent adult probes.
- Linear array probes are typically used for central venous access and work well for epicardial echocardiography (ECE) imaging.
- Image depth is rarely greater than 12 cm for ECE examinations, whereas the optimal depth for epiaortic ultrasound (EAU) is often in the range of 8 cm. Surrounding structures can be used to confirm proper probe orientation.
- Images for all EAU and ECE studies should be acquired at the highest possible resolution. ECE images of the mitral valve (MV), in particular, may not have as high a resolution as the corresponding TEE images.
- A standoff is strongly recommended for EAU examinations with a phased array probe. Most manufacturers do not sell a standoff for phased array, but the hard plastic or rubber component of a disposable airway circuit reservoir bag can be used on some probes.
- Linear array probes do not require a standoff. The probe in the sheath can be placed directly on the ascending aorta because the focal zone is not an issue.

Image Acquisition and Optimization

Two operators are required to complete an ECE or EAU examination. The probe operator does not need experience to obtain the images; however, an expert intraoperative echocardiographer with advanced training should be available to guide image acquisition and interpretation.

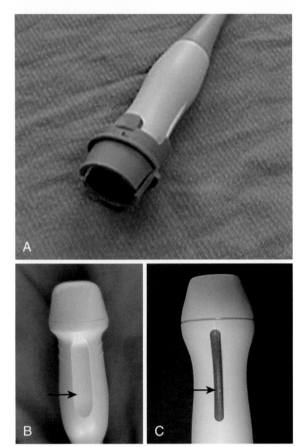

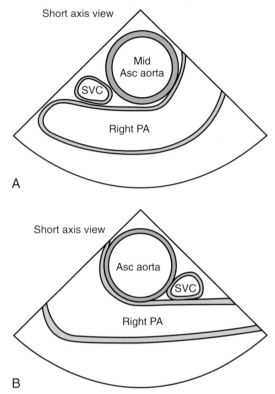

Figure 9-1. High-resolution TTE probe. **A,** Note the applied standoff and the raised mark on the right-hand side of the probe. **B** and **C,** Additional examples of standoffs *(arrows)* are noted.

Figure 9-2. Probe orientation. **A,** The images were acquired with the correct orientation. Asc, ascending. **B,** The probe has been rotated 90 degrees, and the SVC is on the opposite (i.e., incorrectly oriented) side of the screen.

- The images are acquired through an open chest; vigilance is necessary to avoid disturbing the surgical field; and sterile procedure skills are mandatory.
- The probe marker for the phased array transducer cannot be seen easily through the sterile sheath. Therefore, the probe should be marked or on-screen imaging can be used to guide orientation.
- Orientation for the linear array probe can be determined by tapping on one end of the probe while simultaneously reviewing the screen to first determine which side is medial or lateral and then reorienting as needed.
- Artifacts may be present on EUA and ECE images similar to TTE and TEE and other surface ultrasound-based images.
- Filling the chest cavity with warm (body temperature) saline can improve imaging and decrease artifacts, especially side lobes. Avoid overly hot or cold saline that can cause arrhythmias or hypertension.

- Linear array probes have a narrow imaging sector that limits simultaneously viewing of the full width and depth of the adult aorta. Therefore, the examination should be performed twice, once with adequate depth and once with adequate width.
- Phased array probes may permit imaging of the entire aorta with a standoff. However, imaging of the anterior left and right walls of the aorta may be limited if a standoff is not used and may require moving the probe from side to side to obtain complete images.

Maintaining a Sterile Field

Use of a TTE for EAU and ECE imaging requires a sterile sheath to cover the probe and maintain sterility of the surgical field.

- The surgical team should inspect and test the sheath for leaks before inserting the probe.

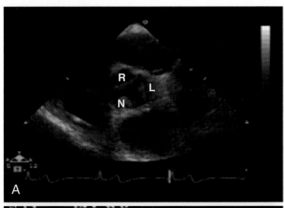

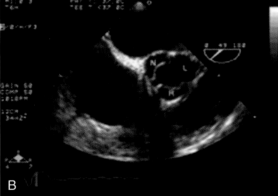

Figure 9-3. **A,** An epicardial AV SAX, with the right coronary cusp closest to the transducer (most anterior). L, left; N, noncoronary cusp; R, right. **B,** An analogous TEE ME AV SAX, with the right coronary cusp farthest from the transducer (most anterior).

- The sterile sheath should be filled with sterile saline or ultrasonic gel by the scrub technician. The echocardiographer at the head of the bed inserts the probe into the sheath opening. The echocardiographer should ensure that the standoff is at an acceptable depth (~1 cm) before inserting the probe (Figure 9-4).
- Air can be trapped in the standoff and will impair optimal image resolution. The probe operator should invert the apparatus under fluid to remove the air.
- Once the examination is complete and the probe is no longer needed, the probe and sheath are removed from the surgical field together before the sheath is discarded.
- Available probes cannot be sterilized to perform these examinations. Therefore, it is important to strictly follow the maintenance instructions provided by the vendor. Probes should not be submersed for long periods of time and should be allowed to dry thoroughly between examinations.

EPIAORTIC ULTRASONOGRAPHY

Prevention of Stroke

Atherosclerosis of the ascending aorta and arch has been associated with perioperative stroke in cardiac surgical patients.

KEY POINTS

- TEE examination of the ascending aorta is not as sensitive or specific as EAU imaging for identifying pathology. A significant portion of the ascending aorta cannot be seen with TEE owing to air-filled bronchi between the esophagus and the aorta, thus preventing ultrasound beam transmission.
- High-grade atherosclerosis of the descending aorta seen on TEE is often associated with an increased risk of ascending aortic disease.
- Cardiac surgical patients are at increased risk of perioperative stroke due to direct manipulation of the ascending aorta and subsequent risk of atherosclerotic embolization.
- Many different techniques are available to the surgeon for managing diseased aortas in order to minimize stroke risk, including changing the cannulation or cross-clamp site or minimizing aortic manipulation.

Standard Views and 12-Segment Nomenclature:

KEY POINTS

- The ascending aorta is divided into three segments: proximal, mid, and distal. The segment adjacent to the right pulmonary artery (PA) is the mid portion. The proximal segment is from the sinotubular junction (STJ) to the PA. The distal segment is from the PA to the takeoff of the innominate artery (Figure 9-5).
- Each segment of the aorta is then divided into four regions: left, right, anterior, and posterior. The right PA is adjacent to the left side, the superior vena cava (SVC) is adjacent to the right side, the anterior wall is closest to the transducer, and the posterior wall is farthest away.
- Determining the location of atherosclerotic plaques using EAU is critical. The aortic cannula is typically placed in the distal ascending aorta, slightly left of anterior, while the cross-clamp is typically placed at the level

Continued

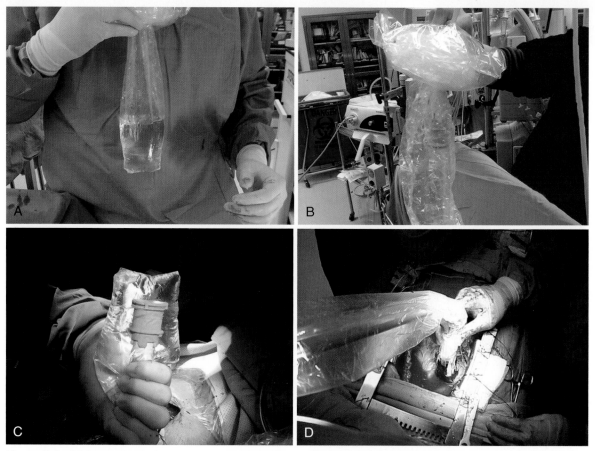

Figure 9-4. **A,** The sterile sheath is filled with saline. **B,** The echocardiographer inserts the probe within the sterile sheath. **C,** The operator inverts the probe within the saline to clear air from inside the standoff. **D,** The operator places the probe on the aorta, angling the probe toward the AV to start imaging.

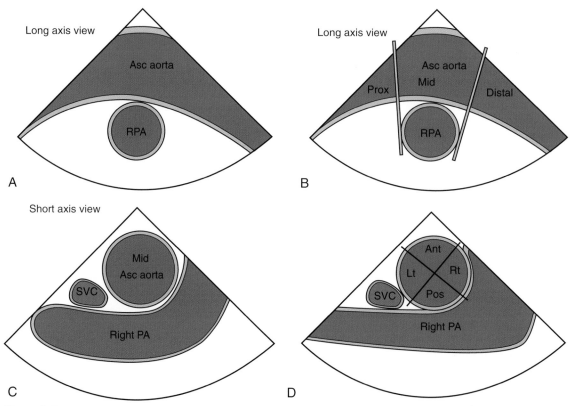

Figure 9-5. **A,** LAX epiaortic images of the ascending aorta. RPA, right pulmonary artery. **B,** Proximal, mid, and distal segmentation of the ascending aorta from a LAX perspective. **C,** SAX epiaortic image of the ascending aorta. **D,** Anterior, left, right, and posterior segmentation of the ascending aorta from a SAX perspective.

Performing an Epiaortic Ultrasonography Examination

- The operator places the sterile sheathed probe on the ascending aorta as proximal as possible. The probe usually needs to be angled to the patient's left and about 20 degrees anterior to direct the ultrasound beam and image toward the AV and through the left ventricular outflow tract (LVOT). AV leaflet motion should not be confused with mobile atheromatous disease.
- The echocardiography probe should be positioned on the aorta perpendicular to blood flow for optimal two-dimensional imaging. The angle is correct if the left-right aortic diameter is equal to the anteroposterior diameter. The probe can be advanced into the proximal aorta past the STJ and a short axis (SAX) image obtained.
- Maintaining proper orientation of the aorta in SAX requires frequent angle orientation changes to the probe. The aorta arises from the AV and changes its orientation in the anterior, lateral, and cephalad planes. Near the mid ascending aorta, less anterior angulation is needed. From the mid segment, slight posterior angulation and rotation toward the midline is needed.
- To obtain the long axis (LAX) view from the mid ascending aortic SAX, the probe should be rotated 90 degrees; with the probe oriented toward the patient's right shoulder. LAX imaging can frequently permit visualization of the entire ascending aorta in one plane. If the entire aorta is not visualized, the probe can be angled downward toward the AV (left side) to image the proximal aorta in LAX. Small angle manipulations will be needed to maintain the proper image orientation, as with SAX imaging. Reversing the angulation will bring the distal ascending aorta and proximal aortic arch into view.
- LAX views should not be used to measure plaque height because oblique angles can over- or underestimate disease severity.

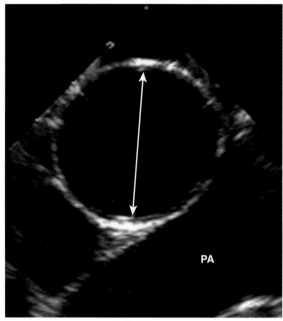

Figure 9-6. Measuring the ascending aortic diameter. The maximum diameter of the aorta should be measured from the inner near-field edge to the inner far-field edge during systole. Note the RPA coursing from right to posterior along the aorta, indicating this is a mid ascending aortic view.

- At a minimum, digital images should be acquired and stored at each level of the ascending aorta in SAX and LAX and incrementally as needed to demonstrate areas of abnormal thickening and atherosclerosis severity.
- The maximum diameter of the aorta should also be measured from the inner near-field edge to the inner far-field edge during systole (Figure 9-6).

Atherosclerosis Grading (Figure 9-7)

- Plaque height is measured from the level of the intimal surface to the maximum point of protrusion into the aorta. Each plaque should be measured individually. A grade should be provided for each of the 12 segments noted previously.
- Overall grading should consider the highest level of disease noted on the EAU examination.
- Numerous grading criteria for atherosclerosis have been published. Five-point grading scales are the most common. Each institution should agree on a preferred grading scale to avoid miscommunication about disease severity.
- The absence of significant aortic atherosclerosis (i.e., "normal") is typically

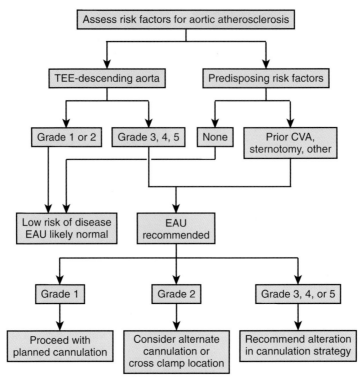

Figure 9-7. A suggested algorithm for the use of EAU in the assessment of ascending aortic atherosclerosis. CVA, cerebrovascular accident.

TABLE 9-1	ATHEROSCLEROSIS GRADING SCALE	
Grade	**Severity**	**Description**
Grade 1	Normal	Normal, no intimal thickening
Grade 2	Mild	Intimal thickening ≤ 3 mm
Grade 3	Moderate	Sessile atheroma > 3 mm but < 5 mm
Grade 4	Severe	Sessile atheroma ≥ 5 mm
Grade 5	Mobile	Protruding atheroma with mobile components

EPICARDIAL ECHOCARDIOGRAPHY

When Transesophageal Echocardiography Is Not an Option

ECE predates TEE for surgical diagnosis and evaluation and, currently, is most often used when a TEE probe cannot be placed or is contraindicated. Table 9-2 lists the recommended ECE views and the corresponding TTE views.

defined as less than 2 mm protrusion into the aortic lumen. The definition of "moderate" is controversial and varies among medical and surgical cohorts owing to the need for aortic manipulation in surgical patients. Evidence seems to suggest that more than 3 mm of plaque height portends increased risk in cardiac surgical patients.

- Severe disease is universally defined as greater than 5 mm protrusion into the aortic lumen (Table 9-1).
- Mobile disease defines any plaque with a mobile component regardless of size.

KEY POINTS
• ECE does not include imaging of structures outside of the immediate surgical field including the descending aorta for diagnosing an aneurysm, Stanford B dissection, or placement of an intra-aortic balloon pump (IABP).
• ECE requires knowledge of TTE imaging planes and anatomy.
• The same probe used for EAU or even a standard TTE probe can also be used for ECE.
• As with all other echocardiographic techniques, a comprehensive ECE is necessary to fully diagnose pathology.

TABLE 9-2 EPICARDIAL AND TRANSESOPHAGEAL ECHOCARDIOGRAPHY VIEW NOMENCLATURE

Epicardial Views	Corresponding TTE View
AV SAX	Parasternal AV SAX
AV LAX	Suprasternal AV LAX
LV basal SAX	Modified parasternal MV basal SAX
LV mid SAX	Parasternal LV mid SAX
LV LAX	Parasternal LAX
Two-chamber	Modified parasternal LAX
RVOT	Parasternal SAX

AV, aortic valve; LAX, long axis; LV, left ventricle; MV, mitral valve; RVOT, right ventricular outflow tract; SAX, short axis.

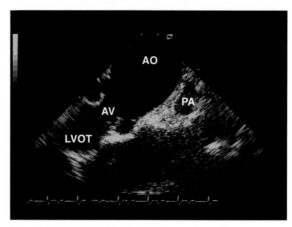

Figure 9-8. ECE AV LAX. This view allows the proper angle to perform spectral Doppler evaluations in addition to CF Doppler. Note the LVOT can be evaluated from this view for dynamic outflow obstruction, subaortic membrane, or other pathologies. AO, aorta.

KEY POINTS—cont'd

Limited examinations, whether owing to time constraints, patient condition, or inability to obtain all images, should be followed with a comprehensive examination as soon as feasible.

Seven Standard Epicardial Echocardiographic Views

- A comprehensive analysis of LV and right ventricle (RV) global and regional function can be assessed from ECE imaging windows.
- The incorporation of Doppler modalities can permit a comprehensive assessment of all four valves for stenosis or regurgitation.
- Machine presets frequently have different Doppler gain and scale settings for TEE and TTE probes. Thus, a thorough review of the settings before obtaining optimal images is necessary to prevent misdiagnosis.

Image Acquisition

Step 1: Aortic Valve Short Axis
(see Figure 9-3)

- Place the probe on the ascending aorta with the transducer marker oriented toward the left shoulder. Angle the probe medial and posterior until the AV is in view. In this SAX view, the right coronary cusp is closest to the transducer, the left cusp is to the right, and the noncoronary cusp is to the left on the monitor.

Step 2: Aortic Valve Long Axis
(Figure 9-8)

- From the AV SAX image, move the probe until the marker is parallel with the aorta and rotate it until the LVOT and the AV leaflets are seen.
- Measurements of the LVOT, annulus, and aortic root can be made from this view.
- In addition, color and spectral Doppler assessment of gradients or regurgitation severity can be performed because the transducer can be placed parallel to blood flow from this view.

Step 3: Left Ventricle Basal Short Axis (Figure 9-9)

- LV epicardial views are obtained through a right ventricular (RV) window. Moving the probe along the length of the RV and changing the angulation and rotation will allow visualization of the MV, subvalvular apparatus, and basilar, mid, and apical LV.
- An epicardial view of the LV will differ from TEE views in that the RV (and tricuspid valve [TV]) are the most anterior structures on the examination.
- When the probe is properly aligned, the MV anterior leaflet will be closest to the transducer and the anterolateral commissure will be on the right.
- Color flow (CF) Doppler evaluation at this level is equivalent to a transgastric (TG) basal TEE view of the MV that demonstrates origin of regurgitant jets and can be used for planimetry and effective regurgitant orifice area calculations.

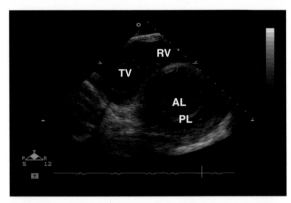

Figure 9-9. ECE LV basal SAX. Note the imaging plane is through the RV, with the anterior leaflet (AL) of the MV as the most anterior structure, similar to the surgical anatomic view of the valve. The TV can usually be seen from this view as well. PL, posterior leaflet.

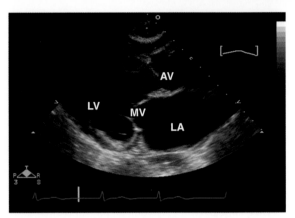

Figure 9-11. ECE LV LAX. This view closely approximates the TTE parasternal LAX view (see Table 9-2). This is the best ECE view for mitral subvalvular apparatus assessment. CF Doppler assessment of the AV, MV, and LVOT can be performed from this view.

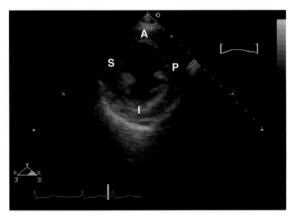

Figure 9-10. ECE LV mid SAX. The regional wall segments are indicated on this image using the 16-segment nomenclature. A, anterior; I, inferior; P, posterior; S, septal.

Step 4: Left Ventricle Mid Short Axis
(Figure 9-10)

- This view allows visualization of the same structures seen on a TG midpapillary LV SAX view and allows assessment of volume status, global and regional wall motion, and chamber size.
- In order to maintain the proper orientation, move and/or angle the probe inferiorly and to the left from the basilar view to obtain the LV mid SAX view.
- The anterolateral papillary muscle will be on the right and the posteromedial will be on the left of the image.
- The anterior wall of the LV will be at the top of the image and the inferior wall will

be on the bottom—opposite to a comparable TEE view.
- Because the medial and lateral orientations are not affected, the left ventricular (LV) septal wall will continue to be on the left side of the image and the lateral wall on the right side.
- Moving the probe laterally will permit visualization of the RV and allow global RV function assessment.

Step 5: Left Ventricle Long Axis
(Figure 9-11)

- This view very closely approximates the TTE parasternal LAX view and provides significant information about ventricular and valvular function. It most closely resembles the TEE midesophageal (ME) LAX view for anatomic characteristics.
- From the LV mid SAX view, rotate the probe toward the patient's right shoulder and angle the probe anteriorly until the image approximates the one shown in Figure 9-10.
- The most commonly seen LV walls are the inferolateral and anterolateral, but anatomic variations among patients may generate images that are not perfectly aligned. If you cannot see the interventricular septum, angle the probe until it is in view to ensure you are labeling the region appropriately.
- Images of the MV may not have the same resolution as TEE views, but the presence of leaflet pathology can still be determined, and a CF Doppler evaluation can be performed. Effective regurgitant orifice area determinations are also possible from this view.

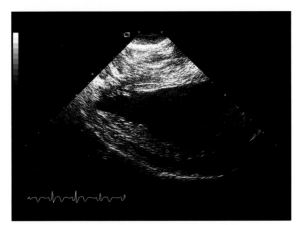

Figure 9-12. ECE two-chamber. As with other ECE views, the anterior wall is adjacent to the transducer and the inferior wall is farthest away. In this image, the LV apex is to the left side of the image and the MV and LA are just off the screen to the right. Moving the probe cephalad can provide a view of the MV that is comparable (but inverted) with a TG LAX image. This LV LAX view allows assessment of LV regional wall motion for the anterior and inferior walls. The LV apex is better seen in this ECE view than in TEE so evaluation of a potential LV apical thrombus should be preferentially performed with TTE preoperatively or ECE imaging intraoperatively.

- AV regurgitation can be assessed with CF Doppler.
- The LVOT can be measured and evidence of dynamic outflow obstruction can be ascertained from this view as well.
- The interventricular septum can be interrogated for defects.
- Rightward angulation of the transducer will allow visualization of the right atrium (RA) and RV as well as CF and spectral Doppler assessment of the TV.

Step 6: Two-Chamber (Figure 9-12)
- The epicardial two-chamber view closely approximates the TEE ME two-chamber view. The LV, MV, and left atrium (LA) can all be evaluated. The LA appendage can frequently be seen as well, potentially allowing assessment for thrombus or air.
- This view is obtained by rotating the probe clockwise and moving it medially across the RV surface until the LV is directly under the transducer.
- LV regional wall motion of the basal and mid segments of the anterior and inferior walls can be assessed.
- This view can be difficult to obtain. Similar to other LV views, careful review of surrounding structures is necessary to ensure correct identification of the wall in question for assessment of abnormalities.

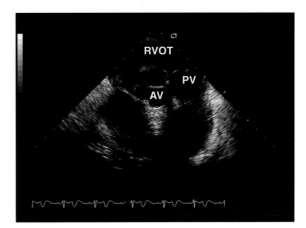

Figure 9-13. ECE right ventricular outflow tract (RVOT) view. This view approximates the TEE ME RV inflow-outflow view and is the hardest of all the ECE views to obtain. A modified examination, evaluating the pulmonic valve (PV) then adjusting the probe to evaluate the tricuspid, may be easier than imaging all structures simultaneously. CF and spectral Doppler evaluation of both valves should be performed from this view.

Step 7: Right Ventricular Outflow Tract (Figure 9-13)
- This view is similar to an inverted ME TEE RV inflow-outflow view. In patients with a normal size RV, this ECE view may be difficult to obtain.
- If the ECE examination is performed in the suggested order, beginning with the ECE two-chamber view, the probe now needs to be moved back toward the RV and the marker needs to be reoriented toward the patient's left shoulder.
- With proper alignment, both the TV and the pulmonic valve (PV) can be assessed with CF and spectral Doppler for the presence of stenosis or regurgitation.
- The main PA can also be seen, allowing evaluation for pulmonary embolus or confirmation of PA catheter placement (see Figure 9-7).

Suggested Readings
Epiaortic
1. Glas KE, Swaminathan M, Reeves ST, et al. Council for Intraoperative Echocardiography of the American Society of Echocardiography. Society of Cardiovascular Anesthesiologists. Society of Thoracic Surgeons. Guidelines for the performance of a comprehensive intraoperative epiaortic ultrasonographic examination: recommendations of the American Society of Echocardiography and the Society of Cardiovascular Anesthesiologists; endorsed by the Society of Thoracic Surgeons. *Anesth Analg.* 2008;106:1376-1378.
2. Davila-Roman VG, Phillips KJ, Daily BB, et al. Intraoperative transesophageal echocardiography and epiaortic ultrasound for assessment of atherosclerosis of the thoracic aorta. *J Am Coll Cardiol.* 1996;28:942-947.

3. Bucerius J, Gummert JF, Borger MA, et al. Stroke after cardiac surgery: A risk factor analysis of 16,184 consecutive adult patients. *Ann Thorac Surg.* 2003;75:472-478.

4. van der Linden J, Hadjinikolaou L, Bergman P, Lindblom D. Postoperative stroke in cardiac surgery is related to the location and extent of atherosclerotic disease in the ascending aorta. *J Am Coll Cardiol.* 2001;38:131-135.

5. Katz ES, Tunick PA, Rusinek H, et al. Protruding aortic atheromas predict stroke in elderly patients undergoing cardiopulmonary bypass: Experience with intraoperative transesophageal echocardiography. *J Am Coll Cardiol.* 1992;20:70-77.

Epicardial

6. Reeves ST, Glas KE, Eltzschig H, Shernan SK. Guidelines for performing a comprehensive epicardial echocardiography examination: Recommendations for the American Society of Echocardiography Council for Intraoperative Echocardiography and the Society of Cardiovascular Anesthesiologists. *Anesth Analg.* 2008;105:22-28.

7. Rosenberger P, Shernan SK, Loffler M, et al. The influence of epiaortic ultrasonography on intraoperative surgical management in 6051 cardiac surgical patients. *Ann Thorac Surg.* 2008;85:548-553.

8. Eltzschig HK, Kallmeyer IJ, Mihaljevic T, et al. A practical approach to a comprehensive epicardial and epiaortic echocardiographic examination. *J Cardiothorac Vasc Anesth.* 2003;17:422-429.

9. Hilberath JN, Shernan SK, Segal S, et al. The feasibility of epicardial echocardiography for measuring aortic valve area by the continuity equation. *Anesth Analg.* 2009;108:17-22.

Masses and Devices

10

Massimiliano Meineri and Patricia Murphy

KEY POINTS

- The knowledge of normal anatomic variants is critical. Incorrect identification of a mass as pathologic may lead to unnecessary diagnostic tests and treatments including surgery.
- In the left atrial appendage (LAA), pectinate muscles may be mistaken for thrombus.
- The "coumadin ridge," if not imaged correctly, may appear as a free-floating structure in the left atrium (LA).
- Lambl's excrescences are degenerative strands on the aortic valve (AV) and are of no clinical significance.
- The transverse pericardial sinus, when fluid-filled, may appear as a distinct vascular structure.

Several normal cardiac structures may mimic abnormal masses. In this section, we describe some of the structures (Table 10-1) that are frequently mistaken for pathologic entities.

RIGHT ATRIUM

Crista Terminalis

- Prominent muscle ridge (Figure 10-1A).
- Junction of the right atrium (RA) and the superior vena cava (SVC).
- Trabeculations of the right atrial appendage (RAA) originate from the crista terminalis.
- Can be misinterpreted as tumor or thrombus.
- Characteristic appearance and position confirm correct identification.
- Best seen in the midesophageal (ME) bicaval view, adjusting the probe depth to display the SVC-RA junction.

Eustachian Valve

- Originates at the junction of the inferior vena cava (IVC) and the RA (see Figure 10-1B).
- Embryologic remnant of the right venous valve.
- Can be misdiagnosed as thrombus.
- Typically appears as a thin and mobile structure attached to the RA wall.
- Can be differentiated from thrombus by its typical location, attachment to the RA, and filamentous appearance.
- Best seen in ME bicaval view, advancing the probe to visualize the IVC-RA junction.

Chiari Network

- Found in 2% to 3% of the patients by transesophageal echocardiography (TEE).
- Vestigial remnant of the IVC valve.
- Fine meshwork of fine fibers that cross the RA (see Figure 10-1C).
- Runs between the eustachian valve and the interatrial septum (IAS).
- Connects the eustachian valve to the thebesian valve at the orifice of the coronary sinus (CS).
- Has no clinical relevance.
- Can be misdiagnosed as thrombus or other atrial mass, or the interatrial septum.
- Typical location and appearance allow correct identification.
- Best seen in the ME four-chamber view by rotating the probe to the right to display the RA and in the ME bicaval view.

Thebesian Valve

- Embryologic remnant of the valve to the CS.
- Prevents regurgitation of blood into the CS.
- May prevent insertion of retrograde cardioplegia cannula in the CS.
- Best seen in the ME four-chamber view by advancing the probe to visualize the CS.
- Can also be visualized in a modified ME bicaval view at 110 degrees adjacent to the septal leaflet of the tricuspid valve (TV).

TABLE 10-1   ANATOMIC VARIANTS

Variant	Differential Diagnosis	Location	Echocardiography Views	Echocardiography Features
Eustachian valve	Thrombus, catheter, vegetation, tumor	RA	ME Bicaval	Thin, mobile membrane at junction of RA and IVC
Chiari network	Thrombus, vegetation	RA	ME 4C ME Bicaval	Filamentous, fenestrated membrane at junction of RA and IVC
Lipomatous hypertrophy of IAS	Tumor, mural thrombus, infiltrative disease	IAS	ME 4C	Dumbbell-shaped hypertrophy of IAS with sparing of fossa ovalis
IAS aneurysm	Thrombus, vegetation	IAS	ME 4C view	Mobile atrial septum with redundancy of 1.5 cm and displacement of 1 cm
Crista terminalis	Thrombus, tumor	RA	ME bicaval	ME bicaval view prominent muscle ridge seen at junction of SVC and RA
Pectinate muscles	Mural thrombus, tumor	RA/LA	ME 4C ME 2C	Parallel muscle ridges on inner surface of both atria. Echo density same as atrial wall
Coumadin ridge	Thrombus	LA	ME 2C	Prominent ridge of tissue at junction of LUPV and LAA
Transverse sinus	Cyst, abscess, aortic dissection	Pericardium	ME LAX	Triangular echo-free space between LA, pulmonary trunk, and ascending aorta
Moderator band	Tumor, thrombus, vegetation	RV	ME 4C	Prominent band in apical one third of RV from free wall to IVS
Lambl's excrescence	Tumor, thrombus, vegetation	AV	ME AV LAX	Thin echogenic strands attached to ventricular side of AV

AV, aortic valve; 4C, four-chamber; IAS, interatrial septum; IVC, inferior vena cava; LA, left atrium; LAA, left atrial appendage; LAX, long axis; LUPV, left upper pulmonary vein; ME, midesophageal; RA, right atrium; RV, right ventricle; SVC, superior vena cava; 2C, two-chamber.

INTERATRIAL SEPTUM

Interatrial Septal Aneurysm

- Prevalence is between 2% and 10%.
- Mobile or redundant septum.
- IAS right-left displacement of more than 1 cm.
- Fixed IAS bulge of more than 1.5 cm (see Figure 10-1D).
- Increased risk of stroke due to thrombus.
- Fifty percent are associated with patent foramen ovale (PFO).
- Characteristic sigmoid shape of IAS.
- May mimic mobile atrial mass.
- Best viewed in the ME four-chamber focusing on the IAS or in the ME bicaval view.

Lipomatous Hypertrophy of the Interatrial Septum

- Infiltration of the atrial septum by adipocytes.
- It normally spares the fossa ovalis.
- Diagnostic thickness criteria are 1.5 to 2.0 cm.
- Echogenic typical "dumbbell" shaped (see Figure 10-1E).
- Characteristic shape differentiates lipomatous hypertrophy from other structures and masses.
- Fatty deposits cause prominent acoustic shadow.
- Best viewed in the ME four-chamber focusing on the IAS or in the ME bicaval view.

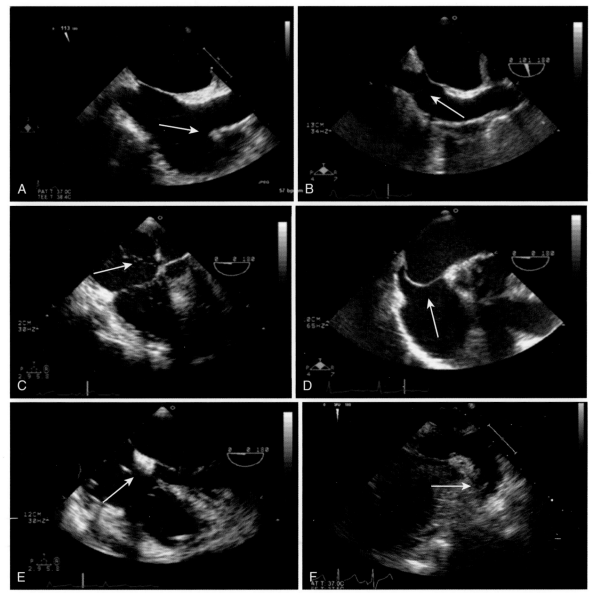

Figure 10-1. Several normal anatomic variants can be mistaken for intracardiac masses. In the RA, we can often distinguish the embryologic remnants *(arrows)*: crista terminalis (**A**) at the junction of the SVC and the RA, eustachian valve (**B**) at the junction of the IVC and the RA, and Chiari network from the eustachian valve to the interatrial septum (**C**). Normal variants affecting the IAS are aneurysmal septum (**D**) and the typically bell-shaped lypomatous septal hypertrophy (**E**). In the LAA, we can often note a regular network of parallel fine muscle fibers known as *pectinate muscles* (**F**).

LEFT ATRIUM

Pectinate Muscles

- Parallel muscular ridges found in both atria.
- Are prominent in the LAA (see Figure 10-1F) and can simulate an LAA thrombus.
- Typically have a tissue characterization similar to muscle.
- Scanning multiple planes is essential to differentiate from thrombus.

- Trabeculations emanate perpendicular from the LAA wall in a regularly spaced pattern (see Figure 10-1F).

Coumadin Ridge

- A prominent muscular ridge formed between the LAA and the left upper pulmonary vein (LUPV) (see Figure 10-1G).

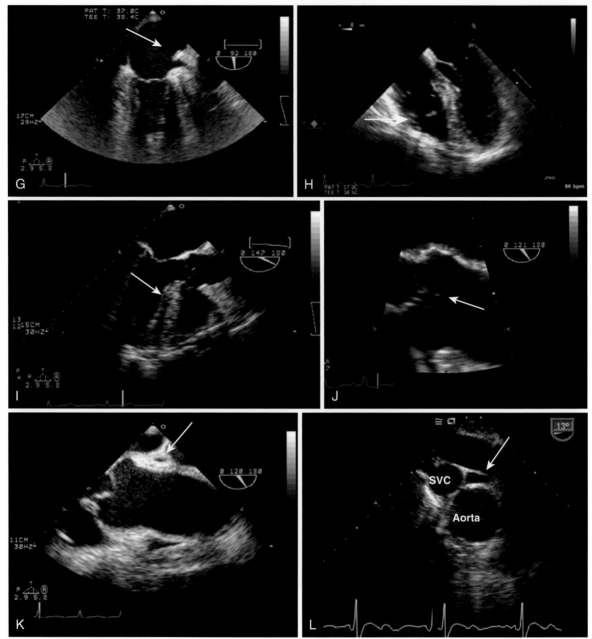

Figure 10-1, cont'd In the LA, the coumadin ridge (**G**), a prominent muscle bridge, that divides the LAA from the LUPV. Within the RV, a transverse muscle ridge, known as the *moderator band* (**H**), characterizes the RV and can be mistaken for thrombus. Distal hypertrophy of the IVS with sigmoidal appearance: normal variant of aging and hypertension (**I**) is typical of longstanding hypertension. Normal filaments attached to the edges of the AV leaflets are the Lambl's excrescences (**J**). They can be mistaken for endocarditic vegetations. The transverse sinus is a pericardial reflection between the ascending aorta and the PA. When expanded by minimal pericardial fluid, it becomes evident in the ME LAX (**K**) and the ascending aorta SAX (**L**) views.

- Linear structure with bulbous ends that give it the "Q-tip sign."
- Historically mistaken for a thrombus and triggered anticoagulation therapy, thus, its name.

- Lack of mobility and characteristic location distinguish it from an abnormal structure.
- Best visualized in the standard ME two-chamber view.

RIGHT VENTRICLE

- *Trabeculations:* muscle bands in the right ventricle (RV).
- *Moderator band:* prominent apical muscle band from septum to the anterior papillary muscle (PM; see Figure 10-1H).
- *PMs.*
- Right ventricular (RV) structures most commonly confused as masses are the RV trabeculations.
- RV is heavily trabeculated, and with right ventricular hypertrophy (RVH) trabeculations, become very prominent.
- Catheters within the RV can appear as small mobile echo densities that resemble intracardiac masses.
- Catheters are echo dense and produce typical reverberations and side lobe artifacts shadowing other structures.

LEFT VENTRICLE

- Several normal structures in the left ventricle (LV) may be mistaken as masses.
- *PMs:* usually two, one in the parachute mitral valve (MV).
- *Aberrant chordae tendinae:* abnormal extra MV chordae without structural function. Typically attached to the MV leaflets or to primary or secondary chordae. Homogeneous in structure, can be thickened compared with other chordae.
- *Distal hypertrophy of the interventricular septum (IVS) with sigmoidal appearance:* normal variant of aging and hypertension (see Figure 10-1I).
- *False tendons:* fine filaments across the left ventricular (LV) near apex.
- If imaged tangentially, PMs can be mistaken for masses.
- The location and attachments of the MV apparatus are distinguishing features of PM.

AORTIC VALVE

- *Nodules of Arantius:* points of coaptation of the AV. Seen at the tip of the AV as small globular thickening.
- *Lambl's excrescences:* degenerative strands on either side of the AV (see Figure 10-1J). Commonly seen in older patients. They have no pathologic implications.
- Lambl's excrescences can be misinterpreted for endocarditis.
- Lambl's excrescences are fine homogeneous filaments attached to the AV closure line of normal AV leaflets.

PERICARDIUM

- Normal pericardium is an echolucent layer with a normal thickness less than 1 mm.
- There is good correlation between TEE and computed tomography (CT) measurements of pericardial thickness.

Transverse Sinus, Fat Pad, Cyst

Transverse Sinus
- A reflection of the pericardium.
- It is a virtual space in absence of any pericardial effusion.
- It is seen as a triangular echo-free space between the ascending aorta, pulmonary trunk, and LA when filled with pericardial fluid.
- May be misinterpreted as a thrombus, cyst, or abscess.
- Pericardial fluid or fat in the transverse sinus can also be misdiagnosed as a mass in the LA
- Best imaged in the ME long axis (LAX) view between the ascending aorta and the right pulmonary artery (PA; see Figure 10-1K).
- Can also be visualized in the ME ascending aorta short axis (SAX) view between the ascending aorta and the PA (see Figure 10-1L).

Fat Pad
- A hypoechoic space anterior to the parietal pericardium. It is most often found adjacent to the RV and the LV apex.
- May be misinterpreted as a pericardial effusion.
- Pericardial fat is slightly more echogenic than an effusion, and it moves in concert with the heart. Pericardial effusion is motionless.

Pericardial Cyst
- Remnant of defect in the embryologic development of the pericardium.
- Normally localized in the right or left costophrenic angle.
- Usually asymptomatic.
- The echo appearance is of a localized echolucent thin-walled spherical structure.
- Differential diagnosis is pericardial effusion and pericardial fat.

TRANSESOPHAGEAL ECHOCARDIOGRAPHY ASSESSMENT OF INTRACARDIAC MASSES

- Cardiac pathologic masses are: thrombus, infective vegetations, or tumor.
- TEE allows superior images of the LA, LAA, RA, and aorta.
- TEE is the gold standard in the diagnosis of vegetations and intracardiac thrombi, although visualization of the ventricular apex may not always be accurate.
- TEE allows differentiation of normal variants (see Table 10-1) and pathology.
- It can guide surgical therapy for intracardiac masses.

Systematic Transesophageal Echocardiography Assessment of Intracardiac Masses

Step 1: Describe shape, size, echodensity.
Step 2: Define number, location, and attachment.
Step 3: Identify coexisting pathology.
Step 4: Assess hemodynamic impact (e.g., flow obstruction).
Step 5: Quantify tissue invasion to determine resectability and its impact on adjacent structures.

Intracardiac Thrombi
- Appear as homogeneous and more echogenic than normal myocardium.
- Sessile or pedunculated; can reach a large size.
- Fresh thrombi are more mobile and friable, thus at higher risk of embolization (see Case 10-3 on the Expert Consult website).

- Older thrombi are more stable, are organized in layers, and may present initially with calcification.
- Predispositions to clot formation are blood stasis, hypercoagulable state, and rough surfaces.
- Can be found in all cardiac chambers. Predisposing factors vary (Table 10-2).
- TEE is indicated when transthoracic echocardiography (TTE) is inconclusive.

Spontaneous Echocardiographic Contrast
- Dense swirling pattern seen in situations of low-flow states resembling smoke (Figure 10-2A) (see Case 10-4 on the Expert Consult website).
- May be a prodrome to clot formation and coexist with thrombi.
- Can be appreciated in the atrial and ventricular cavities during cardiopulmonary bypass (CPB).
- Thick spontaneous contrast in the LA can be confused with thrombus.
- Assess underlying anatomy and valvular and ventricular function.

Left Atrium
- Thrombi present as irregular masses of variable echogenicity that move with the underlying structure.
- LAA is the most common location of intracardiac thrombi (see Figure 10-2B).
- Very often associated with atrial fibrillation.
- LAA thrombi are rare in patients in sinus rhythm.
- LAA must be carefully assessed in the presence of mitral stenosis, LA enlargement, and stagnant flow with spontaneous echocontrast.
- Can be attached to a prosthetic MV and MV annuloplasty rings.

TABLE 10-2	INTRACARDIAC THROMBI			
Chamber	**Location**		**Appearance**	**Other Findings**
LV	Free wall		Sessile In layers	LV wall motion abnormalities LV aneurysm LVAD cannula
LA	LAA		Round	Atrial fibrillation Mitral stenosis Mitral valve prostheses
RV, RA	Free-floating, wires, catheters		Serpiginous	Wires and catheters Deep venous thrombosis Pulmonary embolism

LAA, left atrial appendage; LV, left ventricle; LV, left ventricular; LVAD, left ventricular assist device; RA, right atrium; RV, right ventricle.

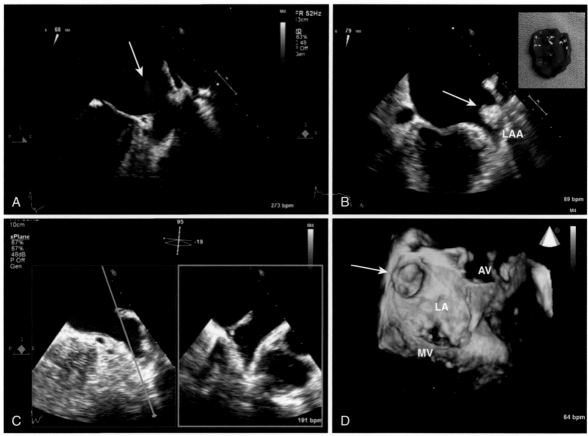

Figure 10-2. **A,** Spontaneous echo contrast indicates stagnant blood flow *(arrow)* and increased risk of thrombus formation. **B,** ME two-chamber view in a patient with LAA thrombus *(arrow)* underwent surgical removal. **C,** 3D TEE assessment of the LAA for thrombi includes X plane mode that allows simultaneous display of two perpendicular planes; in this example, the second plane *(green)* is positioned on the first to cut though the center of the LAA. **D,** Zoom and full-volume modes provide an en face view of the LAA inlet *(arrow)* from the LA.

- TEE is the gold standard in the assessment of LAA.
- Location can help differentiate from tumors because thrombi are rarely attached to the IAS.
- TEE assessment of LAA implies two-dimensional (2D), color flow, and pulse wave (PW) Doppler.
- LAA PW Doppler has a typical biphasic trace. A peak velocity less than 40 cm/s indicates a low-flow risk of thrombus formation.
- 3D TEE allows superior visualization of the LAA using all 3D modalities (see Figure 10-2C and D).

Left Ventricle
- Rare in the absence of severe LV dysfunction.
- LV thrombi coexist with left ventricular wall motion abnormalities, LV dilatation (Figure 10-3C), and aneurysm.
- Attached to the endocardium of the akinetic segment (see Figure 10-3A and B).

- Can be attached to hardware (e.g., left ventricular assist device [LVAD] cannulas).
- Can be surrounded by spontaneous echocontrast.
- Can be sessile or pedunculated.
- Apical thrombi can often be better viewed on TTE.
- Assess underlying ventricular function and presence of hardware.
- Use multiple views and try to visualize the true LV apex.

Inferior Vena Cava, Right Atrium, Right Ventricle
- Appear as irregular masses of variable echogenicity that move with underlying structure.
- Seen in the RA in the presence of venous thromboembolism and pulmonary embolism (Figure 10-4B) (see Case 10-3 on the Expert Consult website).
- Occur on pacer wires and catheters in low-flow states.

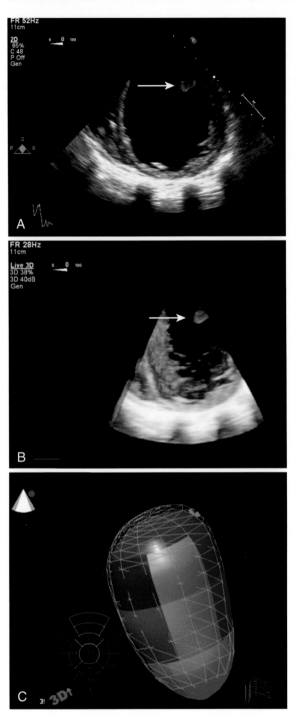

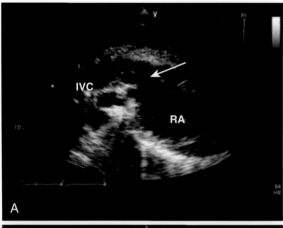

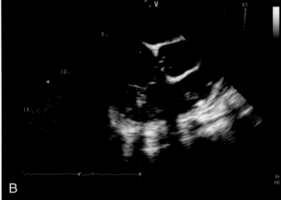

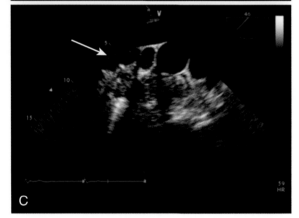

Figure 10-3. Patient presented for an LVAD implant in dilated cardiomyopathy. **A** and **B**, An independently mobile mass *(arrow)* is noted in the LV. **C**, LV function is severely compromised, as shown by end-systolic frame on 3D LV reconstruction.

Figure 10-4. Emergent TEE is performed for cardiac arrest following graft reperfusion after liver transplant. **A**, Modified ME bicaval view displays IVC and IVC-RA junction: thrombotic material *(arrow)* is noticed in the IVC. **B**, ME RV inflow-outflow view shows thrombi in the RV. **C**, Modified ME ascending aorta SAX view shows thrombus *(arrow)* in the distal right PA.

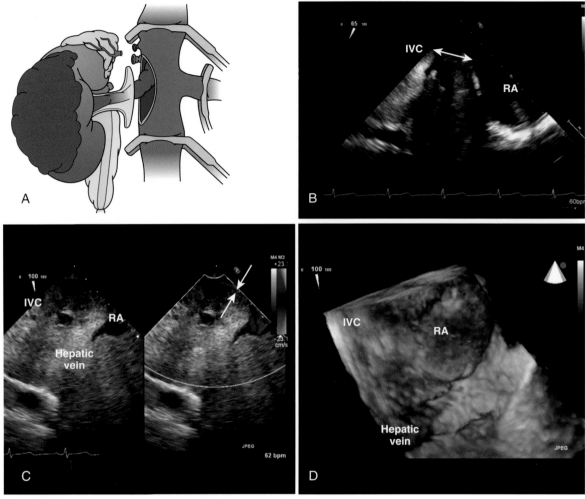

Figure 10-5. Patient with renal cell carcinoma (**A**), scheduled for nephrectomy and IVC thrombectomy. **B,** IVC thrombus is displayed and the distance between the thrombus and the IVC-RA junction is measured *(arrow)*. **C,** IVC flow limitation is displayed by color Doppler. **D,** 3D TEE allowed an en face view of the IVC thrombus from the RA and its relation to the hepatic vein.

- RA thrombi can cross a PFO and result in systemic embolism (see Case 10-3 on the Expert Consult website).
- IVC thrombi are often observed in patients with renal cell carcinoma (Figure 10-5).
- Thrombi in RA are often associated with thrombi in IVC, RV, and PA (see Figure 10-4).
- TEE can visualize the right PA and the proximal left PA; the distal left PA is usually obscured by the left mainstem bronchus.
- The absence of thrombi in the PA by TEE does not exclude pulmonary embolism.
- Assess the right circulation from the IVC to the distal right PA.

Infective Endocarditis
- Infective endocarditis (IE) is a severe condition that carries a 6-month mortality of 25%.

- The diagnosis is based on clinical and echocardiographic data according to the modified Duke Criteria (Table 10-3).
- Positive TTE or TEE is a major criterion.
- TEE is indicated whenever TTE is inconclusive.
- TEE is also indicated in patients with prosthetic valves or elderly patients with valve abnormalities.
- IE can affect normal valves, but it mostly occurs on abnormal cardiac valves.
- Presence of foreign material as well as intravenous drug use increases the risk for IE.
- Advanced forms of IE result in abscess and fistulae, especially when the aortic valve is involved.
- A form of noninfective endocarditis is marantic endocarditis. It may be observed in

TABLE 10-3   MODIFIED DUKE CRITERIA

Major Criteria

Positive TTE or TEE (any of the following)

	• Mass	• Discrete • Echogenic • Independently mobile • Valve or supporting structure • Path of regurgitant jet • Implanted material • Absence of alternative anatomical explanation
	• Periannular abscess • New partial dehiscence of prosthetic valve • New valvular regurgitation	
Positive blood cultures for typical IE microorganism ×2	• Common microorganisms	1. *Streptococcus viridans* 2. *Streptococcus bovis* 3. HACEK group 4. *Staphylococcus aureus* 5. *Enterococcus*

Minor Criteria

IV Drug use
Fever (>38°)

Vascular phenomena	• Embolization • Septic pulmonary infarct • Intracranial hemorrhage • Janeway's lesions
Immunologic phenomena	• Glomerulonephritis • Osler's nodules • Roth's spots • Rheumatoid factor

Positive blood culture ×1 **OR** nontypical microorganism

Diagnosis

	Major Criteria	Minor Criteria
Definite	2 1 0 **OR** Positive pathology	0 3 5
Possible	1 0	1 3

HACEK, haemophilus, aggregatibacter, cardiobacterium hominis, eikenella corrodens, kingella; IE, infective endocarditis; IV, intravenous; TEE, transesophageal echocardiography; TTE, transthoracic echocardiography.

patients with adenocarcinoma and antiphospholipid syndrome. Lesions are very difficult to differentiate from IE.

Vegetations
- Common appearance is as irregular sessile or pedunculated masses.
- In active endocarditis, masses are more soft and friable.
- In chronic IE, they become more stable and dense.
- Fungal endocarditis presents with larger but less invasive vegetations.
- Independently mobile; embolization is not uncommon.

- TEE has a sensitivity of 90% to 100% and a specificity of 88% to 100% in detecting vegetations.
- Each cardiac valve is affected with a different frequency and pattern.

Aortic Valve
- Commonly attached to the ventricular side of the AV (Figure 10-6A and E).
- Predisposing conditions are bicuspid AV, rheumatic deformities, and valve degeneration.
- Vegetations may move back and forth during the cardiac cycle.
- Common evolution is aortic root abscess (see Figure 10-6A and E) and invasion of the intervalvular fibrosa.

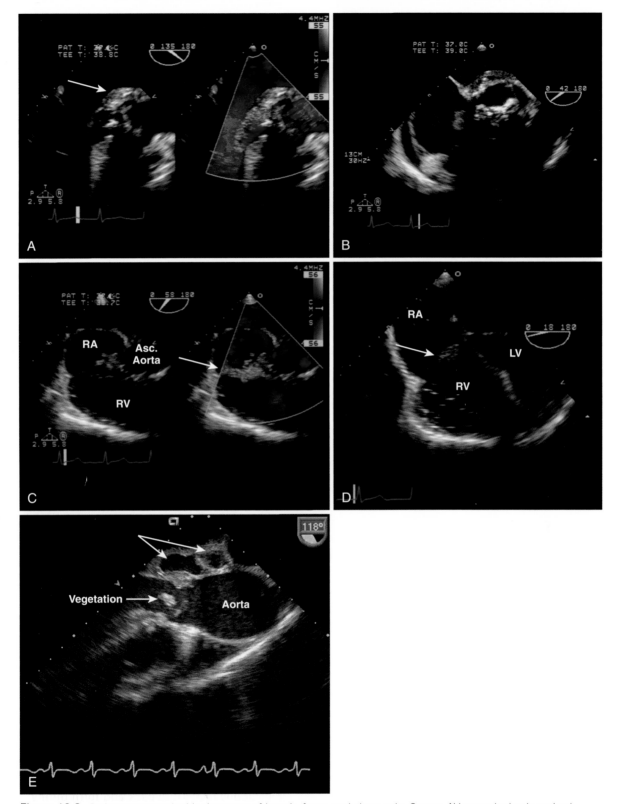

Figure 10-6. Patient presented with shortness of breath, fever, and chest pain. Severe AV regurgitation is noticed
(**A**) on a bicuspid AV (**B**). Large vegetations are attached to the ventricular aspect of the AV. Aortic root is enlarged and
presents an abscess of the sinus of Valsalva (*arrow* in **A**). **C,** Color flow Doppler reveals an aortic root to RA fistula with a
left-to-right shunt. **D,** A large, independently mobile mass is noticed at the base of the TV septal leaflet in proximity to
the exit point of the ascending aorta fistula. The mass indicates spread of infection to the right side of the heart.
Pulmonary valve was spared in this case. **E,** Discrete abscess.

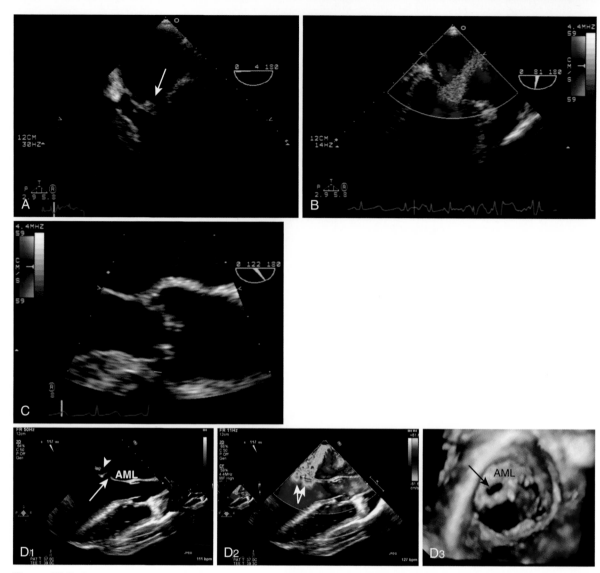

Figure 10-7. Patient scheduled for MV replacement for endocarditis. Vegetations on the atrial aspect of the MV leaflets (*arrow* in **A**) and severe MV regurgitation (**B**) are displayed. All other valves are carefully inspected for vegetations and regurgitant lesions. **C,** The AV is noticed to be thickened. The AV was surgically inspected and found mildly sclerotic and was not replaced. **D,** In another patient with MV endocarditis, central coaptation (*arrowhead*) and a perforation of the anterior mitral leaflet (AML) (*arrow*) are seen. Two areas of proximal flow acceleration are seen on the ventricular side of the valve (*double arrow*). In the right panel, 3D TEE replicating the "surgeons view" of the mitral valve demonstrates the perforation (*arrow*). (**D** courtersy of Jorg Dziersk and Eliot Fagley.)

- In case of aortic regurgitation, vegetations may also be found on the chordae tendinae and the anterior MV leaflet.
- IE on the AV can result in leaflet perforation and aortic regurgitation and are at high risk of embolization.
- Assessment of the AV is performed on multiple views. Zoom is used to better assess the AV leaflets.

Mitral Valve
- Most frequently involved valve in IE.
- Commonly attached to the atrial side of the MV (Figure 10-7A).

- Predisposing conditions are rheumatic heart disease, valve degeneration and calcifications.
- MV IE commonly evolves into leaflet perforation and mitral regurgitation (MR; see Figure 10-7B).
- AV has to be assessed for new AR or leaflet abnormalities (see Figure 10-7C).
- Vegetations on the MV can be distinguished from torn chordae because the latter results in flail of the respective MV segment.

Tricuspid Valve
- Commonly attached to the atrial or the ventricular side of the TV.
- Chordae tendinae can also be affected.

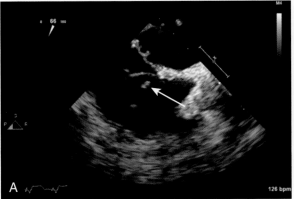 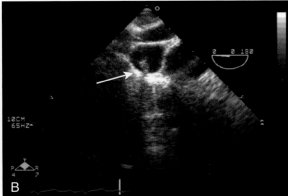

Figure 10-8. In a patient with a recent stroke, a TEE is performed to rule out intracardiac source of emboli. **A,** A small thrombus is noticed in the RA, attached to a permanent pacemaker wire. **B,** A small mass is also noticed surrounding the same wire in the SVC *(arrow).*

- Commonly observed in intravenous drug users.
- Permanent RV catheters such as pacemaker leads are a risk factor (Figure 10-8).
- Result in leaflet perforation and disruption causing tricuspid regurgitation.
- Artifacts from hardware may prevent identification of small vegetations.
- TV can also be involved in presence of ascending aorta-RA (see Figure 10-6D) fistulae as a consequence of AV IE.

Pulmonic Valve
- Less frequently affected by IE.
- In case of involvement of the PV, always suspect congenital heart disease and the presence of intracardiac shunts.

Prosthetic Valves
- Commonly attached to the sewing ring.
- On mechanical valves, it may be difficult to differentiate from pannus.
- IE on prosthetic valves may result in partial dehiscence of the valvular ring and paravalvular regurgitation.
- May cause the destruction of bioprosthetic leaflets and result in valvular regurgitation.
- Vegetations on prosthetic valves are more difficult to identify on TEE owing to echo shadowing from an adjacent valve, especially in patients with concomitant MV and AV prostheses.
- 3D TEE may allow better definition of the number and localization of the vegetations on bioprosthetic valves.

Abscess
- A complication of IE.
- It is defined as a thin-walled cavity containing purulent material as a result of bacterial infiltration.
- A common location is the aortic root as a sequela of AV IE (see Figure 10-6A and E).
- Abscess of the aortic root or the aorta-mitral intravalvular fibrosa may evolve into a

pseudoaneurysm: a recess connected to the aortic root or left ventricular outflow tract (LVOT). Pseudoaneurysms expand during systole and are at risk of rupture.
- On TEE, abscesses appear as echo dense areas in continuity with the valvular plane.
- Abscesses can have a cystic component.
- Abscesses are associated with valvular regurgitation or prosthetic valve dehiscence.
- Abscess of the aortic root are commonly seen in the ME AV LAX view (see Figure 10-6A and E).

Fistulae
- The result of ruptured pseudoaneurysms.
- Aortic root abscesses may rupture into LA, RA, LVOT, or right ventricular outflow tract (RVOT) (see Figure 10-6C).
- Color flow Doppler allows identification of fistulae and may help determine the direction of flow within them.
- Dissemination of infection to downstream structures is common.
- May be single or multiple.

KEY POINTS

- Intracardiac thrombi occur most commonly in the presence of atrial fibrillation, as a consequence of intravascular catheters, and in areas of stagnation such as an aneurysmal LV apex.
- TEE is the standard method to assess the LAA for thrombus before cardioversion. A comprehensive examination of both the LAA and the LA proper is required. This is especially present in patients with rheumatic heart disease.
- "Smoke," or spontaneous echo contrast, indicates a low-flow state and is especially worrisome when it fails to clear from the LAA after several beats.

Continued

TABLE 10-4 PRIMARY CARDIAC TUMOR

	RA	RV	LV	LA	Valves	Pericardium
Benign						
Myxoma				X		
Rhabdomyoma		X	X			
Lipoma	X		X			
Papillary fibroelastoma					X	
Fibroma			X			
Malignant						
Angiosarcoma	X					
Rhabdomyosarcoma	X	X	X	X	X	X
Lymphoma	X	X				
Mesothelioma						X

LA, left atrium; LV, left ventricle; RA, right atrium; RV, right ventricle.

Cardiac Tumors

- Primary cardiac tumors are relatively rare and found in approximately 0.02% of autopsies.
- Only 15% of primary tumors are malignant.
- Metastatic tumors are more common but rarely referred for surgery.
- Intracavitary tumors are typically seen in the atria.
- Intramural tumors are found in the ventricles and infiltrate the ventricular walls.
- Extracardiac tumors are confined to the visceral and parietal pericardium.
- Tumor location may guide diagnosis (Table 10-4).

Benign Primary Cardiac Tumors
Myxoma
- Most common benign tumor in adults.
- Localized in the LA (Figure 10-9A) in 75% of the cases; can also be found in the LV or RV in 5% of cases.
- Usually arises from the IAS with a stalk attached to the fossa ovalis (see Figure 10-9B and C).
- Recurrence after resection is rare.
- Smooth surface, homogeneous consistency.
- Can grow to a very large size (see Figure 10-9D).
- May mask underlying MV pathology and cause MV obstruction.
- Location and appearance allow easy differentiation from other masses.

- ME four-chamber, AV SAX, and bicaval allow assessment of the size and attachment of LA myxomas.

Rhabdomyoma
- Most common in children.
- Localized on the ventricular side of the atrioventricular valves.
- Often multiple.
- Well-circumscribed homogeneous echogenic mass.
- Spontaneous regression with age is common.

Lipoma
- Well-circumscribed, spherical, or elliptical.
- Homogeneous echo-free structure.
- Localized on endocardial surface of the LV or RA.
- Twenty-five percent of cases can be intramyocardial.
- Magnetic resonance imaging (MRI) is the gold standard for definitive diagnosis.

Papillary Fibroelastoma
- Most common primary valve tumor.
- Common localizations in order of frequency are AV (LVOT or ascending aortic aspect), MV (atrial aspect), TV, and PV.
- Can also be attached to chordae tendinae (Figure 10-10).
- Tend to arise in areas of endocardial damage such as valve degeneration or after surgery.
- Six percent are multiple.
- Smooth, lobulated, pedunculated mass.
- May be difficult to differentiate from vegetation.
- Rarely causes valve regurgitation.

Fibroma
- Commonly present as a solitary mass (Figure 10-11).
- Normally affects the ventricular myocardium (see Figure 10-11): IVS, apex, or free wall.

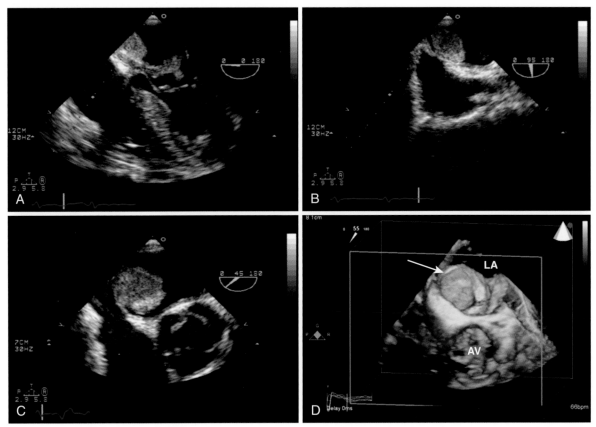

Figure 10-9. Patient with a large left atrial myxoma, scheduled for elective surgical resection. **A,** In the ME four-chamber view, a large mass is noticed in the LA and prolapses through the MV during diastole. **B** and **C,** The attachment of the mass to the IAS is demonstrated in different views. **D,** 3D TEE allows a full view of the mass *(arrow)* and its relation with the surrounding anatomic structures.

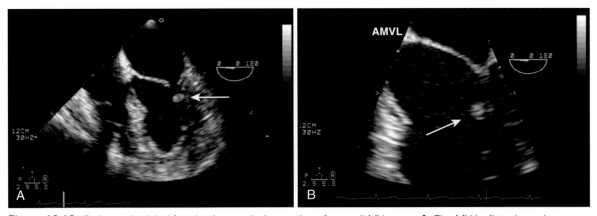

Figure 10-10. Patient scheduled for elective surgical resection of a small MV mass. **A,** The MV leaflets *(arrow)* appear normal on 2D and no regurgitation is noticed. **B,** A small round mass *(arrow)* is attached to the secondary chordae of the posterior MV leaflet. Pathologic examination confirmed the diagnosis of papillary fibroelastoma.

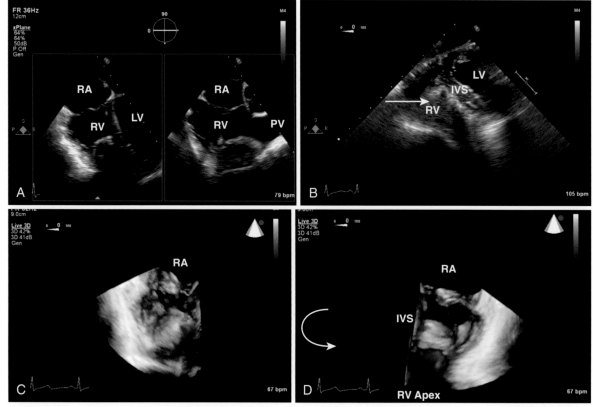

Figure 10-11. Patient presented for elective surgical resection of RV mass. **A,** X planes technology displays simultaneous perpendicular views of the RV. **A** and **B,** A large mass obliterates the distal RV cavity. Live 3D TEE allows rotation of the 3D image. The mass can thus be viewed from the front (**C**) and the back (**D**), allowing better understanding of its relationship with the surrounding structures. The histologic diagnosis was fibroleiomyoma.

- May have central calcification.
- Can be large and present multiple calcifications.
- Difficult to differentiate from rhabdomyoma and apical hypertrophic obstructive cardiomyopathy.

Malignant Primary Cardiac Tumors
- Most malignant cardiac tumors are sarcomas (see Case 10-2 on the Expert Consult website).

Angiosarcoma
- Most common sarcoma in adults.
- Most common localization is the RA (80%), but it can also involve the pericardium.
- Rapid progression, poor prognosis.
- It is an intramural mass that extends to the pericardium and vena cava.
- Hemorrhagic pericardial effusion is common.

Rhabdomyosarcoma
- Second most common sarcoma.
- Multiple locations are common.
- Any cardiac chamber can be involved.
- Obstruction of valve orifices is common.

- Rapid growth, poor prognosis.
- Intracavitary and infiltrative growth.
- Local, valvular, and pericardial invasion.

Lymphoma
- Affects all ages.
- Higher incidence in immunocompromised patients (acquired immunodeficiency syndrome [AIDS] and transplant recipients).
- RA and RV are more commonly involved but it can invade any other structure.
- Presents with myocardial infiltration.
- Lesions appear as nodules.
- Tissue diagnosis is required for certain diagnosis.

Mesothelioma
- A malignant tumor of the pericardium more common in adults.
- Originates from visceral or parietal pericardium.
- MRI is the gold standard for diagnosis.
- On TEE, presents as pericardial thickening and effusion.
- Covers the pericardium and encases the heart.
- Invades the heart only superficially.

Secondary Cardiac Tumors

- More common than primary cardiac tumors.
- Cardiac involvement is by direct extension or intravascular spread.
- Typically involve the epicardium.
- Pericardial effusion is common and tamponade may be the clinical presentation.
- Locations are single or multiple.
- All tumors metastasize to the heart, except tumor of the central nervous system.
- Great majority of secondary cardiac localizations are clinically silent.
- Difficult TEE diagnosis of type. Clinical history should guide identification of primary.

Lung

- Direct and intravascular extension to LA through pulmonary veins.
- Most common in men.

Breast

- Direct extension to the RA and LA.
- Most common in women.

Melanoma

- Highest rate of cardiac metastases of all extracardiac tumors.
- Small multiple metastases are common.
- All cardiac chambers and any cardiac structure can be involved.
- Usual incidental diagnosis.

Renal Cell Carcinoma

Uterine Carcinoma

- Venous extension via the IVC to the RA.
- Large occluding masses in the IVC are common.
- TEE is used to guide surgical resection in the IVC.

Intraoperative Echocardiographic Assessment of Cardiac Tumors

- Intraoperative TEE is commonly used to guide surgical resection of cardiac tumors.

Before Cardiopulmonary Bypass

- Confirm presence of tumor before skin incision and exclude embolization.
- Identify appearance and location of tumor (see Case 10-1 on the Expert Consult website).
- Assess the tumor attachment and resectability.
- Define coexisting pathology requiring correction.
- Complete examination to define underlying structures and function.
- 3D TEE provides superior imaging of cardiac tumors allowing better definition of invasion and attachment.
- Careful assessment of the IVC and SVC guides venous cannulation for CPB.

After Cardiopulmonary Bypass

- Assess impact of resection.
- Confirm successful reconstruction and lack of new shunt or damage to cardiac structures.
- Incomplete resection is not uncommon.
- Assess ventricular function and exclude coronary embolization.
- Underlying pathology can be unmasked by tumor resection.

Key Points
• The most common primary benign cardiac tumors are myxomas. They are typically localized in the LA, have a homogeneous appearance, and grow to very large sizes.
• All malignant primary cardiac tumors are sarcomas. The most common sarcomas in adults are the angiosarcomas. They are typically localized in the RA and have a poor prognosis.
• Secondary metastatic tumors are the most common cardiac tumors. They typically involve the epicardium and present with pericardial effusion. The most common primary sources of cardiac metastasis are the lungs for males and the breasts for females. Malignant melanoma has the highest rate of cardiac metastasis.
• Renal and uterine cancers may extend to the heart by extension via the IVC.
• The aim of intraoperative TEE for cardiac tumors is to confirm the presence of the mass before skin incision, define the invasion of cardiac structures, and assess underlying pathology.
• After resection of the tumor, TEE must exclude incomplete resection, confirm successful reconstruction, and exclude new or residual valvular pathology.

DEVICES FOR CLOSURE OF INTRACARDIAC SHUNTS

Atrial Septal Defect, Patent Foramen Ovale Device Closure

- Device closure of atrial septal defect (ASD) and PFO has become standard of practice.
- ASD closure is normally performed under fluoroscopy in awake patients.
- Intravascular ultrasound has been used to guide ASD location, size, and device deployment.
- TEE likely requires general anesthesia, and it has been successfully used in this clinical setting.

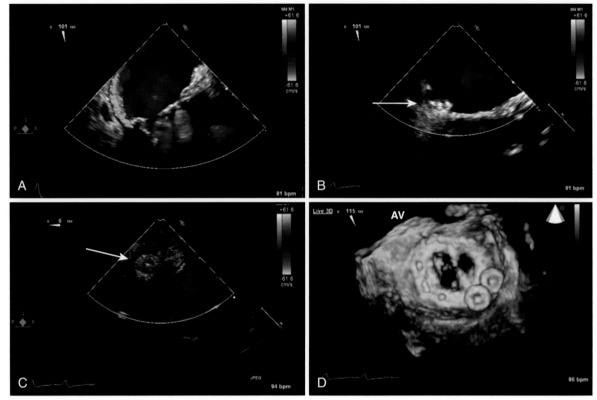

Figure 10-12. **A,** In a patient with an MV bioprosthesis presenting with a large PL, TEE is used to guide percutaneous closure. **B,** Color flow Doppler reveals no residual leak after deployment of two Amplatzer devices *(arrow).* **C,** The device is clearly seen on 2D *(arrow).* **D,** 3D TEE provides an en face view of the MV from the LA and allows easy location of the device along the MV annulus.

Before Deployment

- 2D measurement of the defects.
- Analysis of the geometry of the rim for suitability for device closure (maximum diameter < 4 cm).
- 3D TEE provides an en face view of the septal defect and is very accurate in detecting multiple defects.
- TEE can effectively guide positioning of wires across the defect and display deployment of the device.

After Deployment

- Assess stability of the deployed device.
- Assess residual leaks.
- Exclude iatrogenic valvular damage.
- Infection, dislodgment, and erosion into adjacent structures are common long-term complications of IAS devices.
- If present, IAS devices are removed during open heart surgery for other pathologies because manipulation of the heart may cause dislodgment and perforation of adjacent structures.

Mitral Valve Paravalvular Leak Device Closure

- Paravalvular leaks (PLs) are a common complication after prosthetic valve implant.
- PLs accounting for mild regurgitation are not clinically significant but may cause hemolysis.
- Percutaneous closure of MV PLs is becoming the treatment of choice (Figure 10-12).
- TEE is used to guide device positioning and deployment, and it is complementary to fluoroscopy.

Before Deployment

- Localization of the leak and confirmation of severity.
- 3D TEE provides an en face view of the MV in the surgical view and allows prompt location of the PL
- 3D TEE also allows assessment of the leak geometry and provides precise measurements of the defect.
- TEE can effectively guide positioning of wires across the leak before device deployment.

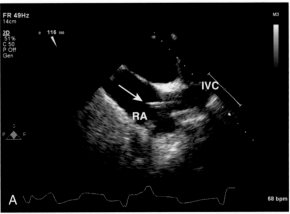 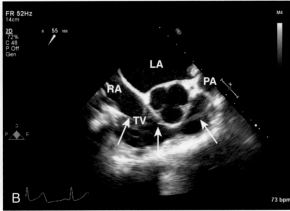

Figure 10-13. **A,** ME bicaval view is used to confirm presence of Seldinger wire *(arrow)* in the SVC before cannulation of the internal jugular vein. **B,** ME RV inflow-outflow view can be used to guide positioning of the PAC *(arrows)* in the PA.

- During deployment, TEE can assess the impact of the device on the prosthetic valve.

After Deployment
- Assess stability of the deployed device.
- Assess residual leaks.
- Exclude valve malfunction.
- The device may prevent complete closure of mechanical leaflets and result in severe intravalvular regurgitation.

CENTRAL VENOUS CATHETERS

- TEE can effectively locate the wire in the SVC.
- TEE can exclude presence of persistent left SVC and contraindicate left-sided cannulation.
- In cases of persistent left SVC, agitated saline contrast injected in a left arm peripheral vein will reach the RA though the CS.
- ME bicaval view is used to visualize the advancement of the wire into the SVC (Figure 10-13A).
- ME bicaval view allows visualization of the tip of the catheter in respect of the SVC to RA junction.
- Correct central venous catheter (CVC) tip position is approximately 1 cm from the SVC-RA junction.

PULMONARY ARTERY CATHETER

- TEE may be used to locate the wire in the SVC.
- ME bicaval view angulated to show the TV is used to guide the PA catheter through the TV.

- ME RV inflow-outflow view is used to guide advancement of the PAC into the PA (see Figure 10-13B).

CARDIOPULMONARY BYPASS

- The use of CPB was first described by Dennis and coworkers in 1951.[14]
- It allows performing open heart surgery on a bloodless surgical field and a still heart.
- The basic CPB comprises a venous cannula, reservoir, pump, oxygenator, and arterial cannula.
- The blood is passively drained by gravity through the venous cannula into the venous reservoir. A mechanical pump pumps the blood from the venous reservoir through the oxygenator back into the patient's arterial circulation.
- The heart is arrested in diastole by injecting a cardioplegic solution into the coronary arteries.

Venous Cannulas

- Different types of venous cannulas can be used, depending on the surgical procedure that is performed.
- Peripheral cannulation is performed through the femoral or the internal jugular veins or both and is used for minimally invasive cardiac surgery (Figure 10-14A). Venous cannulas are advanced into the RA (see Figure 10-14B and G).
- Central cannulation can be single or double.

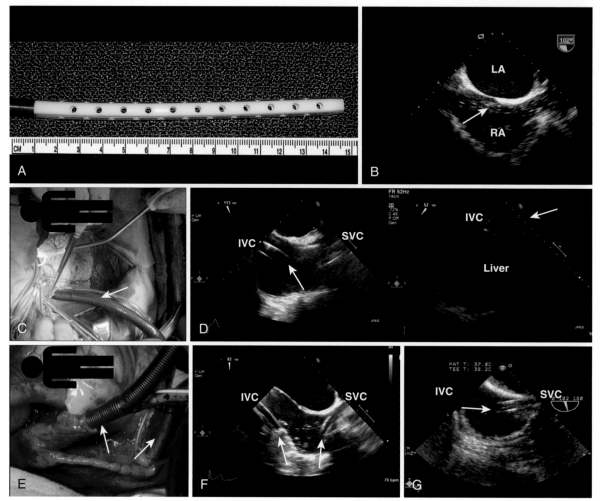

Figure 10-14. **A,** Minimally invasive cardiac surgery is often performed using a long femoral venous cannula. **B,** The cannula is advanced under TEE guidance to the RA and positioned just below the SVC-RA junction. In the ME bicaval view, the cannula can be seen in the RA *(arrow)*. **C,** A double-stage venous cannula is inserted in the RA and advanced to the IVC to provide venous return for CPB. **D,** Advancing the probe to follow the cannula and assess the correct position in the IVC. **E,** Double venous cannulation with single-stage cannulas is used to divert blood flow from the RA and allow a bloodless surgical field. **F,** ME bicaval view allows visualization of the IVC and SVC cannulas. **G,** Jugular vein cannulation is performed for minimally invasive cardiac surgery. In the ME bicaval view, the tip of the venous cannula *(arrow)* can be identified in the RA.

- Single cannulation (see Figure 10-14A) is performed using a two-stage cannula with an opening at the tip and side holes at 5 to 10 cm from the tip. When correctly positioned, the tip is sitting in the IVC and the side ports in the RA. This technique is normally used for surgery on the aorta and AV and well as for coronary artery bypass grafts.
- For surgery on the atrioventricular valves, double cannulation (see Figure 10-14D) is usually performed to effectively deviate all venous blood from the atria. Two single-stage cannulas (without side holes) are inserted in the IVC and in the SVC.

- The ME bicaval view is used to visualize venous cannulas (see Figure 10-14B, F, and G).
- From the ME bicaval view, the TEE probe is advanced to follow the venous cannula into the IVC (see Figure 10-14D).
- TEE can detect malpositioning of the venous cannula into the hepatic veins resulting in poor venous drainage.[16]
- When peripheral cannulation is performed, the ME bicaval view is commonly used to confirm correct positioning of the tip on venous cannulas in the RA (see Figure 10-14B, F, and G).

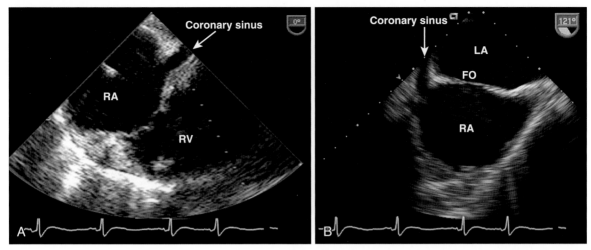

Figure 10-15. **A,** The CS is seen in a modified ME four-chamber view advancing the probe to visualize the long axis of the CS *(arrow)* draining into the RA. **B,** A modified ME bicaval view is commonly used to guide CS cannulation. In this view, the TV and the CS *(arrow)* are simultaneously seen. FO, fossa ovalis.

Left Ventricular Vent

- LV vent is placed in the right upper pulmonary vein (RUPV) and advanced into the LV.
- It is used to drain blood from the LV during AV and MV surgery.
- LV vent is commonly seen entering the LA via the RUPV, and is appreciated in most of the ME views displaying the LA.

Coronary Sinus Catheter

- Cannulation of the CS is performed to provide retrograde cardioplegia during CPB.
- It normally is performed after sternotomy with a cannula inserted into the RA.
- For minimally invasive cardiac surgery, a CS cardioplegia cannula is placed percutaneously using a special catheter in the internal jugular vein.
- TEE has been successfully used to guide positioning of CS catheters during both open and minimally invasive surgery.
- A prominent thebesian valve and a small CS make CS cannulation very difficult.
- Possible complications include CS rupture and insufficient cardioplegia resulting in postoperative ventricular dysfunction.
- CS is commonly seen in a modified four-chamber view obtained from a standard four-chamber view by advancing the probe and retroflexing it. The CS is visualized in its long axis, draining into the RA (Figure 10-15A).

- To guide positioning of CS cannulas, a modified bicaval view at 110 degrees is normally used. The CS is seen in its SAX adjacent to the septal leaflet of the TV (see Figure 10-15B).
- Once the catheter is in place, its position should be reconfirmed using the modified four-chamber view.
- LV pressure trace transmission to the CS catheter should be obtained to confirm placement.
- Fluoroscopy and venography are used during minimally invasive surgery to confirm correct position.

Arterial Cannulas

- The arterial cannula is commonly positioned in the ascending aorta or the proximal aortic arch.
- Retrograde perfusion through the femoral artery is used in specific conditions when direct cannulation of the ascending aorta is contraindicated such as dissection and ascending aortic aneurysms.
- In these circumstances, the axillary artery may be cannulated to provide forward flow.
- For minimally invasive surgery, a long aortic cannula is advanced from the femoral artery into the ascending aorta to provide antegrade flow through a lumen proximal to the aortic endoclamp balloon.
- Aortic cannula can be seen in the ME AV LAX view by withdrawing the probe and

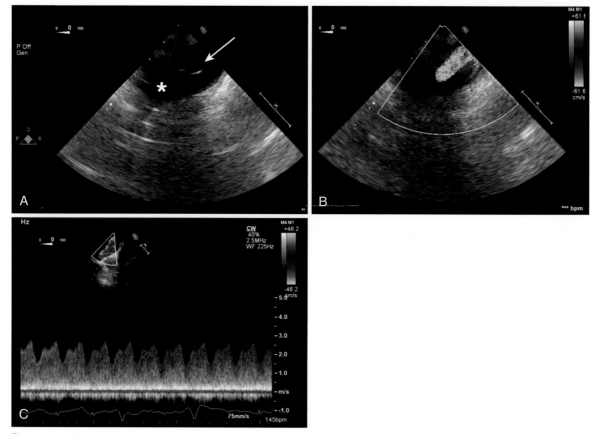

Figure 10-16. **A,** The tip of the arterial cannula *(arrow)* can often be seen in the proximal arch *(asterisk)* in the UE aortic arch LAX view. **B,** Color flow Doppler is used to display continuous flow from the cannula. **C,** Flow velocity and pattern can be assessed using continuous wave Doppler.

increasing the interrogation angle to visualize as much of the ascending aorta as possible.

- The tip of the aortic cannula can commonly be seen in the proximal arch by using the upper esophageal (UE) aortic arch LAX view (Figure 10-16A).
- TEE can identify the aortic cannula, confirm flow using color flow Doppler (see Figure 10-16B), and exclude aortic dissection.
- Continuous wave Doppler can be used to measure the flow velocity in the aortic cannula (see Figure 10-16C).
- In case of aortic dissection and femoral or axillary cannulation, ME thoracic aorta LAX and SAX views are used to confirm perfusion of the true lumen.
- After removal of aortic cannula, ME AV LAX, UE aortic arch LAX, and ME thoracic aorta LAX and SAX views can help rule out aortic dissection.
- ME AV LAX view is also used to visualize ascending aortic plaque and guide cannulation of normal tissue.

KEY POINTS

- TEE is commonly used to guide device closure of ASDs and PLs. 2D and 3D TEE allow precise localization and measurement of the defects for sizing. TEE is also used to guide wire positioning and assess the final result of the procedure.
- TEE is commonly used in the operating room to aid positioning of CVCs. TEE allows confirmation of venous cannulation, continuous visualization of the wire, and guidance for the final positioning of the catheter tip.
- TEE can guide correct positioning of venous cannulas and ensure adequate venous return for CPB. TEE is very useful to assess aortic plaque, guide aortic cannulation, and promptly detect complications at cannulation and decannulation of the aorta.
- Port access systems and minimally invasive approaches rely on TEE guidance for correct positioning of CS catheters for delivery of cardioplegia solution.

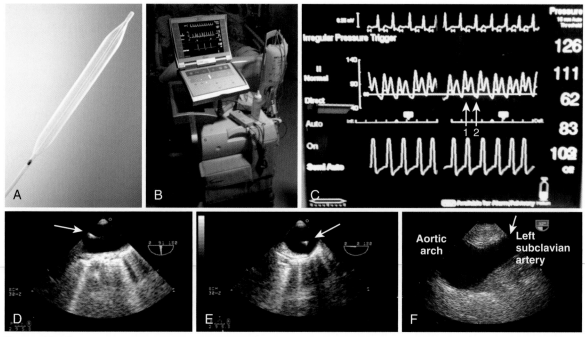

Figure 10-17. **A,** IABP is a catheter-mounted balloon. The controller (**B**) inflates the balloon at the dicrotic notch (**C1**) and deflates it at the isovolumic phase of systole (**C2**). The electrocardiogram (ECG) or the invasive arterial pressure can trigger IABP inflation. TEE can easily image the IABP catheter in the thoracic aorta. The IABP catheter *(arrows)* can be visualized in its LAX (**D**) or SAX (**E**) view. **F,** TEE is used to assess good positioning of the IABP, ensuring its tip is distal to the left subclavian artery *(arrow)*. **A,** *Courtesy of Datascope.*

Intra-aortic Balloon Pump

- Intra-aortic balloon pump (IABP) is a catheter-mounted balloon of 30 to 50 mL and is used to improve coronary perfusion and diminish LV afterload (Figure 10-17A and B).
- Positioned percutaneously through the femoral artery to the thoracic aorta.
- Inflates at the dicrotic notch and deflates in the early isovolumic phase of systole (see Figure 10-17C).
- Preoperative insertion is indicated in patients with severely impaired LV function.
- Also inserted in the presence of acute ventricular septal defect (VSD) and MR post myocardial infarction.

Baseline Assessment
- Define LV and RV function.
- AV insufficiency prevents increases in coronary perfusion with inflation of the IABP.
- Severe aortic insufficiency is an absolute contraindication to IABP insertion.
- Atherosclerotic plaques of the thoracic aorta should be assessed because they can be disrupted by IABP.

- In case of severe peripheral vascular disease, IABP can be inserted intraoperatively in the distal aortic arch and the driveline passed above the sternal notch.
- Aortic dissection and thoracic aneurysms are absolute contraindications to IABP positioning.

Positioning
- Confirm position of the guidewire in the thoracic aorta before catheter advancement to avoid placement in the venous system or the contralateral iliac artery.
- Localize the IABP tip distal to the left subclavian artery.
- ME descending aorta SAX view and ME descending aorta LAX views are normally used to visualize wire and IABP.

Post Positioning
- Assess correct positioning of the IABP distal to the origin of the left subclavian artery (see Figure 10-17F). To do so: identify the IAPB tip in the descending aorta LAX view. Hold the TEE probe handle with one hand and pinch the probe with the other hand at the

patient's teeth. Withdraw the probe until the UE aortic arch LAX view is obtained. The distance from the finger pinching the probe and the patient's teeth is a good estimate of the distance between the tip of the IAPB and the aortic arch.
- When correctly positioned, the tip of the IABP lies a few centimeters distal to the origin of the left subclavian artery.
- Confirm correct function of IABP with visualization of inflation and deflation of the balloon (see Figure 10-17D and E).
- Exclude complications (e.g., balloon perforation, aortic dissection).
- Exclude new or worsening AV insufficiency and dynamic LVOT obstruction.
- Monitor change in LV function after initiation of IABP.

Weaning
- TEE allows direct assessment of LV and RV function during weaning.
- Normally, the IABP is weaned from 1:1 to 1:2 mode after a few hours and then to 1:3 if hemodynamically stable.
- IABP at 1:3 provides minimal hemodynamic support.

Ventricular Assist Devices

Assessment of Left Ventricular Assist Device Placement
(Figures 10-18 and 10-19)
- Ventricular assist devices (VADs) provide mechanical support to the left (LVAD), the right (RVAD), or both (BiVAD) ventricles (see Case 10-4 on the Expert Consult website).
- VADs are used as a bridge to transplant or recovery or as a destination therapy.
- RVAD and BiVAD are not commonly used for mid- and long-term treatment.
- VADs can be classified based on the type of flow provided, the duration of support, and the location of the pump (Table 10-5).

Cannulation
- The inflow cannula brings blood into the device.
- The outflow cannula brings blood from the device back into the circulation.
- For LVAD, the inflow cannula is usually at the apex of the LV and the outflow cannula in the aorta.
- In LVAD, the inflow cannula may also be attached to the LA either directly or through one of the pulmonary veins.

- For RVAD, the inflow cannula drains blood from the RA, with outflow going to the PA.

Baseline
- Confirm LV dysfunction and/or RV dysfunction.
- Assess RV function and tricuspid regurgitation.
- If there is moderate or severe RV dysfunction that has not been medically addressed (i.e., high central venous pressure [CVP]), reconsideration may be appropriate; however, if this is not the case, then LVAD insertion can probably proceed with the caveat that RVAD placement may be necessary if the unloading provided to the RV by the LVAD is not sufficient.
- Assess for PFO or ASD using color flow Doppler and agitated saline contrast with concomitant Valsalva maneuver. These abnormalities must be corrected at the time of LVAD placement to prevent a postoperative right-to-left shunt. Similarly, the presence of a VSD must be corrected at the time of LVAD placement.
- Quantify aortic insufficiency. Any degree of aortic insufficiency more than mild requires treatment. Moderate and severe AV insufficiency causes a short circuit of the blood stream within the VAD and lack of flow distal to the ascending aorta. If there is minimal chance of myocardial recovery, oversewing the AV is an acceptable practice. In all other cases, AV replacement with a bioprosthetic prosthesis should be performed.
- In patients with a dilated and aneurysmal LV, identify intracavitary thrombi.
- Rule out the presence of LA thrombi.
- Assess the presence of aortic atheroma (ascending, transverse, or descending aorta) to guide outflow cannula positioning.

Weaning from Cardiopulmonary Bypass

- TEE confirms identification of the true LV apex showing invagination when the surgeon presses on the site identified for cannulation.
- Confirm the position of the inflow cannula through the entire myocardial thickness.
- The tip of the inflow cannula should be pointing toward the MV and not toward the IVS.
- Complete and careful deairing of all heart chambers should be obtained before activating the LVAD.

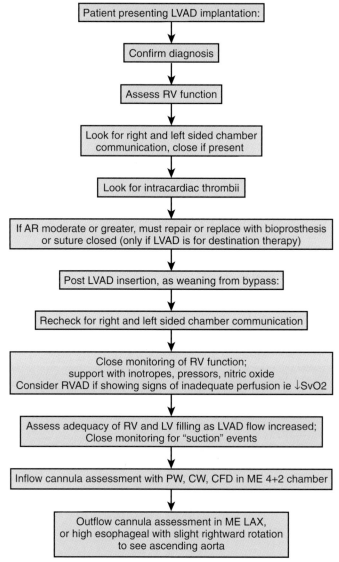

Figure 10-18. Assessment of LVAD placement. SvO₂, venous oxygen saturation.

- LVAD inflow cannula is usually well visualized in the ME four-chamber and two-chamber views. These views also allow Doppler measurement of flow.
- LVAD outflow cannula can be seen in the ME LAX view. The same view allows Doppler measurement of flows.

Post Implant
- Confirm absence of PFO; active emptying of the LV may cause opening of previously closed PFOs.
- Assess RV size and function. A failing RV would result in low preload to the LVAD and low output.

- Identify new or worsened tricuspid regurgitation and estimate RV systolic pressures.
- Color Doppler assessment of flow through the inflow (see Figure 10-19A) and outflow (see Figure 10-19C) cannulas.
- Continuous wave Doppler measurement of gradients in the inflow (see Figure 10-19B) and outflow (see Figure 10-19D) cannulas. Peak velocities are usually around 1 meter per second.
- Confirm LV decompression.
- A closed AV through the entire cardiac cycle is a sign of lack of native ejection and effective LV unloading.

TABLE 10-5   VENTRICULAR ASSIST DEVICES

Type	Term*		Flow		Valves†				Extra	Pump‡		RVAD	BiVAD
	Short	Long	Pulsatile	Continuous	Mech	Bio	PUR	No	Extra	Abdo	Med	RVAD	BiVAD
BVS 5000 Abiomed	X		X				X		X			X	X
VAS Thoratec	X		X		X				X			X	X
HeartMate Thoratec		X	X			X				X			
Novacor WorldHeart		X	X			X				X			
HeartMate II Thoratec		X		X				X			X		
Jarvic 2000 Nasa		X		X				X			X		
LVAD HeartWare		X		X				X			X		
DuraHeart Terumo		X		X				X		X			

*Term: short, <7 days; long, >7 days.
†Valves = VAD internal valves.
‡Pump = pump location.
Abdo: abdominal preperitoneal pouch; Bio, biological; BiVAD, biventricular assist device; Extra, extracorporeal; Mech, mechanical; Med, mediastinal; No, none; PUR, polyurethane; RVAD: right ventricular assist device.

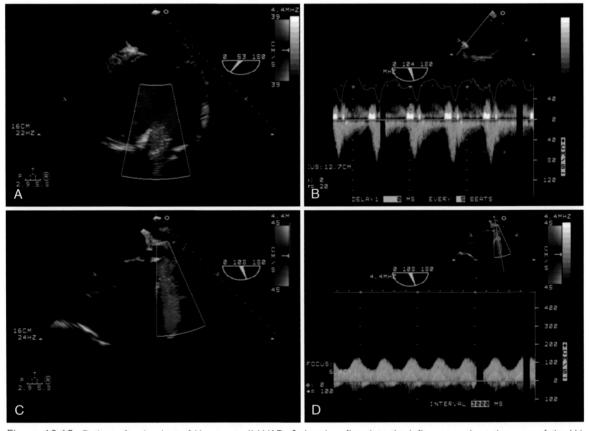

Figure 10-19. Patient after implant of Heartmate II LVAD. **A,** Laminar flow into the inflow cannula at the apex of the LV is displayed on color flow Doppler. Flow through the inflow cannula is measured using continuous wave (CW) Doppler. **B,** The CW spectral wave displays pulsatility due to residual LV contraction and augmentation of flow through the LVAD inflow cannula. **C,** Laminar flow is demonstrated by color flow Doppler from the LVAD outflow cannula into the ascending aorta. **D,** CW Doppler confirms normal flow velocities.

- Reassess AV insufficiency.
- Complete TEE examination should confirm LV unloading and adequate RV function in uneventful LVAD implant.

Postoperative Low Device Output and Common Complications

- TEE is useful in the differential diagnosis of low device output.
- Hypovolemia results in empty LV and collapse of the ventricle around the LVAD inflow cannula.
- RV dilatation and hypokinesis may be secondary to the effects of CPB or because of increased venous return due to LVAD performance. RV dilatation is commonly seen in the ME four-chamber view.
- Pericardial effusion causing tamponade is not uncommon after LVAD implant due to the higher risk of bleeding in these patient populations.
- Sudden hypoxia after LVAD implant may be due to a reopened PFO with right-to-left shunt.
- Inflow cannula obstruction would result in high gradient and turbulent flow.
- Outflow cannula obstruction would result in a high gradient and turbulent flow.
- Device thrombosis would result in increased inflow or outflow gradients.
- Pulmonary embolism may be the cause of RV failure.
- In pulsatile devices, prosthetic valve failure is not uncommon. Although the valves cannot be seen by TEE, flow reversal or high gradients can be detected by spectral and color flow Doppler.
- Complete TEE examination can promptly exclude most causes of low device flow.

Weaning

- TEE allows prompt assessment of RV and LV function during weaning of the VAD.
- For long-term LVADs, TTE is usually preferred to TEE.

EXTRACORPOREAL MEMBRANE OXYGENATION

- Extracorporeal membrane oxygenation (ECMO) comprises a centrifugal pump, a membrane oxygenator, and an arterial and a venous cannula.
- A form of temporary circulatory and respiratory support normally indicated for up to 10 days.

Cannulation

- Cannulation for ECMO can be central or peripheral.
- In case of central cannulation, cannulas are placed in the same fashion as for CPB.
- CPB cannulas are often left in place and the CPB circuits switched to the ECMO.
- For central cannulation, the venous cannula is in the RA and the arterial cannula is in the ascending aorta.
- Peripheral cannulation can be performed with surgical dissection of the vessels or using percutaneous technique.
- In adults, the femoral vein and artery are used. A long venous cannula advanced to the RA is commonly used.
- In case of poor venous drainage, a second venous cannula can be placed in the jugular vein.
- In children, the internal jugular and the carotid artery are used. The venous cannula is advanced to the RA.

Insertion

- Confirm correct position of cannulas (Figure 10-20A and C).
- Assess flow in arterial and venous cannulas with color flow Doppler (see Figure 10-20B and D).
- Venous cannulas are seen in the RA in the modified ME bicaval view (see Figure 10-20A).
- In case of percutaneous cannulation, TEE can guide wire placement and positioning of cannulas.
- TEE is very sensitive in detecting air in the cardiac chambers and should guide careful deairing before initiation of ECMO.
- The arterial catheter is not seen when peripheral cannulation is used but can be seen if placed in the ascending aorta. Color flow Doppler interrogation of the thoracic aorta should confirm continuous laminar flow.
- Always exclude aortic dissection.
- TEE allows optimization of venous drainage by assessing chamber size and distention.
- TEE can immediately assess LV and RV decompression when ECMO is initiated.
- A complete assessment includes new or worsening AV and MV regurgitation.

Post Implant Monitoring

- TEE guides fluid management by assessing chamber size and distention.
- Common complications that lead to low flows and hypotension can be detected by TEE and

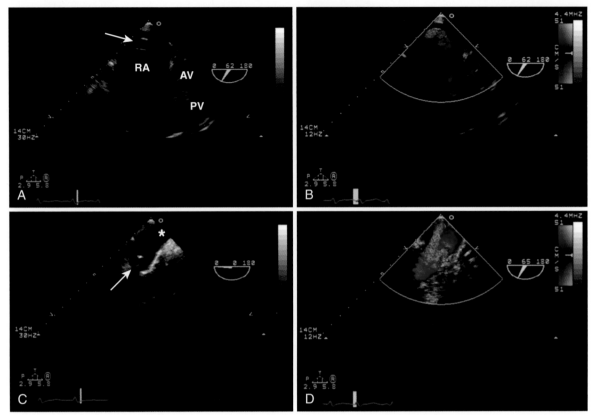

Figure 10-20. A patient is placed on ECMO after failing to wean from CPB. **A,** The ECMO venous cannula is seen in the RA *(arrow)*. **B,** Flow is confirmed with color flow Doppler. **C,** The outflow cannula *(arrow)* is seen in the arch. The *asterisk* indicates the distal arch. **D,** A narrow, continuous, mildly turbulent flow from the arterial cannula is seen on color flow Doppler.

include low filling, tamponade, thrombi, and dislodgment of cannulas.

Weaning

- TEE allows direct assessment of RV and LV function during weaning of ECMO and assessment of myocardial recovery.
- TEE also provides direct measurement of cardiac output in this circumstance when thermodilution is not entirely reliable.

KEY POINTS

- During insertion of IABP, TEE allows visualization of the guidewire in the thoracic aorta and the IABP tip in the correct position distal to the subclavian artery. TEE can also detect absolute contraindications to IABP insertion (e.g., severe aortic insufficiency) and promptly detect complications (e.g., aortic dissection). TEE has also been useful in

---

KEY POINTS—cont'd

assessing ventricular function after insertion and during weaning.
- TEE is a useful tool to assist LVAD implant. The focus of TEE examination at baseline is to quantify aortic regurgitation, look for communication between left- and right-sided chambers (ASD, VSD), assess for left-sided thrombi, and determine RV function. After LVAD insertion TEE is used to interrogate adequate flow in the VAD cannulas, assess ventricular filling, look for impending "suction" events, and continue to monitor RV function. TEE is also used to detect postoperative complications (e.g., tamponade) and ventricular function during weaning.
- During ECMO insertion, TEE is used to assess ventricular function and shunts at baseline and guide positioning of the venous cannulas. After initiation of ECMO flow, TEE provides optimal monitoring of ventricular filling and may guide fluid management. TEE assessment of ventricular function is also very useful during weaning.

Suggested Readings

1. Goldman JH, Foster E. Transesophageal echocardiographic (TEE) evaluation of intracardiac and pericardial masses. *Cardiol Clin*. 2000;18:849-860.
   Nice review of TEE imaging of masses.

2. Kerut EK, Norfleet WT, Plotnick GD, Giles TD. Patent foramen ovale: A review of associated conditions and the impact of physiological size. *J Am Coll Cardiol*. 2001;38:613-623.
   Nice clinical and pathologic comparison of the properties and unique characteristics of LV thrombus.

3. Schneider B, Zienkiewicz T, Jansen V, et al. Diagnosis of patent foramen ovale by transesophageal echocardiography and correlation with autopsy findings. *Am J Cardiol*. 1996;77:1202-1209.
   Details the utility of 3D echocardiography in evaluating the LAA for thrombus.

4. Ling LH, Oh JK, Tei C, et al. Pericardial thickness measured with transesophageal echocardiography: Feasibility and potential clinical usefulness. *J Am Coll Cardiol*. 1997;29:1317-1323.
   An excellent clinical and imaging reference for IE.

5. Durand M, Lamarche Y, Denault A. Pericardial tamponade. *Can J Anaesth*. 2009;56:443-448.
   A nice descriptive paper outlining the early experience with percutaneous cardiac interventions.

6. Srichai MB, Junor C, Rodriguez LL, et al. Clinical, imaging, and pathological characteristics of left ventricular thrombus: A comparison of contrast-enhanced magnetic resonance imaging, transthoracic echocardiography, and transesophageal echocardiography with surgical or pathological validation. *Am Heart J*. 2006;152:75-84.

7. Karakus G, Kodali V, Inamdar V, et al. Comparative assessment of left atrial appendage by transesophageal and combined two- and three-dimensional transthoracic echocardiography. *Echocardiography*. 2008;25:918-924.
   These two papers describe the utility of TEE in the placement of cardiac cannulas when operative exposure is limited.

8. Durack DT, Lukes AS, Bright DK. New criteria for diagnosis of infective endocarditis: Utilization of specific echocardiographic findings. Duke Endocarditis Service. *Am J Med*. 1994;96:200-209.
   Beautifully illustrated review of continuous flow LVADs and what to look for in the echocardiographic examination.

9. Cheitlin MD, Armstrong WF, Aurigemma GP, et al. ACC/AHA/ASE 2003 guideline update for the clinical application of echocardiography: summary article: A report of the American College of Cardiology/American Heart Association Task Force on Practice Guidelines (ACC/AHA/ASE Committee to Update the 1997 Guidelines for the Clinical Application of Echocardiography). *Circulation*. 2003;108:1146-1162.

10. Bayer AS, Bolger AF, Taubert KA, et al. Diagnosis and management of infective endocarditis and its complications. *Circulation*. 1998;98:2936-2948.

11. Shapiro LM. Cardiac tumours: Diagnosis and management. *Heart*. 2001;85:218-222.

12. Balzer J, Kuhl H, Rassaf T, et al. Real-time transesophageal three-dimensional echocardiography for guidance of percutaneous cardiac interventions: first experience. *Clin Res Cardiol*. 2008;97:565-574.

13. Biner S, Rafique AM, Kar S, Siegel RJ. Live three-dimensional transesophageal echocardiography-guided transcatheter closure of a mitral paraprosthetic leak by Amplatzer occluder. *J Am Soc Echocardiogr*. 2008;21:1282e7-1282e9.

14. Dennis C, Spreng DS Jr, Nelson GE, et al. Development of a pump-oxygenator to replace the heart and lungs: An apparatus applicable to human patients, and application to one case. *Ann Surg*. 1951;134:709-721.

15. Applebaum RM, Cutler WM, Bhardwaj N, et al. Utility of transesophageal echocardiography during port-access minimally invasive cardiac surgery. *Am J Cardiol*. 1998;82:183-188.

16. Kirkeby-Garstad I, Tromsdal A, Sellevold OF, et al. Guiding surgical cannulation of the inferior vena cava with transesophageal echocardiography. *Anesth Analg*. 2003;96:1288-1293, table of contents.

17. Lebon JS, Couture P, Rochon AG, et al. The endovascular coronary sinus catheter in minimally invasive mitral and tricuspid valve surgery: A case series. *J Cardiothorac Vasc Anesth*. 2010;24:746-751.

18. Varadarajan B, Karski J, Vegas A, Heinrich L. A rare complication of intra-aortic balloon pump placement. *J Cardiothorac Vasc Anesth*. 2005;19:259-260.

19. Deng MC, Edwards LB, Hertz MI, et al. Mechanical circulatory support device database of the International Society for Heart and Lung Transplantation: Third annual report—2005. *J Heart Lung Transplant*. 2005;24:1182-1187.

20. Rose EA, Gelijns AC, Moskowitz AJ, et al. Long-term use of a left ventricular assist device for end-stage heart failure. *N Engl J Med*. 2001;345:1435-1443.

21. Vegas A. Assisting the failing heart. *Anesthesiol Clin*. 2008;26:539-564.

Intraoperative Echocardiography for Heart and Lung Transplantation

11

Mark Edwards and James Drew

BACKGROUND

- Heart, lung, and heart-lung transplantation have become well-established therapies for suitable patients with end-stage cardiac and pulmonary disease. There are currently over 200 centers performing heart transplants and over 120 centers performing lung transplants worldwide who report their results to the International Society for Heart and Lung Transplantation.
- This chapter provides an overview of intraoperative echocardiography for donor heart retrieval procedures, heart transplants, and lung transplants. Fewer than 100 heart-lung transplants are currently performed worldwide each year. The principles of echocardiography described in this chapter can be applied to heart-lung transplantation, but the technique is not specifically discussed further.
- In most transplant centers, echocardiography is used routinely throughout the perioperative period for patients undergoing heart or lung transplantation.
- Transesophageal echocardiography (TEE) is used intraoperatively for both diagnosis and monitoring.
- In particular, echocardiographic assessment of the right ventricle (RV) is of fundamental importance during both heart and lung transplant procedures because both procedures impose risks of acute right ventricular (RV) failure.
  - TEE is used both to detect changes in RV function and to monitor therapy instituted to reverse RV dysfunction.
  - In the intraoperative setting, most RV assessment is qualitative. Owing to the complex geometry of the RV, and with rapid changes in RV volumes and function occurring during transplant procedures, quantitative assessment of RV function is difficult.
- Refer to Chapter 6 for detailed assessment of echocardiographic imaging of the RV.

HEART TRANSPLANT: DONOR ECHOCARDIOGRAPHY

Background

- The optimal way to assess the suitability of a donor heart for transplantation remains controversial, but echocardiography is commonly used.

Overview of Echocardiographic Approach

- A baseline transesophageal echocardiography (TTE) study is usually undertaken as part of donor assessment.
- TEE may be used to supplement TTE imaging. Retrieval teams from some transplant programs utilize TEE during the retrieval procedure.

Anatomic Imaging and Physiologic Data: Acquisition, Analysis, and Pitfalls

- Baseline echocardiogram as part of donor assessment
  - Typically, a TTE study is undertaken with emphasis on the assessment of global and segmental left ventricular (LV) function, LV wall thickness, RV function, and valvular function.
  - Because the donor is intubated and ventilated, TTE image quality may be suboptimal and some views may be unobtainable.

- LV size and function: Current consensus guidelines suggest that a heart is not suitable for transplantation if there are echocardiographic findings of discrete wall motion abnormalities, a left ventricular ejection fraction (LVEF) less than 40% despite optimization of hemodynamics with inotropes, or severe LV hypertrophy.
- Valvular function. Ideally, no significant valve lesions should be present. Bench repair before implantation of diseased mitral valves and repair or replacement of donor aortic valves have been reported. A normally functioning bicuspid aortic valve is not a contraindication to transplantation. As discussed later, some centers routinely perform bench tricuspid valve (TV) annuloplasty during heart transplant procedures.
- TEE use during the organ retrieval procedure
  - Use of TEE can aid decision making if there is doubt about the suitability of the heart for retrieval (e.g., in the setting of borderline LV function or an increase in vasopressor/inotrope therapy during the interval between acceptance as a suitable heart for retrieval and before commencement of the retrieval operation).
  - Compared with TTE, TEE may provide better images and more clearly define anatomy (e.g., if there is doubt about the severity or mechanism of a valvular lesion).
  - Monitoring with TEE is useful to assist with optimizing hemodynamic management during the retrieval procedure by assisting with fluid management (e.g., assessing changes in LV end-diastolic area in response to fluid administration) and assessing the response of LV and RV function to changes in inotrope doses.
  - If TEE is used, it is also important to assess the donor heart for the presence of a patent foramen ovale (PFO) (see later) and common congenital problems such as atrial septal defect (ASD) or persistent left superior vena cava (SVC).
  - At the author's institution, a cardiac anesthesiologist is part of the retrieval team. When there is any doubt about the suitability of the donor heart for transplantation, a portable echocardiography machine and TEE probe are taken on the retrieval and a TEE study is performed before commencing the retrieval procedure. TEE findings are taken into consideration when the final assessment of suitability of the heart for retrieval is made.
- Results of echocardiograms undertaken on the donor heart should be communicated to the implanting team, with particular emphasis on global and segmental LV function, RV function, significant valvular lesions, and the presence of a PFO.

KEY POINTS: INTRAOPERATIVE TRANSESOPHAGEAL ECHOCARDIOGRAPHY ASSESSMENT OF THE DONOR HEART

- LV: global and segmental function, wall thickness, intravascular volume state.
- RV: global function.
- Valvular function: assess all valves. If abnormalities are present, the mechanism should be ascertained and severity should be assessed.
- Atrial septum: PFO assessment.
- Other: note significant congenital problems (e.g., ASD, persistent left SVC).
- Notify retrieval team and also implanting team of findings.

HEART TRANSPLANT: RECIPIENT ECHOCARDIOGRAPHY

Background

- During the surgical procedure, recipient cardiectomy is followed by implantation of the allograft.
  - Typically, bicaval venous cannulation and distal ascending aortic cannulation, just proximal to the origin of the innominate artery, are established, following which cardiopulmonary bypass (CPB) is initiated.
  - The most common surgical technique used for implantation is the bicaval anastomotic technique. The right atrium (RA) is completely excised. A cuff of left atrium (LA) and lengths of SVC and inferior vena cava (IVC) from the native heart and great vessels are left in situ. The native aorta and pulmonary artery (PA) are divided, and cardiectomy is then completed.
  - The allograft LA is anastomosed to the remaining recipient left atrial (LA) cuff. End-to-end anastomoses of the IVC and SVC are performed followed by an end-to-end PA anastomosis. Finally, the aortic anastomosis is performed.
  - The biatrial implant technique, which historically was most commonly used, is currently used less frequently than the bicaval technique.

Overview of the Echocardiographic Approach

- In the absence of contraindications, TEE is used routinely.
- Epiaortic ultrasound may be used to assess the ascending aorta before aortic cannulation.

Anatomic Imaging and Physiologic Data: Acquisition, Analysis, and Pitfalls

Before Cardiopulmonary Bypass

- A limited amount of useful information is obtained with the pre-CPB TEE.

  Step 1: Image the left atrial appendage (LAA) and the LV apex and examine for thrombus
  - The LAA is best visualized in the midesophageal (ME) two-chamber view.
  - Findings that increase the likelihood of thrombus include the presence of an enlarged LA, atrial fibrillation, the presence of spontaneous echo contrast in the LA and LAA, and low pulsed wave (PW) Doppler velocities in the LAA (e.g., <20 cm/s sampled 1 cm from the orifice of the LAA).
  - The presence of significant mitral regurgitation (MR) tends to lessen the likelihood of thrombus in the LAA. Pectinate muscles may be confused with LAA thrombus.
  - Because the heart is often dilated in patients undergoing heart transplantation, imaging of the LV apex may be suboptimal. The probe frequency should be reduced to optimize ultrasound beam penetration.
  - In patients with a left ventricular assist device (LVAD) in situ, the area around the inflow cannula in the LV apex should be assessed for thrombus, and inflow cannula velocities should be measured. Elevated velocities on spectral Doppler imaging may indicate partial inflow obstruction by thrombus. Epicardial echocardiography may be used to image the inflow cannula if TEE views are suboptimal.
  - The finding of a thrombus should prompt the surgeon to minimize manipulation of the heart to avoid dislodging the thrombus. In addition, the surgeon may elect to cross-clamp the aorta early after establishing CPB in order to reduce the chance of embolus.

  Step 2: Image the aorta for the presence of atheroma, especially in older patients
  - TEE and surgical digital palpation are of limited value for assessing the ascending aorta. Epiaortic ultrasound can be used to locate aortic cannulation and cross-clamp sites that are free of atheroma.
  - The presence of severe atheroma in the descending aorta is a relative contraindication to the placement of an intra-aortic balloon pump (IABP), should this be necessary after allograft implantation.

  Step 3: Image the pleural spaces
  - Both pleural spaces should be assessed for the presence of significant fluid collections, which if present, should be drained by the surgeon.

Weaning from Cardiopulmonary Bypass and after Cardiopulmonary Bypass

- If the information is available, the findings of the donor echocardiogram should be noted.
- Once the heart is filled and ejection is established, an assessment of the adequacy of deairing, LV and RV systolic function, and valvular function should be made before separation from CPB.
- After separation from CPB, a complete TEE examination should be performed with focus on the assessment of systolic LV and RV function, valvular function, and an assessment of the atrial septum and the surgical anastomoses.
  - Assessment of the surgical anastomoses is of less importance than during lung transplantation.
- Primary graft dysfunction may be a result of LV, RV, or biventricular dysfunction. RV dysfunction is the most common cause.
- In the presence of significant primary graft dysfunction, TEE is helpful to assess changes in ventricular function in response to medical therapy (e.g., inotropes or pulmonary vasodilators), and to assist with positioning of mechanical support devices (e.g., IABP, right ventricular assist device [RVAD] or LVAD, or venoarterial extracorporeal membrane oxygenation [ECMO]), should they prove necessary.
- It may be necessary to use nonstandard transducer rotation to obtain standard two-dimensional (2D) echocardiography views.
  - The donor heart is usually smaller than the explanted heart and it often sits in a more medial, clockwise-rotated position in the chest.

Step 1: Assess for Deairing

- Before weaning from CPB, there is often a significant amount of air present on the left side of the heart.
  - Typical sites of accumulation include the pulmonary veins, atrial septum, the LAA,

the midapical ventricular septum, and the LV apex.

- Although TEE is very sensitive for detecting air, it is difficult to adequately detect air until the heart is full and LV ejection is established.
- Adequate deairing lessens the chance of RV dysfunction from air embolism into the anteriorly positioned right coronary artery.

Step 2: Assess Left Ventricular Function

- An assessment of global and segmental LV function should be made utilizing the ME and transgastric (TG) LV views. Diastolic function should be assessed using PW Doppler of mitral inflow velocities, pulmonary vein velocities, and mitral annular tissue Doppler imaging. In addition, LV wall thickness should be assessed.
- LV systolic function and assessment of LV preload.
  - Although LV systolic function is often assessed subjectively, it is helpful to measure fractional area change or formal LVEF to allow comparisons over time (see Chapter 6).
  - LV systolic function may be impaired in the immediate post-CPB period owing to the effects of brain death on the allograft as well as the effects of imperfect myocardial preservation. This should improve over the hours after implant.
  - Serial visual assessments and measurements such as LV end-diastolic area, measured in the TG mid short axis (SAX) view, can be used to assess LV preload to help guide fluid administration and titrate vasoactive medications.
  - LV wall thickness may be increased, most likely due to myocardial edema. This should resolve over time.
- LV diastolic function.
  - Diastolic dysfunction is common post-transplant and can range from impaired relaxation to restrictive filling. These changes may persist for days to weeks.
- Segmental wall motion abnormalities.
  - As is common in post-CPB assessments, particularly in the presence of ventricular pacing, a "flat" ventricular septum or paradoxical ventricular septal motion is often seen. If abnormal septal motion is present, careful assessment of RV function should be undertaken to exclude RV dysfunction as the cause of the abnormal septal motion.
  - Persistent, discrete segmental wall motion abnormalities, especially in the distribution of a specific coronary artery, are abnormal.

Step 3: Assess Right Ventricular Function

- A thorough initial assessment of RV systolic function should be made and then ongoing serial assessments should be made as necessary in response to changes in the clinical state of the patient.
  - Typically, qualitative assessment is made via visual assessments of ME RV views. Quantitative imaging may be useful if time allows.
  - Impaired RV function is common at separation from CPB and during the first hours after allograft implant. Potential etiologies are listed in Box 11-1.
- Echocardiographic manifestations of acute RV impairment are outlined in Box 11-2. In the setting of acute RV impairment, TEE should be used to assess changes in RV function in response to therapeutic maneuvers.
- In the presence of significant tricuspid regurgitation (TR), RV function may appear less impaired than it actually is (i.e., significant TR "flatters" the RV).

BOX 11-1 Potential Etiologies of Right Ventricular Impairment during Separation from Cardiopulmonary Bypass and the Early Post-Cardiopulmonary Bypass Period in Heart Transplant Patients

- The effects of brain death on the donor RV.
- Suboptimal myocardial protection during retrieval, transport, and implantation.
- The imposition of elevated recipient PA pressures and PVR on an allograft previously exposed to normal PA pressures and PVR.
- Donor-recipient size mismatch (smaller donor heart to larger recipient).
- Air embolus to the anteriorly positioned right coronary artery.
- Mechanical obstruction to RV outflow at the level of PA anastomosis.

PA, pulmonary artery; PVR, pulmonary vascular resistance; RV, right ventricle; RV, right ventricular.

BOX 11-2 Echocardiographic Features of Acute Right Ventricular Impairment

- RV dilatation.
- Impaired RV systolic function.
- Leftward shift and flattening of the ventricular septum, with a D-shaped LV cavity and paradoxical septal motion.
- The left ventricle may appear small and underfilled.
- Onset of, or worsening of preexisting, TR.

LV, left ventricular; RV, right ventricular; TR, tricuspid regurgitation.

- RV compression resulting in significant worsening of RV function can result from chest closure, particularly in the setting of myocardial edema or lung dysfunction requiring high levels of positive end-expiratory pressure. It is the author's practice to leave the TEE probe in situ after the chest is closed to reassess RV function.

Step 4: Assess Valvular Function

- Standard 2D and color flow Doppler imaging of the valves should be undertaken. In the presence of abnormalities, the mechanism should be ascertained.
- The most common lesions in the perioperative period are TR and mitral regurgitation (MR).
- TR
  - TR is the most common valve lesion seen in the post-CPB period.
    - Mild TR occurs commonly. Moderate or severe TR is less common (Figure 11-1).

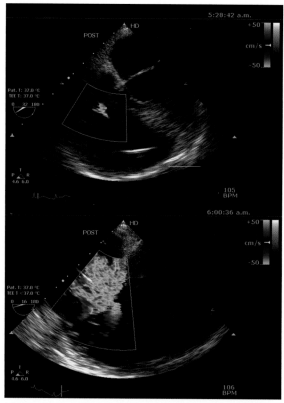

Figure 11-1. TR occurring after separation from CPB in a heart transplant patient. These ME four-chamber still-frame images, with the transducer turned to the right to focus on the TV demonstrate worsening TR after sternal closure. **Top,** After separation from CPB (taken at 0528 hr), there is trivial TR. **Bottom,** After sternal closure (taken at 0600 hr), there is severe TR. In addition to worsening TR, there was also deterioration in RV function.

- The leaflets are usually morphologically normal with annular dilatation as the mechanism (i.e., functional TR).
- Potential causes include
  - Use of biatrial rather than bicaval implantation technique.
  - Allograft RV dysfunction.
  - Size mismatch between donor and recipient hearts.
  - Myocardial edema.
  - Volume overload.
- Worsening TR typically indicates deteriorating RV function.
- Some centers use prophylactic TV repair, which is performed on the donor heart before implantation. TV repair has been shown to reduce intraoperative TR, late TR, and in one series, long-term cardiac-related mortality.
- MR
  - Trivial or mild MR is often seen and may be related to being present in the donor heart, to changes in LA geometry at implantation, or to transient segmental wall motion abnormalities affecting the inferior LV wall.
  - In the presence of significant MR, ascertaining the mechanism is important because surgical intervention may be appropriate.
  - LV function may appear less impaired than it actually is (i.e., significant MR "flatters" the LV) in the presence of significant MR.
  - Worsening functional MR typically indicates deteriorating LV function.
- Other valves
  - It is rare to find significant lesions of the aortic valve or pulmonic valve.

Step 5: Assess the Atria

- The LA often appears enlarged, with an "hourglass" shape and an echo-dense, suture line ridge across the mid part of the atrium (Figure 11-2). If the ridge is mobile or pedunculated, LA thrombus should be considered.
- There may be an echo-free space behind the neo-LA, which is native LA tissue.
- Excessive donor atrial tissue, if present, can prolapse and cause an acquired cor triatriatum which can, rarely, lead to obstruction to mitral valve inflow.
- No RA anastomosis occurs with the bicaval technique. The RA anastomosis is seldom seen with the biatrial implant technique.

Step 6: Assess the Caval Anastomoses

- The caval anastomoses can be assessed using 2D and color flow Doppler imaging by moving the probe from the ME bicaval view.

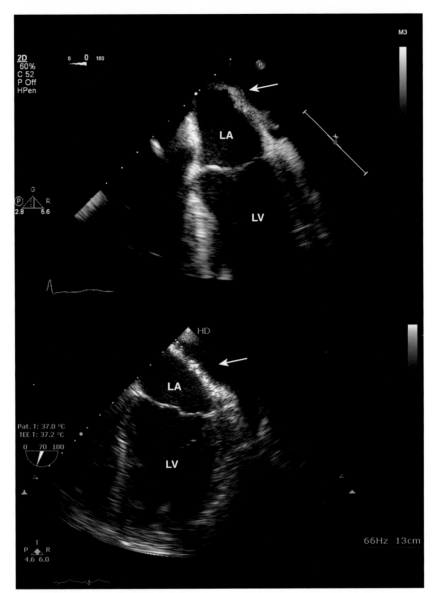

Figure 11-2. LA suture line after heart transplantation. In these post-CPB images of two different patients, an echogenic line, caused by the LA suture line, is demonstrated in the LA *(arrows)*. **Top,** An ME four-chamber view. **Bottom,** An ME two-chamber view.

- The probe should be withdrawn and rotated to keep the image aligned with the SVC.
- The probe should be advanced and rotated to keep the image aligned with the IVC.
- The presence of narrowing at the anastomosis on 2D imaging or turbulent flow on color flow Doppler imaging may alert the operator to stenosis at the anastomosis.

Step 7: Assess the Pulmonary Veins
- During the recipient cardiectomy, the pulmonary veins are retained as part of the native LA cuff.

- All four veins can be inspected with 2D, color flow, and PW Doppler imaging.
- If abnormal flow patterns are present, they are most likely to be caused by problems with the LA anastomosis causing distortion of the pulmonary veins.

Step 8: Assess the Pulmonary Artery and Aorta
- The PA anastomosis is best assessed using 2D, color flow, and spectral Doppler imaging in the ME ascending aortic SAX view or the upper esophageal aortic arch SAX view. Epicardial echocardiography can be used if these views are suboptimal.

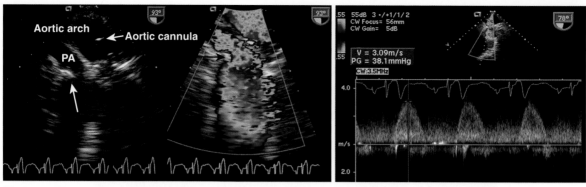

Figure 11-3. In this patient who had just received a heart transplant, a large discrepancy was found between his RV and PA systolic pressures. **Left,** TEE revealed redundant tissue *(arrow)* in the main PA, with color Doppler showing marked turbulence. **Right,** CW Doppler showed a gradient across the obstruction of 38 mm Hg. The anastomosis was revised with a normalization of right-sided pressures.

- Redundancy in the PA at the anastomosis can lead to kinking of the vessel, causing obstruction to RV outflow and RV failure. With TEE, distortion can be visualized on 2D imaging. In addition, there is turbulence on color flow Doppler imaging and elevated velocities with spectral Doppler imaging (Figure 11-3).
- Aortic anastomosis—Rarely visualized with TEE.

Step 9: Check for Patent Foramen Ovale

- The atrial septum should be assessed for the presence of a PFO, even if no PFO was found during the donor retrieval procedure.
- Elevated right-sided pressures after implantation, which is common, can result in right-to-left shunting across a previously undetected PFO and contribute to hypoxia.
- In addition, should ventricular function deteriorate and LVAD implantation be required, it is important to know if a PFO is present.

KEY POINTS: POST-CARDIOPULMONARY BYPASS TRANSESOPHAGEAL ECHOCARDIOGRAPHY ASSESSMENT DURING HEART TRANSPLANT

- A complete TEE study should be performed, and then serial assessments of LV and RV function.
- If primary graft dysfunction occurs, the most common manifestation is acute RV failure. LV failure and biventricular failure both occur but are less common.
- Segmental wall motion abnormalities in the distribution of a coronary artery are abnormal.
- The most common valvular abnormality is functional TR, which can range from mild

---

KEY POINTS: POST-CARDIOPULMONARY BYPASS TRANSESOPHAGEAL ECHOCARDIOGRAPHY ASSESSMENT DURING HEART TRANSPLANT—cont'd

(common) to severe (uncommon). Prophylactic TV annuloplasty is performed at some transplant centers.
- Worsening TR is often a marker of deteriorating RV function. Furthermore, TR tends to mask the severity of RV dysfunction by making RV function appear better than it actually is.
- Anastomoses should be assessed, but significant anastomotic problems are uncommon.
- RV function should be reassessed once the chest is closed. RV function can deteriorate with the compression from sternal closure.

Step 10: What to Assess Just Prior to Chest Closure

- The pericardium and pleural spaces should be assessed to exclude the presence of significant collections of blood.
  - The allograft is typically smaller than the explanted heart, so there is usually space around the heart to allow fluid to collect.

LUNG TRANSPLANT: RECIPIENT ECHOCARDIOGRAPHY

Background

- Lung transplant procedures may be single or bilateral.
  - Single lung transplants (SLTs) are undertaken via a lateral thoracotomy with a pneumonectomy then implantation of the

lung allograft with anastomoses at the proximal main bronchus, pulmonary veins, and proximal PA.

- Bilateral lung transplants (BLTs) are usually completed as sequential SLTs via a thoracosternotomy (clamshell) incision.
- Historically, SLTs were a more common procedure than BLTs, but over recent years, there has been a steady increase in the frequency of BLTs, and they now account for more than 70% of lung transplants.
- Use of CPB varies depending on the transplant center. Some use CPB routinely, others rarely.
  - In most centers, elective CPB is used in cases in which there is significant pulmonary hypertension (e.g., recipients with primary pulmonary hypertension) or when a patient with impaired RV function is thought unlikely to tolerate the increased RV afterload induced by PA clamping.
  - If CPB is not used routinely, it must be immediately available in case significant cardiac or pulmonary decompensation occurs during the procedure.
- Patients undergoing lung transplantation usually have minimal cardiopulmonary reserve.
  - Depending on their underlying disease, they usually have at least some degree of pulmonary hypertension and RV impairment.
  - In addition, the transplant procedure itself imposes a significant physiologic strain on the recipient due to need for one-lung ventilation, significant surgical manipulation of the heart and great vessels, and variable degrees of reperfusion injury to the transplanted lungs.
  - Older patients (typically those with chronic obstructive pulmonary disease) may have cardiac comorbidities such as coronary artery disease as well as cardiac effects of other disorders such as hypertension.

Overview of Echocardiographic Approach

- In the absence of contraindications, TEE is commonly used during BLT procedures, and sometimes in SLT procedures to monitor cardiac function and to evaluate surgical anastomoses. At the author's institution, TEE is used routinely for all lung transplant procedures.

- If CPB is used, epiaortic ultrasound may be used to assess the ascending aorta for atheroma before aortic cannulation.
- Epicardial echocardiography may be used to assist with the assessment of anastomoses (pulmonary veins and PAs) if TEE imaging is suboptimal or to confirm significant abnormal findings on TEE that may require surgical revision.

Anatomic Imaging and Physiologic Data

Acquisition, Analysis, and Pitfalls: Initial Assessment after Anesthetic Induction

- Time and clinical condition of the patient permitting, a complete baseline TEE study with 2D, color, and spectral Doppler imaging is performed.
  - In the event of cardiovascular instability after anesthetic induction, TEE can be used to diagnose or rule out cardiovascular causes such as acute RV failure.
- It is particularly important to image and assess the following:
  - LV
    - Global and segmental function, and wall thickness.
    - Most patients have normal LV systolic function. Those with significant LV dysfunction may tolerate the operative procedure poorly, especially without CPB.
  - RV
    - RV global function, size, and wall thickness.
    - The heart should be assessed for signs of pressure and/or volume overload by evaluating the ventricular septum (Figure 11-4).
    - Depending on the underlying disease process, variable degrees of RV hypertrophy (end-diastolic wall thickness >5 mm) and RV systolic impairment, are typically present.
  - Valvular function
    - A baseline assessment of valvular function, particularly of the tricuspid valve, should be performed.
    - An assessment of the mechanism and severity of TR is important. A degree of TR is often present. TR is usually functional, due to annular dilatation as a result of elevated pulmonary vascular resistance and RV dysfunction. Refer to

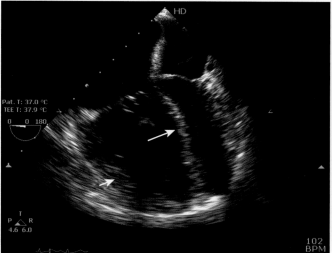
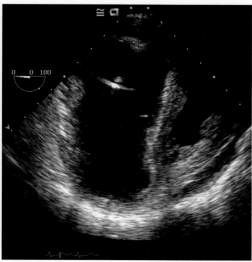

Figure 11-4. RV pressure overload demonstrated by abnormal position of the ventricular septum in a patient undergoing lung transplant for primary pulmonary hypertension. **Left,** In this ME four-chamber image, captured near end-systole, the ventricular septum is curved toward the LV and away from the RV *(large arrow)*. In addition, the RV is dilated and the free wall is hypertrophied *(small arrow)*. The LV cavity appears compressed. The atrial septum is bowed toward the LA, signifying high right atrial (RA) pressure. **Right,** A TG image illustrating a "D" shaped septum, typical of RV pressure overload.

Chapter 4 for a detailed discussion of the assessment of TR.

- In the presence of significant TR, RV systolic function appears better than it actually is.
- An attempt to measure PA systolic pressure using CW Doppler of the TR jet should be undertaken. Using TEE, it is often difficult to capture a complete Doppler envelope, which can lead to underestimation of PA pressure.
- Atrial septum
  - Best assessed in the ME four-chamber view and the bicaval view.
  - The position of the atrial septum should be assessed.
  - Normally, the septum bows toward the RA, expect for a brief reversal during midsystole when it transiently bows toward the LA.
  - In those patients with elevated RA pressure or significant TR, the septum typically bows toward the LA throughout the cardiac cycle.
  - The presence of a PFO should be sought with color flow Doppler imaging and (sometimes) a contrast study using agitated saline.
  - Color flow Doppler images should be assessed with the Nyquist limit at 50 to 60 cm/s, and also at 20 to 30 cm/s if no flow across the septum is seen at 50 to 60 cm/s. It is the practice of the authors

to complete a contrast study using agitated saline if no PFO is present with color flow Doppler imaging.

- The presence of a significant right-to-left shunt at baseline requires consideration of repair of the PFO, which entails the use of CPB.
- As with heart transplant patients, with higher right-sided pressures after implant, worsening of a right-to-left shunt with resultant significant hypoxemia may occur.
- Pulmonary veins
  - Imaging of all four pulmonary veins with 2D and color flow Doppler imaging should be undertaken. Baseline velocities should be measured using PW Doppler with the cursor sample volume set at 2 mm and positioned 1 cm into each vein.

Acquisition, Analysis and Pitfalls: Native Lung Explant and Allograft Implant (No Cardiopulmonary Bypass)

- TEE is used as a monitor to assess changes in RV function, TR, LV filling, and deairing.
- To assess RV function, the ME four-chamber view, with the probe turned to the right to optimize images of the RV, is generally the most useful view.
- One-lung ventilation and especially clamping of the PA tends to increase RV afterload,

which may lead to acute RV failure (see Box 11-2).

- In addition, ventricular septal shift toward the LV may impair LV diastolic filling resulting in low cardiac output. On TEE, the LV usually appears underfilled, with unchanged systolic function.
- Along with the clinical state of the patient and hemodynamic data, TEE findings of deteriorating RV function and worsening TR may contribute to a decision to institute CPB emergently.
- TEE should be used to assess deairing when PA anastomoses are unclamped.
  - Transient hypotension is very common with unclamping and is usually caused by vasodilatation from release of ischemic metabolites from the graft.
  - Air is sometimes present in the LV at this stage and has been reported to cause hemodynamic instability due to embolus to the anteriorly positioned right coronary artery.
- After allograft implantation, the pulmonary venous and PA anastomoses should be examined.
  - Figure 11-5 shows the relationship between the LA cuff and the pulmonary veins, both from the donor organ.
  - It is important to undertake a detailed assessment of the pulmonary veins because stenotic pulmonary vein anastomoses can result in venous hypertension in the lung

draining toward the stenosed vein causing pulmonary edema, primary graft dysfunction, and potentially, pulmonary infarction.

- The pulmonary veins should be examined with 2D and color Doppler imaging, and velocities should be recorded using PW and, if necessary, continuous wave (CW) Doppler (Figure 11-6).
- Using 2D imaging, the diameter of the anastomoses should be assessed.
- It is not possible to state 2D diameters that are acceptable, but a value greater than 5 mm appears to be acceptable, and measurements of less than 2.5 mm have a high frequency of clinical sequelae.
- Comparing the anastomotic site with the native upstream vessel can provide a useful comparison.
- Color flow Doppler typically demonstrates aliased flow due to turbulence if stenosis is present.
- Normal PW Doppler velocities are less than 75 cm/s.
- It is not uncommon in lung transplant patients to have flows of up to 120 cm/s or even higher without any clinical sequelae. However with narrowed veins, turbulent flow, and high velocities in the setting of clinical problems, surgical revision may be necessary.
- If flow velocities are high, CW Doppler may need to be used for accurate measurement.
- In BLT, velocities should be measured after the second lung has been implanted because they may be artefactually high after first lung implant because the entire cardiac output is going through one side.
- Velocities need to be considered in the context of cardiac output. High cardiac output will result in higher velocities.
- Pulmonary vein thrombosis has also been reported to occur. Thrombi ranged from nonocclusive, mobile thrombi to occlusive thrombi. Although typically seen on 2D imaging, they may be associated with elevated flow velocities.
- Epicardial echocardiography can be used to assess pulmonary vein anastomoses when TEE imaging has been suboptimal.
- The right PA anastomosis can usually be visualized with TEE, but the left is often not seen.
  - The ME ascending aortic SAX view (with gentle anteflexion of the transducer)

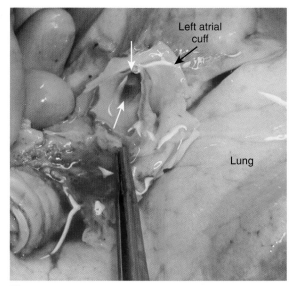

Figure 11-5. The donor lung. The *white arrows* show the orifices of the pulmonary veins surrounded by the LA cuff.

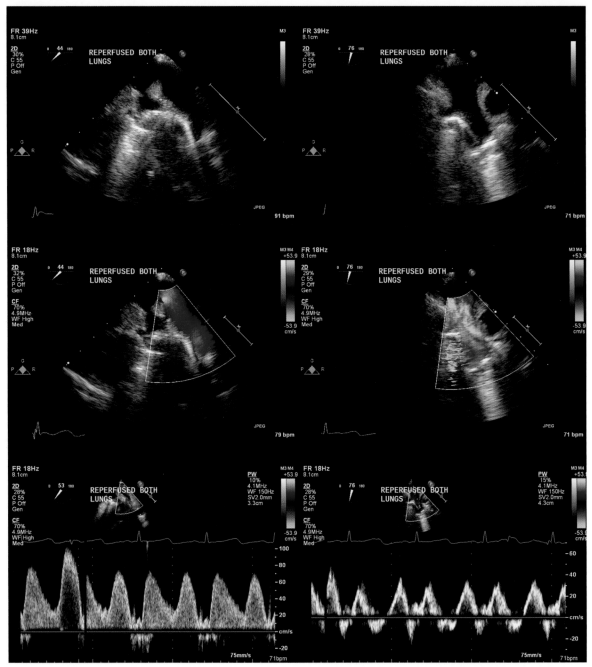

Figure 11-6. Assessment of the pulmonary veins in a lung transplant patient. These images demonstrate typical, acceptable left and right pulmonary vein anastomoses. Each side is assessed with 2D imaging **(top)**, color flow Doppler **(middle)**, and PW Doppler **(bottom)**.

usually provides the best view of the right PA (Figure 11-7).

- Using color flow Doppler, it is common to see turbulent flow at this anastomosis. Presumably, this is due to size mismatch and technical features of the anastomosis. However, it is rare to need surgical revision.

- If there is concern about the anastomosis, epicardial echocardiography can be used for 2D imaging and to obtain spectral Doppler velocities.

- Before chest closure, LV filling and systolic function, RV function, and TR severity should be reassessed.

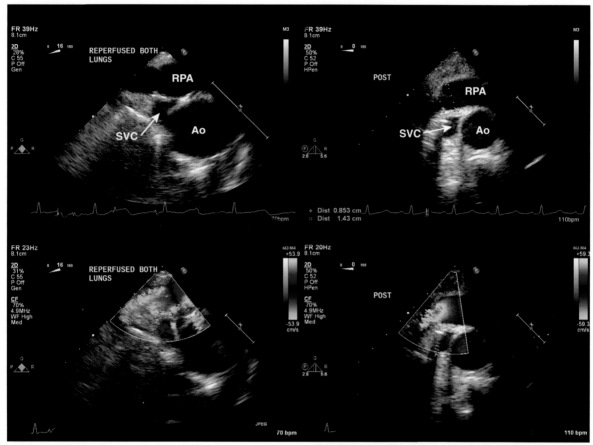

Figure 11-7. Right PA anastomosis in two lung transplant patients. ME ascending aortic SAX views demonstrate the right pulmonary artery (RPA) anastomosis. **Left,** A typical anastomosis. The anastomosis is clearly visible in the right PA on 2D imaging **(top)** as an insignificant narrowing of the vessel. There is minimal turbulent flow with color flow Doppler imaging **(bottom). Right,** A narrow anastomosis. The anastomosis appears significantly narrowed on 2D imaging **(top),** and there is turbulent flow present on color flow Doppler imaging **(bottom).** The narrow anastomosis was thought to be due to size mismatch between a small recipient and a larger donor. Ao, ascending aorta.

- The pleural spaces and pericardial space should be assessed to ensure there are no fluid collections amenable to surgical drainage.
- It is also the authors routine practice to reassess RV function and TR after the chest is closed, particularly in patients with prior RV dysfunction, because there is sometimes a tamponade effect from chest closure (especially if the implanted lungs are a large size relative to the patient's chest cavity), resulting in deterioration of RV function.
- In the presence of increased preoperative pulmonary vascular resistance and RV hypertrophy, post implantation right ventricular outflow tract obstruction may occur. This is a result of the now normalized pulmonary vascular resistance and is accentuated by hypovolemia (Figure 11-8).

KEY POINTS: TRANSESOPHAGEAL ECHOCARDIOGRAPHY ASSESSMENT POST-IMPLANTATION LUNG TRANSPLANT

- LV function. New problems are uncommon.
- RV function. Sequential assessment is important. Reassess after chest closure because RV function can deteriorate.
- Valvular function. Reassess TR, especially if RV function has changed.
- Anastomoses (Figure 11-9)
  - Pulmonary veins: evaluate left- and right-sided veins after reperfusion (after both lungs are reperfused in BLT). Assess dimensions (2D imaging) and flow patterns (color flow and spectral Doppler) to rule out obstruction. Echocardiographic signs of obstruction include narrow vessel diameter on 2D imaging (e.g., <0.5 cm), elevated flow velocities (e.g., >100-140 cm/s), and turbulence on color flow imaging,

Continued

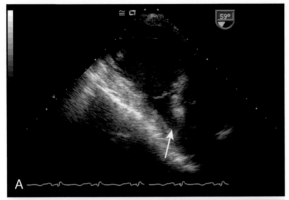

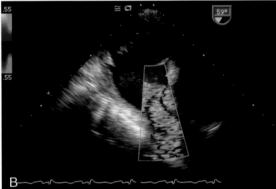

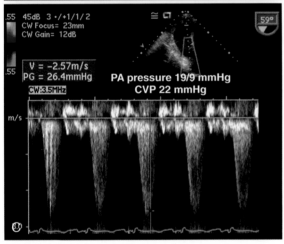

Figure 11-8. In this patient after BLT, hypotension developed. TEE revealed a normal pulmonic valve. A TG right ventricular outflow tract (RVOT) image was obtained, revealing systolic narrowing of the RVOT (*arrow* in **A**) with color Doppler evidence of turbulence (**B**). **C,** CW Doppler showed a gradient across the RVOT of 26 mm Hg. Intravascular volume was administered and the situation resolved. CVP, central venous pressure.

KEY POINTS: TRANSESOPHAGEAL ECHOCARDIOGRAPHY ASSESSMENT POST-IMPLANTATION LUNG TRANSPLANT—cont'd

particularly if associated with pulmonary edema.
- Pulmonary artery: Some narrowing is commonly seen at the right-sided anastomosis, which is usually of no clinical consequence. The left-sided anastomosis is generally not visible with TEE, because of interposition of the left mainstem bronchus between the esophagus and the left PA.
- Pleural and pericardial spaces should be assessed for drainable collections before chest closure.

Acquisition, Analysis, and Pitfalls: Procedure Performed with Cardiopulmonary Bypass

- The pre-bypass assessment should be undertaken as for part A discussed previously (see "Acquisition, Analysis, and Pitfalls: Initial Assessment after Anesthetic Induction"). In addition, epiaortic ultrasound may be used in older patients to assess the ascending aorta for the presence of atheroma and to select a suitable cannulation site.
- TEE assessment in the post-CPB period is outlined in Box 11-3.
- The pleural and pericardial spaces should be assessed post-CPB, because bleeding is usually more significant in patients whose procedure is undertaken utilizing CPB. The pericardium may be left open, in which case, bleeding will tend to accumulate in the pleural cavities.

BOX 11-3 Transesophageal Echocardiography Assessment in Lung Transplant Patients after Cardiopulmonary Bypass

- LV global and segmental function.
- RV systolic function.
- Valvular function—particularly changes in TR.
- Anastomoses—pulmonary veins and pulmonary arteries.
- Pleural and pericardial spaces.

LV, left ventricular; RV, right ventricular; TR, tricuspid regurgitation.

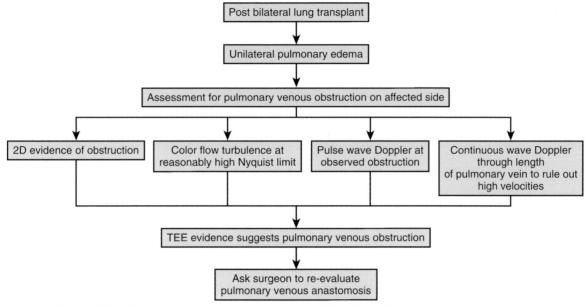

Figure 11-9. Flow chart in the investigation of a post-BLT patient with unilateral pulmonary edema.

Suggested Readings

1. Stehlik J, Edwards LB, Kucheryavaya AY, et al. The Registry of the International Society for Heart and Lung Transplantation: Twenty-seventh official adult heart transplant report—2010. *J Heart Lung Transplant.* 2010;29:1089-1103.

2. Christie JD, Edwards LB, Kucheryavaya AY, et al. The Registry of the International Society for Heart and Lung Transplantation: Twenty-seventh official adult lung and heart-lung transplant report—2010. *J Heart Lung Transplant.* 2010;29:1104-1118.
   These articles summarize a large database of heart and lung transplant procedures and are a useful reference.

3. Venkateswaran RV, Townend JN, Wilson IC, et al. Echocardiography in the potential heart donor. *Transplantation.* 2010;89:894-901.
   Excellent review of what to look for in assessing a donor heart for transplant suitability.

4. Asante-Korang A. Echocardiographic evaluation before and after cardiac transplantation. *Cardiol Young.* 2004;14(Suppl 1):88-92.

5. Romano P, Mangion JM. The role of intraoperative transesophageal echocardiography in heart. *Echocardiography.* 2002;19:599-604.
   Two nice reviews of what to look for in children and adults after cardiac transplantation.

6. Chumnanvej S, Wood MJ, MacGillivray TE, Melo MF. Perioperative echocardiographic examination for ventricular assist device implantation. *Anesth Analg.* 2007;105:583-601.

7. Augoustides JG. Perioperative echocardiographic assessment of left ventricular assist device implantation: Additional causes of inflow cannula obstruction. *Anesth Analg.* 2008;106:673-674.
   Two nice reviews of the specifics in the examination of patients with assist devices.

8. Michel-Cherqui M, Brusset A, Liu N, et al. Intraoperative transesophageal echocardiographic assessment of vascular anastomoses in lung transplantation. A report on 18 cases. *Chest.* 1997;111:1229-1235.

9. Huang YC, Cheng YJ, Lin YH, et al. Graft failure caused by pulmonary venous obstruction diagnosed by intraoperative transesophageal echocardiography during lung transplantation. *Anesth Analg.* 2000;91:558-560.

10. Myles PS, Marasco S. Misleading turbulent flow through pulmonary venous anastomoses during lung transplantation. *Anesth Analg.* 2008;107:1504-1505.

11. McIlroy DR, Sesto AC, Buckland MR. Pulmonary vein thrombosis, lung transplantation, and intraoperative transesophageal echocardiography. *J Cardiothorac Vasc Anesth.* 2006;20:712-715.
   Four articles that summarize the problems with pulmonary venous anastomoses after lung transplantation.

Pericardial Disease

Peter von Homeyer

12

INTRODUCTION

Background

- The human pericardium is a double-layered sac around the heart, covering most of the surface of the heart and extending on to the proximal portion of the great vessels.
- The inner serous layer of the pericardium is attached to the myocardium, forming the visceral pericardium or epicardium.
- It reflects at the level of the great vessels and turns into the parietal pericardium, which is a fibroserous layer.
- Two sinuses are formed in the posterior pericardial cavity: The (upper) transverse sinus lies anterior to the superior vena cava and posterior to the pulmonary artery and ascending aorta. The (lower) oblique sinus lies posterior and inferior to the heart; the sinus is bounded by the reflection lines of both the left and the right pulmonary veins (Figure 12-1).
- Normal pericardial thickness is approximately 1 to 2 mm. Between the two layers, a small fluid collection of up to 30 mL is considered a normal finding. The pericardial fluid resembles an ultrafiltrate of plasma.
- The pericardium protects and restrains the heart as well as reduces friction. It isolates the heart from other structures in the mediastinum.
- A number of cardiac and systemic diseases involve the pericardial tissue, often with significant clinical consequences.
- Pericardial disease can impair cardiac chamber filling, especially on the thin-walled and low pressure right side of the heart, where constraint can decrease compliance.
- Usually, right ventricular (RV) compliance is greater than left ventricular (LV) compliance, and equalization can exaggerate the phenomenon of ventricular interdependence.
- Intrapericardial pressure is generally similar to intrapleural pressure, varying from approximately −6 mm Hg during inspiration to approximately −3 mm Hg at the end of expiration.
- When intrapericardial pressure drops during inspiration, RV filling and tricuspid inflow are enhanced.
- At the same time, the interventricular septum shifts to the left side of the heart, decreasing LV filling and transmitral flow; the opposite relationship is true for spontaneous exhalation.

Overview of Echocardiographic Approach

- Echocardiography is the most sensitive and specific method for evaluation of pericardial effusion (PE).
- Diagnostic echocardiography of the pericardium involves multiple views to fully understand the degree and localization of pericardial disease.
- Two-dimensional (2D) echocardiography is used for anatomic imaging of the pericardium and pericardial space (Figure 12-2).
- Transthoracic echocardiography (TTE) is the primary method in suspected pericardial disease, although in some cases, transesophageal views provide better images. The midesophageal (ME) four-chamber view, the ME RV inflow-outflow view, and the transgastric (TG) midpapillary short axis view are useful for anatomic imaging.
- M-mode echocardiography can be helpful for the diagnosis of PEs and interrogation of septal motion.
- Spectral Doppler echocardiography is used to interrogate cardiac chamber filling, hepatic and pulmonary vein flows, and overall diastolic function.
- Measurement of inferior vena cava (IVC) size and respiratory variation can be used to reconfirm pericardial disease in the setting of elevated RV filling pressures.

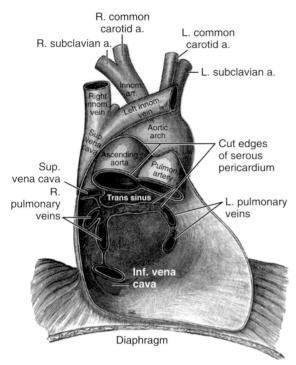

R. common carotid a.

R. subclavian a.

L. common carotid a.

L. subclavian a.

Innom. art.

Right innom. vein

Left innom. vein

Aortic arch

Cut edges of serous pericardium

Sup. vena cava

Ascending aorta

Pulmon. artery

Sup. vena cava

R. pulmonary veins

Trans sinus

L. pulmonary veins

Inf. vena cava

Diaphragm

Figure 12-1. Normal pericardial anatomy. *From Gray H. Anatomy of the Human Body. Philadelphia: Lea & Febiger, 1918; Bartleby.com, 2000.*

KEY POINTS

- Pericardium is a double-layered sac surrounding the human heart.
- Normal thickness is 1 to 2 mm; a fluid collection of up to 30 mL is normal.
- Several cardiac and systemic diseases can involve the pericardium, the most common being pericarditis, PE with or without cardiac tamponade, and constrictive pericarditis.
- The most important clinical endpoint of pericardial disease is impaired cardiac chamber filling.
- On 2D echocardiography, the pericardium is shown as a bright linear echo image surrounding the heart.
- One should acquire images using different views to visualize the whole pericardial sac.
- In addition, M-mode and spectral Doppler echocardiography measurements can be useful to confirm and clarify the diagnosis of specific pericardial diseases.

PERICARDIAL EFFUSION

Background

- A PE is an abnormal fluid collection in the pericardial space.
- A wide variety of diseases can cause PEs, but most commonly, this is seen after cardiac

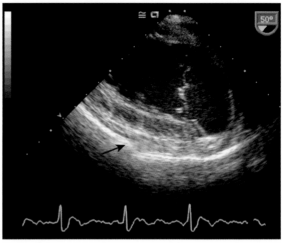

Figure 12-2. Normal echocardiographic appearance of the pericardium *(arrow).*

surgery, in congestive heart failure, acute type A aortic dissections, and end-stage renal disease (Table 12-1).

- PEs become a clinical syndrome as soon as the fluid accumulation causes an increase in intrapericardial pressure and the patient develops symptoms.
- The rate of how fast fluid accumulates in the pericardial space is important. An effusion that is caused by a slow increase in pericardial fluid can become quite large before clinical symptoms occur. Conversely, relatively small fluid collections can cause cardiac tamponade when developing rapidly.
- When the patient is in a supine position, PEs are initially located posterior to the heart. As more pericardial fluid accumulates, the effusion is surrounding the heart and can cause cardiac tamponade (see "Cardiac Tamponade"). Loculated effusions are also possible, especially after cardiac surgery.

Overview of Echocardiographic Approach

- The sensitivity and specificity of echocardiography for the diagnosis of PE are very high.
- On 2D images, a PE will appear as an echo-free space between both pericardial layers (Figure 12-3). This is the most useful imaging modality for the diagnosis of effusions.
- Transesophageal echocardiography (TEE) is especially useful for detection of posterior effusions and in the postoperative setting where retrosternal hematoma can impair transthoracic image quality.

TABLE 12-1 OVERVIEW OF PERICARDIAL DISEASE ETIOLOGIES AND ASSOCIATED SYNDROMES

Etiology	Clinical Endpoints
Idiopathic	
Infectious	
Bacterial	Acute pericarditis
Tuberculous	Acute pericarditis, constrictive pericarditis
Viral	Acute pericarditis
Parasitic	Acute pericarditis
Connective tissue disease	
Systemic lupus erythematosus	Pericarditis, pericardial effusion
Scleroderma	Pericarditis
Rheumatoid arthritis	Pericarditis, pericardial effusion
Wegener's granulomatosis	Pericarditis, pericardial effusion
Post-myocardial infarction	
Dressler's syndrome	Acute pericarditis, pericardial effusion
Ventricular rupture	Pericardial effusion, cardiac tamponade
Metabolic	
Uremia	Pericardial effusion
Myxedema	Pericardial effusion
Trauma	Pericardial effusion, cardiac tamponade
Postradiation	Acute pericarditis, constrictive pericarditis
Postoperatively after cardiac surgery	Pericardial effusion, cardiac tamponade, constrictive pericarditis
Neoplastic	
Primary pericardial and cardiac tumors	Pericardial effusion, cardiac tamponade
Metastatic disease	Pericardial effusion, cardiac tamponade
Congestive heart failure	Pericardial effusion
Aortic dissection, left ventricular rupture	Pericardial effusion, cardiac tamponade
Postoperatively after cardiac catheter or electrophysiologic procedures	Pericardial effusion, cardiac tamponade

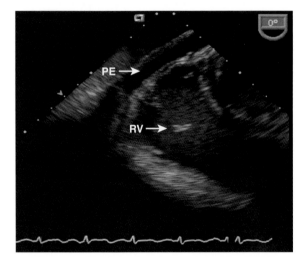

Figure 12-3. 2D echocardiographic image of a small to moderate PE.

- M-mode echocardiography can be useful as an additional tool for the detection of smaller effusions.
- In large PEs, spectral Doppler echocardiography should be considered to assess for markers of possible cardiac tamponade (see "Cardiac Tamponade").

Anatomic Imaging

Step 1: 2D Image Acquisition
- 2D echocardiography will show an echo-free space between the visceral and the parietal pericardium.
- Different views should be obtained in order to appreciate the extent of the PE (Table 12-2).
- M-mode echocardiography images are best acquired using the parasternal long axis view in TTE imaging and the TG mid short axis view in TEE.

TABLE 12-2 TRANSTHORACIC VERSUS TRANSESOPHAGEAL ECHOCARDIOGRAPHY VIEWS FOR THE IMAGING OF PERICARDIAL EFFUSIONS

	TTE	TEE
Useful echocardiographic views	Parasternal long axis Parasternal short axis Apical four-chamber subcostal	ME four-chamber ME RV inflow-outflow Transgastric mid short axis
Benefits and limits	Less invasive technique Poor image quality after cardiac surgery	Better detection of posterior effusion More invasive

ME, midesophageal; RV, right ventricular; TEE, transesophageal echocardiography; TTE, transthoracic echocardiography.

TABLE 12-3 ECHOCARDIOGRAPHIC GRADING OF PERICARDIAL EFFUSIONS

	Location of the Effusion	Distance between Pericardial Layers
Small	Posterior only	<0.5 cm
Moderate	Anterior and posterior	0.5-2 cm
Large	Anterior and posterior	>2 cm

- In some instances, saline contrast can help to discriminate the pericardial space from the heart itself.

Step 2: Image Analysis
- The measured distance between both pericardial layers is used to grade PEs (Table 12-3).
- Although grading scales are neither standardized nor validated, there is obvious correlation between the measured distance and the pericardial fluid volume. This has to be put into the perspective of the patient's clinical presentation.
- More exact measurements estimating pericardial fluid are impractical and not clinically relevant.

Pitfalls
- Surrounding PEs are hard to miss, and generally easy to diagnose, but localized PEs can be more difficult to identify and also have a more complex differential diagnosis, such as intrapericardial hematoma or pericardial mass.
- Hemorrhagic PE may appear more echogenic than a PE caused by serous fluid.
- Not only large circumferential effusions can cause the clinical picture of cardiac tamponade. In some cases, localized PEs can cause a tamponade-like picture, although not

compressing all of the cardiac chambers (Figure 12-4).
- An echo-free space only anterior to the heart is most commonly epicardial fat, and not fluid.

Pericardial versus Pleural Effusion

- Not every echo-free space around the heart is a PE. Differential diagnoses include pleural effusions, and a dilated descending thoracic aorta. On occasion a massively dilated left atrium (LA) may be mistaken for a pericardial effusion.
- Left-sided pleural effusions are visualized as echo-free spaces posterolateral to the descending thoracic aorta on the left (Figure 12-5). The partially collapsed lung is often visualized.
- In contrast, PEs are generally found between the descending thoracic aorta and the LA (Figure 12-6A). On occasion, an effusion may be first appreciated surrounding the left atrial appendage (LAA; see Figure 12-6B).
- Right-sided pleural effusions appear as echo-free spaces adjacent to the right atrium (RA). As opposed to PEs, right-sided pleural effusions are bounded inferiorly to the convex-shaped dome of the diaphragm adjacent to the liver. Similarly to the left side, the partially collapsed lung is often visualized (Figure 12-7).

KEY POINTS

- Echocardiography is the method of choice for the diagnosis of PE.
- A PE appears as an echo-free space surrounding the heart.
- Small PEs are mostly located posterior to the heart.
- The most common cause for PE is recent cardiac surgery.

Continued

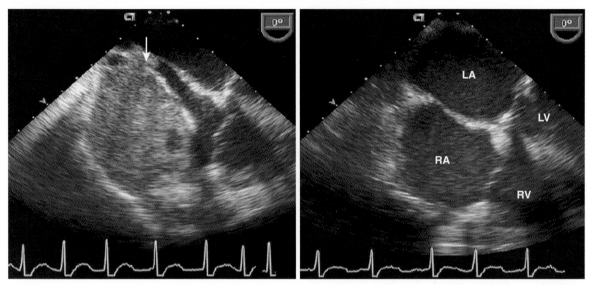

Figure 12-4. Posterior intrapericardial hematoma. Compression of the RA (**left,** *arrow*) and after surgical relief (**right**).

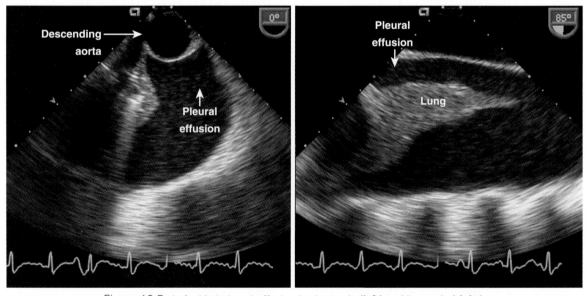

Figure 12-5. Left-sided pleural effusion in short axis (**left**) and long axis (**right**).

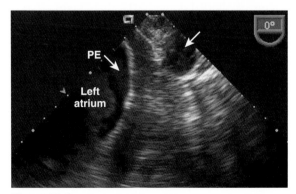

Figure 12-6. PE insinuated between the descending aorta *(arrow)* and the LA.

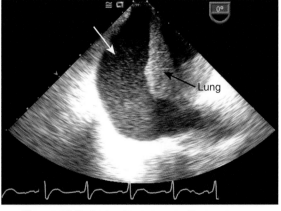

Figure 12-7. Right-sided pleural effusion *(arrow)*.

CARDIAC TAMPONADE

Background

- The pericardium can be somewhat stretched but can accommodate only a limited amount of fluid.
- Whenever there is a rapid or massive collection of pericardial fluid, the pressure inside the pericardium increases and will eventually overcome the intracardiac pressure, leading to impaired cardiac chamber filling.
- Thin-walled chambers on the right side of the heart are usually affected first, unless there is loculated pericardial hematoma adjacent to the left heart causing localized compression.
- As the intrapericardial pressure rises, venous pressures increase in order to maintain cardiac chamber filling.
- The clinical picture includes tachycardia, elevated right atrial (RA) pressure as well as systemic hypotension and decreased cardiac output.
- Pulsus paradoxus is an exaggerated clinical sign of impaired LV filling during inspiration causing a decrease in systolic arterial blood pressure. Patients may feel dizzy and complain of chest pain.
- Blood accumulation in the pericardium is the most common etiology for cardiac tamponade, but clot, exudates, or pus can also be the cause.

Overview of Echocardiographic Approach

- Echocardiography is the key imaging technique in the emergent clinical setting of suspected cardiac tamponade (Figure 12-8).
- Anatomic echocardiographic imaging modalities used are similar to the diagnosis of PE (see "Pericardial Effusion").
- Spectral Doppler echocardiography is critical in the diagnosis of tamponade, but image acquisition should not delay treatment of this life-threatening syndrome.

Anatomic Imaging

Step 1: Image Acquisition
- 2D imaging will confirm the presence of a PE that is usually moderate or large in size (Figure 12-9).
- Images should be acquired using multiple views to evaluate the extent of the effusion and confirm chamber compression.
- 2D echocardiography is used to visualize the IVC and hepatic veins.
- M-mode echocardiography of the interventricular septum can be helpful in some cases.

Step 2: Image Analysis
- The presence of a moderate to large PE is a classic finding in patients with cardiac tamponade.
- The RA shows inversion or collapse in systole. This is usually an early sign due to the thin wall and low pressure of the RA (Figure 12-10).
- A more specific and later sign is RV diastolic collapse. This can be best seen at the level of the right ventricular outflow tract (RVOT; Figure 12-11).
- There is exaggeration of the phenomenon of ventricular interdependence, which results from an increase in RV volume and pressure during inspiration and a leftward shift of the interventricular septum in the first diastole after inspiration. As well, the LA pressure is more dramatically lowered in inspiration. The result is reduced LV filling and systemic hypotension (pulsus paradoxus). Normalization of septal motion and decrease in RV volume is seen in the first diastole after expiration.
- There is IVC plethora, which is defined as a dilated IVC (>2 cm) with a less than 50% inspiratory diameter reduction (Figure 12-12). This is a sensitive, but not a very specific, sign.

Pitfalls
- Absence of a PE in the clinical setting of suspected cardiac tamponade is a diagnostic challenge. This is a trigger for extensive anatomic imaging. Especially after cardiac surgery, loculated effusion or hematoma can cause a tamponade-like syndrome with compression of sometimes only one cardiac chamber (i.e., the LA).
- If echocardiography shows no PE whatsoever, the hemodynamic compromise is probably not due to cardiac tamponade. Conversely, if a patient with a typical hemodynamic pattern suspicious for cardiac tamponade has a

POST CARDIAC SURGERY-HYPOTENSION IN THE ICU

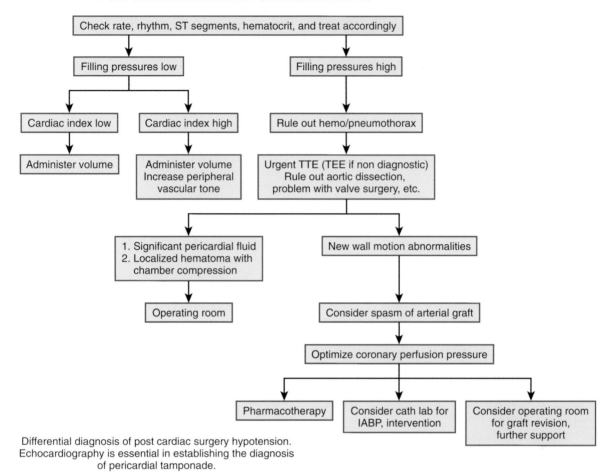

Differential diagnosis of post cardiac surgery hypotension.
Echocardiography is essential in establishing the diagnosis
of pericardial tamponade.

Figure 12-8. Differential diagnosis of post cardiac surgery hypotension. Echocardiography is essential in establishing the diagnosis of pericardial tamponade. IABP, intra-aortic balloon pump; ICU, intensive care unit.

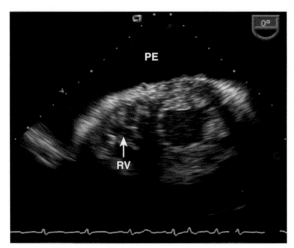

Figure 12-9. Large PE in a patient with clinical symptoms of cardiac tamponade. The RV is collapsed in early diastole when intracavitary pressure is at its lowest.

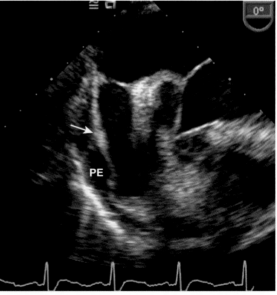

Figure 12-10. RA systolic collapse *(arrow)*.

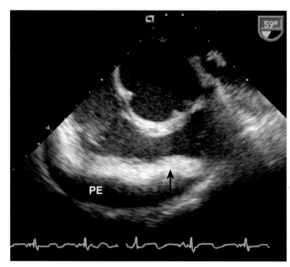

Figure 12-11. RVOT diastolic collapse *(arrow)*.

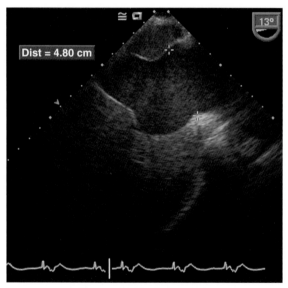

Figure 12-12. Dilated IVC.

measurements of IVC respiratory variations are clinically meaningless.

Step 1: Acquisition of Physiologic Data

- Spectral Doppler echocardiography is used to measure inflow velocities through the mitral and tricuspid valves by pulsed wave Doppler.
- These measurements can be done using the ME four-chamber view in TEE or an apical four-chamber view in TTE. The Doppler sample should be placed at the leaflet tips, and the sample size should be 3 to 5 mm.
- The examination should also include recording of pulsed wave Doppler flow in the pulmonary and hepatic veins.
- Tissue Doppler imaging and color M-mode of transmitral inflow are additional means of gathering physiologic data for the diagnosis of cardiac tamponade.
- In some cases, comparison of aortic and pulmonic velocity time integrals can be helpful. This will require TG long axis views and upper esophageal aortic arch short axis views in TEE, respectively.

Step 2: Analysis of Physiologic Data

- Spectral Doppler recordings will demonstrate exaggerated respiratory changes in diastolic filling of the ventricles.
- This will result in increased transtricuspid and decreased transmitral flow velocities during spontaneous inspiration.
- Respiratory variations can also be seen in aortic and pulmonic velocity time integral measurements.
- Tissue Doppler imaging of the mitral annular velocity (E′) will show a reduction in the presence of cardiac tamponade. There is usually no respiratory variation seen with this type of measurement.

Pitfalls

- Common problems in spectral Doppler imaging can alter findings and potentially make the diagnosis more difficult. The most important problem is an incorrect angle between the Doppler beam and the flow sample of interest.
- Differentiation of tamponade physiology from normal respiratory changes can be difficult, but generally, respiratory changes in flow velocities of more than 25% are considered abnormal.
- In the intraoperative setting with the patient being mechanically ventilated, the classic picture of exaggerated respiratory variation of ventricular volumes and filling is offset and

moderate to large PE, this virtually always confirms the diagnosis.

- There are idiopathic hemodynamically insignificant large PEs that do not result in tamponade physiology. Conversely, low-pressure cardiac tamponade exists where even a small increase in pericardial pressure (and volume) produces the full clinical picture, particularly in patients who are hypovolemic.
- Evaluation of respiratory changes of IVC size is a sensitive, but not a very specific, sign. Dilatation greater than 2 cm and loss of respiratory variation simply reflect elevated RA pressures regardless of cause. In the mechanically ventilated patient,

does not contribute to the diagnosis of cardiac tamponade.

- Although spectral Doppler findings in cardiac tamponade overlap with the findings in pericardial constriction, the difference between the two is the presence or, in the latter case, absence of a significant PE. There is, however, the rare case of so-called effusive-constrictive pericarditis that includes both pericardial thickening and effusion.

Alternative Approaches

- Even though echocardiography is an excellent modality to visualize PE, in some cases, it can be difficult to differentiate effusion from adjacent structures and cavities.
- Computed tomography (CT) and magnetic resonance imaging (MRI) might be of diagnostic help if there is a question of pericardial tumor or cyst (see "Other Pericardial Diseases").
- Diagnostic pericardiocentesis can be indicated whenever there is the suspicion of infectious or malignant PE. This can be a diagnostic as well as a therapeutic procedure at the same time (see "Surgical Considerations").

KEY POINTS

- Because echocardiography is the preferred method to diagnose a PE, it is also an invaluable tool in the diagnosis of cardiac tamponade.
- Classic echocardiographic findings in tamponade physiology include RA systolic collapse, RV diastolic collapse, and respiratory changes in ventricular volumes leading to a leftward shift of the interventricular septum with spontaneous inspiration.
- Although 2D echocardiography is the modality of choice, spectral Doppler can be useful for diagnosis confirmation, but should not delay treatment.
- However, cardiac tamponade is a clinical diagnosis with a typical hemodynamic pattern and cannot be based solely on echocardiographic findings.

CONSTRICTIVE PERICARDITIS

Background

- Constrictive pericarditis is a disease involving chronic fibrotic changes to the pericardium, pericardial thickening, and fusion of both pericardial layers.

TABLE 12-4   PATHOPHYSIOLOGY OF PERICARDIAL CONSTRICTION

1	High atrial pressures increase early filling of the ventricles
2	Ventricular filling is quickly offset by the constriction resulting in a rapid rise of the intraventricular pressure in diastole
3	RV systolic pressure is only mildly elevated, whereas RV diastolic pressures are markedly increased (usually more than one third of systolic pressure)
4	In classic constrictive pericarditis, there is equalization and elevation of diastolic pressures in all cardiac chambers
5	Ventricular volume is limited by pericardial constraint
6	Increased early diastolic RV filling goes along with decreased early diastolic LV filling, which is referred to as exaggerated ventricular interdependence

LV, left ventricular; RV, right ventricular.

- This can occur as a consequence of virtually any pericardial injury or disease, but the most common etiologies today are prior cardiac surgery and radiation of the mediastinum. The incidence of constrictive pericarditis after cardiac surgery is reported to be approximately 0.3%. Historically, infectious diseases, particularly tuberculosis, have been a major cause of constrictive pericarditis (see Table 12-1).
- Pathophysiologically, pericardial constriction causes a biventricular decrease of compliance and diastolic dysfunction (Table 12-4).
- During cardiac catheterization, the ventricular pressure loops show a typical dip-and-plateau pattern or square-root sign indicating an elevated early-diastolic pressure plateau (Figure 12-13).
- As opposed to cardiac tamponade, in which there is filling impairment throughout diastole, in constrictive pericarditis, early filling is usually normal or enhanced.
- The clinical endpoint of pericardial constriction is decreased diastolic filling of the ventricles due to the thick and inelastic pericardium encasing the heart. This goes along with systemic venous congestion and reduced cardiac output.
- Clinical symptoms often develop over months, and patients present with fatigue, dyspnea, peripheral edema, and ascites.
- It is important to recognize constrictive pericarditis, because it is likely curable by surgery. Also, it is important to differentiate it

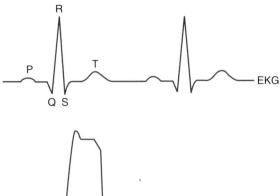

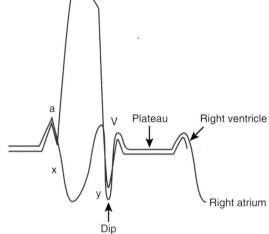

Figure 12-13. Dip-and-plateau pattern of ventricular pressure loops in the setting of pericardial constriction.

from other conditions in which ventricular filling is impaired (i.e., restrictive cardiomyopathy).

Overview of Echocardiographic Approach

- Echocardiography is a useful imaging technique for the diagnosis of constrictive pericarditis.
- TTE and TEE can complement each other for better image quality.
- Spectral Doppler echocardiography is of paramount importance for the diagnosis and differential diagnosis of pericardial constriction.
- Ancillary techniques include M-mode, tissue Doppler imaging, and color M-mode.

Anatomic Imaging

Step 1: Image Acquisition
- 2D echocardiography can be used to assess pericardial thickening. TEE is reported to be more useful in imaging pericardial thickness.

- Again, images should be acquired using multiple views in order to appreciate the extent of pericardial disease.
- M-mode of the interventricular septum can be helpful in some cases.
- The IVC should also be assessed for size and respiratory variation.

Step 2: Image Analysis
- Thickened pericardium will appear brighter than normal pericardium.
- Pericardial thickening and calcification can be ubiquitous or loculated.
- LV size and function are generally normal in patients with constrictive pericarditis.
- Atrial dimensions are often increased due to chronically elevated filling pressures.
- The IVC is usually dilated (>2 cm) because of elevated RA pressures.
- M-mode echocardiography will show the so-called septal bounce, which is the echocardiographic correlate of the dip-and-plateau sign on the LV pressure tracing, and appears as abrupt posterior motion of the septum in early diastole.

Pitfalls
- Reverberation artifacts from calcified pericardium are not uncommon and can potentially affect measurements.
- Even TEE is far from being exact in terms of measuring pericardial thickness. Other imaging techniques such as CT are more accurate in evaluating the magnitude of pericardial thickening.
- Although reports have demonstrated that the septal bounce is a consistent echocardiographic sign of constrictive pericarditis, this finding can be very subtle and also blunted in the setting of mechanical ventilation.
- Similarly, respiratory variations of IVC size are of no diagnostic value in mechanically ventilated patients.
- Echocardiographic findings of constrictive pericarditis and cardiac tamponade can have a lot in common, but in constriction, there is usually no PE, unless it is a (rare) case of effusive-constrictive pericarditis.

Step 1: Acquisition of Physiologic Data
- Spectral Doppler imaging should include pulsed wave Doppler interrogation of mitral and tricuspid inflow as well as hepatic and pulmonary vein flows.
- Any echocardiographic view yielding an appropriate line-up of the Doppler beam and

TABLE 12-5 COMPARISON OF CONSTRICTIVE PERICARDITIS AND RESTRICTIVE CARDIOMYOPATHY

	Constrictive Pericarditis	Restrictive Cardiomyopathy
Hemodynamics		
RA pressure	Elevated	Elevated
Pulmonary artery pressures	Mildly elevated	At least moderately elevated
2D		
	Pericardial thickening and fusion of both layers, no effusion	LV hypertrophy, normal systolic function
	Septal bounce	Usually normal septal motion
Spectral Doppler		
	Transmitral and transtricuspid inflow E > a Increased E-wave velocity Shortened deceleration time Respiratory variation of E-wave velocity and IVRT	Transmitral and transtricuspid inflow E < A (early stage) E >> A (late stage) No respiratory variations
	Pulmonary veins Blunted S-wave, large D-wave	
	Hepatic veins Large A-wave Prominent y descent	
Tissue Doppler		
	E' > 8 cm/s	E' < 8 cm/s
Color M-mode		
	Flow propagation > 45 cm/s	Flow propagation < 45 cm/s

IVRT, isovolumic relaxation time; LV, left ventricular; RA, right atrial; 2D, two-dimensional.

the flow sample can be used (i.e., an apical four-chamber view with TTE imaging). Correct placement of the sample volume at the level of the leaflet tips is important.
- Tissue Doppler of the septal mitral annulus and color M-mode of the mitral inflow will complete the physiologic echocardiography examination.

Step 2: Analysis of Physiologic Data
- E-wave velocity of transmitral inflow is increased and deceleration time is shortened (Table 12-5).
- The classic Doppler finding is enhanced changes in transmitral and transtricuspid inflow velocities with respiration. Mitral inflow is reduced, and tricuspid inflow is increased during spontaneous inspiration, whereas the opposite is the case with spontaneous exhalation. Isovolumic relaxation time (IVRT) is prolonged during spontaneous inspiration and will become shorter with expiration.
- Pulmonary vein flow velocities will also change throughout the respiratory cycle. There is systolic blunting and a prominent D-wave, consistent with pronounced early diastolic filling.

- Interrogation of hepatic vein flow usually shows prominent A-waves, and also deep y descents. This is indicative of rapid early diastolic filling in the presence of high RA pressures (A-wave) and a sudden dip in atrial pressure with ventricular filling (y descent). Flow velocities increase with spontaneous inspiration.
- Tissue Doppler imaging of the septal mitral annulus is normal or even increased (>8 cm/s) because there is no intrinsic myocardial disease and rapid early filling. Flow propagation velocity by color M-mode will also show normal results (>45 cm/s).

Pitfalls
- Reports demonstrated that up to 25% of patients lack those classic respiratory variations. This can be the case when there is concomitant intrinsic heart disease leading to ventricular dysfunction and markedly elevated filling pressures.
- Spectral Doppler interrogations are obviously more difficult in patients with atrial fibrillation. One has to use multiple beats to obtain a reliable picture of respiratory variations.

- In the intraoperative examination, respiratory changes will be blunted in the setting of mechanical ventilation.
- Tissue Doppler imaging of the lateral mitral annulus can be abnormal because of pericardial adhesion of the lateral wall. Therefore, tissue Doppler measurement should be performed interrogating the septal mitral annulus.

Differential Diagnosis of Constrictive Pericarditis

- Restrictive cardiomyopathy is a challenging differential diagnosis.
- In contrast to constrictive pericarditis, restrictive cardiomyopathy is an intrinsic heart disease characterized by ventricular noncompliance, higher degrees of diastolic dysfunction, and relatively normal systolic function. Possible etiologies include cardiac amyloidosis, sarcoidosis, or radiation.
- Hence, 2D and M-mode echocardiography are unreliable measures to differentiate because, in both diseases, the findings include normal chamber size and normal systolic function. Pericardial thickening and septal motion can also be somewhat difficult to assess.
- Spectral Doppler echocardiography is a key for successful differential diagnosis (see Table 12-5), and most importantly, patients with restrictive cardiomyopathy lack the classic respiratory variability of ventricular filling seen in patients with constrictive pericarditis.
- Tissue Doppler imaging is another tool to investigate whether there is "true" diastolic dysfunction or filling abnormality caused by pericardial constraint. Patients with restrictive cardiomyopathy will show reduced E′ velocities, whereas in constriction, E′ velocity is normal or even increased.

Alternative Approaches

- Several other imaging modalities are able to confirm the diagnosis of constrictive pericarditis whenever a comprehensive echocardiographic examination is inconclusive.
- Echocardiographic spectral Doppler measurements can be inaccurate owing to poor image quality and acquisition, or respiratory variations can be blunted by mechanical ventilation.
- Cardiac catheterization is an alternative diagnostic procedure to show the hemodynamic consequences of constriction,

although complete equalization of diastolic pressures is not a consistent finding.
- Pericardial calcification can be seen on a regular chest x-ray, but for the exact evaluation of pericardial thickening, CT and MRI are the most definitive diagnostic tools (Figure 12-14).
- Endomyocardial biopsy may be needed to differentiate restrictive cardiomyopathy from constrictive pericarditis.

KEY POINTS

- Constrictive pericarditis is characterized by pericardial thickening and fusion and is most commonly a consequence of prior cardiac surgery or radiation to the mediastinum.
- The pathophysiologic mechanism is decreased biventricular compliance. A rapid early filling is followed by an abrupt filling impairment due to the constraint of an inelastic pericardium.
- 2D echocardiography can be used to detect and measure pericardial thickness; however, other imaging techniques like CT or MRI are more accurate.
- The hallmark of pericardial constriction is the reciprocal respiratory changes in ventricular inflow during spontaneous inspiration measured by pulsed wave Doppler echocardiography.
- Differentiation of pericardial constriction and restriction caused by intrinsic heart disease can be difficult and involves comprehensive echocardiography and other diagnostic studies. This is highly important because constrictive pericarditis is a disease that is surgically treatable whereas restrictive cardiomyopathy is treated medically.

OTHER PERICARDIAL DISEASES

Acute Pericarditis

- Acute pericarditis is an inflammatory disease of the pericardium and has numerous potential causes (see Table 12-1).
- The clinical picture shows chest pain, changes on the electrocardiogram, and pericardial friction rub on auscultation.
- The echocardiographic signs include PE and possible pericardial thickening. 2D imaging using multiple views can show the extent of the disease.
- However, these findings can be subtle or even absent, making an echocardiographic diagnosis somewhat difficult.
- Acute pericarditis is a clinical diagnosis, and echocardiography can serve as a tool to

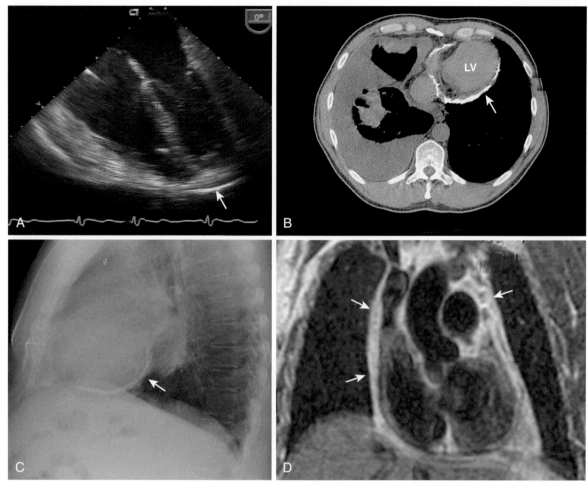

Figure 12-14. Thickened and calcified pericardium *(arrows)* seen with TEE (**A**), CT scan (**B**), chest x-ray (**C**), and MRI (**D**).

identify PE and to detect possible complications such as cardiac tamponade.

Epicardial Fat

- Epicardial fat is ubiquitously found on the surface of the heart. It serves as a visceral fat reserve for the heart, and its embryologic origin is brown adipose tissue.
- Owing to the close proximity of epicardial fat and the myocardium, metabolic, inflammatory and hormonal interactions are present. Although it serves as a buffer and energy reserve, detrimental effects on the coronary vasculature have been described.
- Epicardial fat thickness strongly correlates with diabetes, atherosclerosis, and coronary artery disease. 2D echocardiography is a very capable and inexpensive tool to measure epicardial fat thickness. There are no established normal values yet, but studies suggest the upper limit to be about 7 mm.

- TTE using the parasternal windows is the preferable ultrasound technique. Epicardial fat is visualized as an echo-free space anterior to the heart and can be mistaken for an anterior PE. However, there are usually some fine echoes found inside the epicardial fat pad, and in some cases, the fat can even have a hyperechoic appearance.

Congenital Absence of the Pericardium

- Congenital malformations of the pericardium are rare and are often first diagnosed when patients undergo cardiac or thoracic surgical procedures for other reasons.
- Partial or complete absence of the pericardium is the most common abnormality.
- Studies have demonstrated that complete absence of the pericardium is virtually always asymptomatic, but partial absence

can cause clinical symptoms ranging from chest pain to potentially life-threatening myocardial ischemia or arrhythmias caused by herniation or incarceration of cardiac structures.

- CT or MRI is most commonly used for the diagnosis of congenital absence, but reports have shown that echocardiography can be successfully used to make this diagnosis.
- 2D TTE imaging is the modality of choice, and changing the patient's position during the examination can verify cardiac hypermobility, which is a highly suggestive sign for absence of the pericardium.

Pericardial Cysts and Tumors

- Pericardial cysts are congenital abnormalities but, in some cases, can be acquired after cardiothoracic surgical procedures.
- The typical position is the cardiophrenic angles; they contain water-like fluid and are variable in size.
- These cysts are usually incidental findings, but some patients develop symptoms that are caused by cardiac chamber compression.
- 2D echocardiography is the best noninvasive method for diagnosis of pericardial cysts. Color Doppler echocardiography can help to delineate cysts from blood vessels and cardiac chambers.
- Differentiation among pericardial cysts, effusion, and epicardial fat can be challenging in some cases.
- Pericardial tumors are rare. The most common primary tumors are mesotheliomas.
- The diagnosis is often made in advanced disease when tumor compression of cardiac chambers or significant PE is present.
- In this setting, 2D echocardiography can be used to both detect a PE as well as the actual tumor. In some cases, TEE might be more useful depending on the tumor location.
- Cysts and tumors causing clinical symptoms can be treated surgically with a pericardial window or a pericardiectomy.

SURGICAL CONSIDERATIONS

Pericardiocentesis

- Pericardiocentesis can be performed using local anesthesia at the patient's bedside or in the setting of a cardiac catheterization suite.

- It is usually done when there is suspected PE causing clinical symptoms to confirm the diagnosis and provide an immediate treatment option.
- In some cases, diagnostic pericardiocentesis is used as a truly diagnostic method in order to acquire pericardial fluid samples for bacteriologic or cytologic analysis.
- The approach is transcutaneous from the left xiphocostal area. Once pericardial fluid is aspirated with the needle, a pressure line should be attached to measure intrapericardial pressure. If necessary, a drain can be placed to continue drainage until clinical symptoms of tamponade resolve.
- Echocardiography can increase the success rate and decrease complications of percutaneous pericardiocentesis, and should, therefore, be used to guide this procedure.
- TTE imaging is the preferred method to visualize the effusion, define the optimal anatomic location for needle placement, confirm that the needle tip is inside the pericardial space, ensure adequate fluid drainage, and guide the subsequent placement of a pericardial drain.

Pericardial Window

- A pericardial window or partial pericardiectomy is performed to drain fluid into the pleural or peritoneal compartments in patients with recurring PE.
- This procedure usually requires general anesthesia; operative approaches are thoracoscopic, via an anterior thoracotomy or through a subxiphoid incision.
- After fluid is released, a drain is usually left in the pericardial space. The surgeon will excise enough pericardium to make it an effective fluid drain, but excising too much leads to the potential problem of cardiac prolapse or herniation.
- TEE should be used to confirm adequate drainage of the PE.

Pericardiectomy

- Pericardiectomy is the standard surgical treatment for chronic pericardial constriction.
- Precise preoperative workup is necessary, as mentioned previously, to properly delineate pericardial constriction and intrinsic myocardial diseases that are subject to medical therapy (see "Constrictive Pericarditis").

- It is a technically challenging operation, and the surgeon will encounter dense adhesions, calcifications, and sometimes, myocardial infiltration.
- The standard approach is a median sternotomy, and in some cases, cardiopulmonary bypass is necessary. A left anterior thoracotomy is an alternative surgical approach.
- The general goal is excision of the whole pericardium from one phrenic nerve to the other. In some cases, total excision, especially posterior to the heart, is not feasible and a partial pericardiectomy is performed.
- The LV is preferentially unroofed first in order to avoid the sudden increase in LV volume and pressure that often results if the RV is unroofed first.
- In most of the cases, a substantial decrease in filling pressures can be seen early after the procedure.
- Nonetheless, operative mortality is reported to be as high as 20%, and long-term outcome is largely dependent on the etiology of constrictive pericarditis. Whereas pericardiectomy for idiopathic constrictive pericarditis has an excellent long-term outcome, outcomes in patients undergoing this procedure for postsurgical or postradiation constrictive pericarditis are reported to be poor.
- TEE can be helpful in these cases for hemodynamic monitoring purposes and evaluation of ventricular function throughout the procedure.

Suggested Readings

1. Goldstein JA. Cardiac tamponade, constrictive pericarditis, and restrictive cardiomyopathy. *Curr Probl Cardiol.* 2004;29:503-567.
   A comprehensive review of the normal anatomy and function of the human pericardium. The pathophysiology and clinical diagnosis of cardiac tamponade and pericardial constriction are meticulously described and illustrated with a number of useful figures.
2. Khandaker MH, Espinosa RE, Nishimura RA, et al. Pericardial disease: Diagnosis and management. *Mayo Clin Proc.* 2010;85:572-593.
   A nicely illustrated overview on the clinical management of pericardial disease including several flow charts and diagnostic algorithms.
3. Wann S, Passen E. Echocardiography in pericardial disease. *J Am Soc Echocardiogr.* 2008;21:7-13.
   A concise review on pericardial diseases with the focus on echocardiography as the diagnostic method. It contains explanations of different imaging techniques, matching illustrations, and echocardiographic images.
4. D'Cruz IA, Kanuru N. Echocardiography of serous effusions adjacent to the heart. *Echocardiography.* 2001;18:445-456.
   This article is dedicated to the anatomic imaging and differentiation of pericardial effusion, pleural effusions, and ascites using echocardiography.
5. Reddy PS. Spectrum of hemodynamic changes in cardiac tamponade. *Am J Cardiol.* 1990;66:1487-1491.
   This study in 77 patients with pericardial effusion is a great example for the hemodynamic impact of tamponade with respect to pressure equalization and the response to pericardiocentesis.
6. Yared K, Baggish AL, Picard MH, et al. Multimodality imaging of pericardial disease. *J Am Coll Cardiol Imaging.* 2010;3:650-660.
   A good review looking at different imaging modalities for the diagnosis of pericardial diseases. An emphasis is put on the comparison of echocardiography with other imaging studies.
7. Hatle LK, Appleton CP, Popp RL. Differentiation of constrictive pericarditis and restrictive cardiomyopathy by Doppler echocardiography. *Circulation.* 1989;79:357-370.
   An excellent study focused on the pathophysiology of pericardial constriction. Patients with constrictive pericarditis showed respiratory variation of ventricular inflow velocities, whereas patients with restrictive cardiomyopathy did not. These findings are also illustrated using ventricular pressure tracings.
8. Schwefer M, Aschenbach R, Heidemann J, et al. Constrictive pericarditis, still a diagnostic challenge: Comprehensive review of clinical management. *Eur J Cardiothorac Surg.* 2009;36:502-510.
   A review of the pathophysiology and clinical presentation of constrictive pericarditis, but the focus is on the clinical management, especially the surgical aspects of pericardiectomy and associated outcomes.

Index

Note: Page numbers followed by f refer to figures; page numbers followed by t refer to tables; page numbers followed by b refer to boxes.

3